HOMOEOPATHIC
Materia Medica

THE AUTHORS

Dr. S.K. Ranjan, was born on 25 August 1976 has primary education to the D.A.V. Inter Collage Banda, U.P. He was first admitted in 1999 C.P.M.T. batch to the Himalaya Institute of Medical Science, Dehradun, Uttarakhand for M.B.B.S. course where he stood only 6th month. Then he was transferred from National Homoeopathic Medical Collage Lucknow to Government Lal Bahadur Shastri Homoeopathic Medical Collage & Hospital Allahabad, U.P., India. President-Homoeo Friends Charitable and Research Society of India. He is now actively engaged as a many research work on Homoeopathy. President-Ayush Care Research Society of India.

Dr. F.A. Zaidee, born 1979, was graduated from Allahabad University. He did not completed his M.Sc. (Botany) because he was selected in C.P.M.T. (U.P.).

Primary education to the G.I.C. Allahabad (U.P.).

Chief Secretary–Homoeo-Friends Charitable and Research Society of India.

Member–Ayush Care Research Society of India.

Consultant Physician–Shri Sai Nath Postgraduate Institute of Homoeopathy and Hospital, Allahabad (U.P.).

He is now actively engaged many research work on Homoeopathy such as–Hepatitis AIIMS, New Delhi and HIV/AIDS, California University.

HOMOEOPATHIC
Materia Medica
— With Multiple Choice Questions —

by

Dr. S.K. Ranjan
B.H.M.S.
Government L.B.S. Homoeopathic Medical College, Allahabad (U.P.)
President
Homeo-Friends Charitable & Research Society of India
Ayush Care Research Society of India

Dr. F.A. Zaidee
B.Sc., B.H.M.S.
Government L.B.S. Homoeopathic Medical College, Allahabad (U.P.)
Chief Secretary
Homeo-Friends Charitable & Research Society of India
Member
Ayush Care Research Society of India

2025

Daya Publishing House®
A Division of
Astral International Pvt. Ltd.
New Delhi – 110 002

First Edition 2025

ISBN 978-81-7035-453-6 (PB)

Published by : **Daya Publishing House®**
A Division of
Astral International Pvt. Ltd.
– ISO 9001:2008 Certified Company –
4761-61/23, Ansari Road, Darya Ganj
New Delhi - 110 002
Phone: 011-4354 9197, 2327 8134
E-mail: info@astralint.com
Website: www.astralint.com

Laser Typesetting : **Classic Computer Services**

Printed at : **Replika Press Pvt. Ltd.**

"ॐ अज्ञान तिमिरान्धस्य ज्ञानाज्जन शलाकया।
चक्षुरून्मीलितं येन तस्मै श्री गुरूवे नमः"।।

DEDICATED TO
OUR RESPECTED SIR

DR. S.M. SINGH

Govt. LAL BAHADUR SHASTRI HOMOEOPATHIC MEDICAL COLLEGE & HOSPITAL

PHAPHAMAU – ALLAHABAD, U.P. – INDIA

Phone: 05322647486

Affiliated to University of Agra

FOREWORD

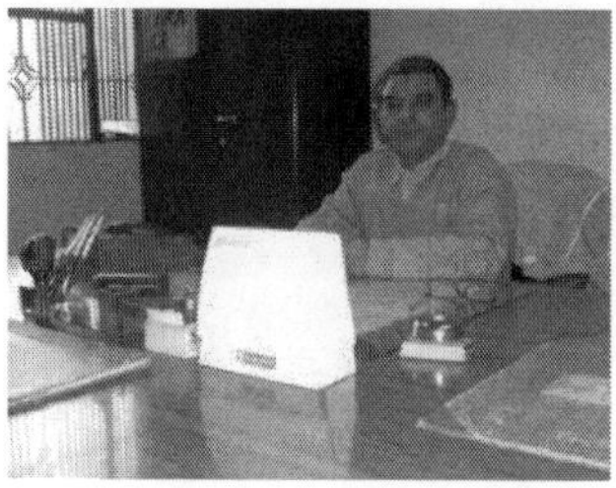

Dr. H.C. RAI

ACTG.-PRINCIPAL

It is a great delight for me to write a foreword to this book on materia medica. I am extremely glad to note that the authors have ventured to write the book at such a young age . Shailendra Kumar Ranjan & Firoz Ahamad Zaidee are devoted students of our college. The authors have tried theirs best to cover all the essential point which are very useful to understand the Homoeopathic Medicine.This book would be of immense help to students of Homoeopathy and even the Physicians.

May God bless theirs success in every thing and their plans.

6.12.05

Dr. H.C. Rai
(Actg.- Principal)
Govt. L. B. S. Homoeopathic
Medical College & Hospital
Phaphamau – Allahabad, U.P. – INDIA

Principal
Govt. L.B.S.H. Medical College
& Hospital, Al: .abad

Preface

This book of Materia Medica has been mainly written with a purpose to cover different type of examinations of Homoeopathic Medical students and as an aid to the Practising Homoeopathic physicians. We have deepen the grand Characteristics of medicine in a special style. So new title of this book has given "Homoeopathic Materia Medica.

We hope that our endeavour should be of help to Homoeopathic Medical students, teaching community and all homoeopathic physicians.

This book is dedicated to Dr. S.M. Singh, who are our respected sir and guide to every aspects of our professional and education life.

We are thankful to the entire teachers staff of Govt. L.B.S. Homoeopathic Medical College, Allahabad (U.P.)- India, especially- Dr. H.C. Rai (Principal), Dr. M.L. Shukla (Ex. Principal), Dr. T.N. Singh, Dr. B.B. Singh, Dr. R.N. Verma, Dr. A.K. Mishra, Dr. H.N. Dixit, Dr. H.P. Tripathi, Dr. N.K. Lal, Dr. C.B. Srivastava, Dr. Pyare Lal, Dr. S.P. Singh and Dr. G.D. Tripathi.

We are thankful to the whole students of Govt. L.B.S. Homoeopathic Medical College, Allahabad (U.P.)- India, especially- Dr. Sandeep Shukla, Dr. Vinod Rao, Dr. Jitendra Singh, Dr. Sadanand Verma, Dr. Arun Yadav, Dr. Ashish Dixit, Dr. Porwal and also thankful to the Homoeopathic Medical Students of other Colleges, especially Dr. Awadhesh Rana, Dr. Ashish Verma, Dr. Somil Rastogi, Dr. O.P. Singh, Dr. Sailesh Singh, Dr. Jitendra Verma and Dr. Umesh Yadav, Dr. Nikhil Saxena.

Our special thanks to Dr. Ratnakar Singh, Dr. Vikash Kannaujia, Dr. R. K. Nirmal, Dr. S.K. Shukla, Dr. K.K. Srivastava, Dr. Amit Anand, Mr. Devendra Gautam (Librarian) and Mr. V. K. Jaiswal.

We should like to deeply thank everyone who has participated in any way in the Publication of this "HOMOEOPATHIC MATERIA MEDICA."

We hope our efforts would meet the expectations of the students. We should greatly welcome and appreciate suggestions, comments and criticism from the students, teachers and Homoeopathic Practiceners to help me to improve the book further.

Ranjan & Zaidee

Contents

Students Must Remember

Physical Classification	*Symbol*	*Therapeutic Picture of Drug*
CONSTITUTION	C_N	C_{N-1}; C_{N-2}; C_{N-3} ......
MIND	M_D	M_{D-1}; M_{D-2}; M_{D-3} ......
HEAD	H_D	H_{D-1}; H_{D-2}; H_{D-3} ......
SENSE ORGANS [Eye; Nose; Ear]	SO	SO_1; SO_2; SO_3 ......
NERVOUS SYSTEM	NS	NS_1; NS_2; NS_3 ......
DIGESTIVE SYSTEM [Mouth; Tongue; Pharynx; Stomach; Intestine; Abdomen; Rectum etc.]	DS	DS_1; DS_2; DS_3 ......
CARDIO-VASCULAR SYSTEM [Blood; Heart; Arteries; Veins etc.]	CVS	CVS_1; CVS_2; CVS_3 ......
RESPIRATORY SYSTEM [Throat; Lungs; Pleura etc.]	RS	RS_1; RS_2; RS_3 ......
FEMALE GENITAL SYSTEM [Ovary; Uterus; Vagina; Vulva; Mammae etc.]	FGS	FGS_1; FGS_2; FGS_3 ......
MALE GENITAL SYSTEM	MGS	MGS_1; MGS_2; MGS_3 ......
URINARY SYSTEM	US	US_1; US_2; US_3 ......

Physical Classification	*Symbol*	*Therapeutic Picture of Drug*
➲ **LOCOMOTORY SYSTEM**	LS	LS_1; LS_2; LS_3 ....
➲ **BACK**	B_K	B_{K-1}; B_{K-2}; B_{K-3} ....
➲ **SKIN**	S_N	S_{K-1}; S_{N-2}; S_{N-3} ....
➲ **FEVER**	F_R	F_{R-1}; F_{R-2}; F_{R-3} ....
➲ **PHYSICAL GENERALS**	PG	PG_1; PG_2; PG_3

The Great Homeopaths

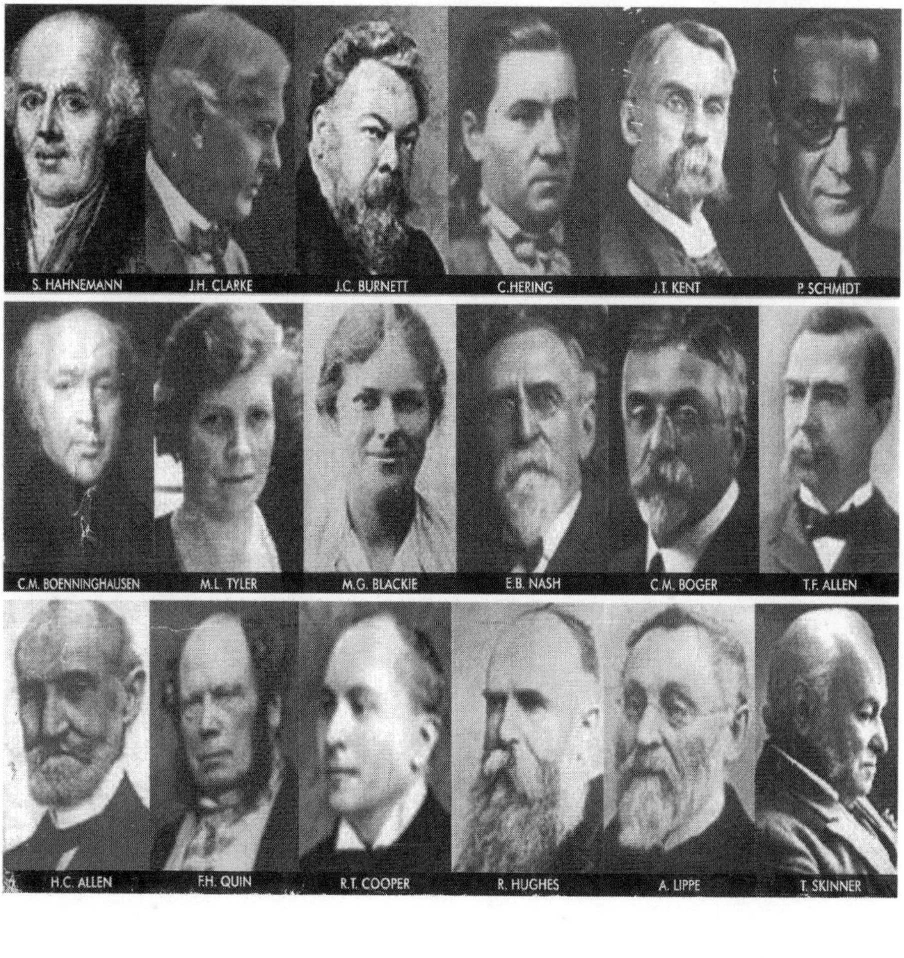

Abrotanum

- PROVED BY: Cushing Devennter Gatchell.
- FAMILY/KINGDOM: Compositae.
- COMMON NAME: Southern Wood [Ladys Love].
- MIASM: Psora.
- RELATION COLD/HEAT: Chilly.
- TEMPERAMENT: Cruel & inhuman.
- DIATHESIS: tubercular.
- SOURCE: Tincture of fresh leaves & stems.
- SPHERES OF ACTION: GIT, Nerves, mind, fibrous tissue and serous membrane.
- SUMMARY OF INDICATIONS: Constipation alternating with diarrhoea-emaciation, marasmus and debility in children, due to constitutional or behaviorial disorders.

THERAPEUTIC PICTURE OF DRUG

C_{N-1} ➲ Child is emaciated, especially more marked in lower extremities.

C_{N-2} ➲ Child is old looking face; face pale and wrinkled.

C_{N-3} ➲ Skin of child is flabby and hangs loose in folds.

C_{N-4} ➲ Child head is very weak and the child can not hold it up.

M_{D-1} ➲ Feeble, dull.

M_{D-2} ➲ Indolence, aversion to bodily motion.

M_{D-3} ➲ Anxious, depressed.

M_{D-4} ➲ Child cross, depressed, very Peevish.

M_{D-5} ➲ Child or adult is ill–natured, irritable, cross and despondent; violent, behaves inhumanily; like being cruel.

DS_1 ➲ Hard lumps in different parts of abdomen.

DS_2 ➲ Food Passes undigested.

DS_3 ➲ Aliments from Suddenly Checked diarrhoea or other secretions, malnutrition defective digestion and absorption.

- DS_4 ➲ Alternate diarrhoea and constipation.
- RS_1 ➲ Cold air causes raw feeling.
- RS_2 ➲ Pressing sensation remains in affected side,. Impeding free breathing. (Pleurisy).
- FGS_1 ➲ Darting in left ovary; twitching in both ovaries,
- FGS_2 ➲ Dysmenorrhoea or suppressed menses.
- FGS_3 ➲ Blood and moisture oozing from navel of the newborn.
- MGS_1 ➲ Hydrocele of children.
- LS_1 ➲ Aching from shoulder–joints to elbows.
- LS_2 ➲ Aching in fingers, first right then lift side.
- LS_3 ➲ Pricking and coldness of finger tips.
- LS_4 ➲ Numb sensation in fingers.
- LS_5 ➲ Legs emaciated.
- LS_6 ➲ Stitching, tearing, itching in old footsore.
- LS_7 ➲ Darwin in ankle joint.
- LS_8 ➲ Inability to move. (Rheumatism)
- LS_9 ➲ Back and limbs sore and lame, worse mornings awaking
- S_{N-1} ➲ Itching chilblains.
- PG_1 ➲ Ravenous hunger; emaciation while eating well.

Modalities

Aggravation

- ➲ Cold air.
- ➲ Checked secretions.

Amelioration

- ➲ Motion.

Relations

➲ COMPARE:	With Nux–Vom. and Agar. In chilblans.
➲ FOLLOWS WELL:	In pleurisy, after Aco. Bryo & Bary–Carb.

Aceticum Acidum

- PROVED BY: C. Hering.
- DURATION: 14–20 days.
- COMMON NAME: Vinegar.
- FAMILY/KINGDOM: Chemical .
- RELATION COLD/HEAT: Cold (kent).
- MIASM: Psora, Siphilis & Sycosis.
- DIATHESIS: Haemorrhagic.
- TEMPERAMENT: Irritable.
- SOURCE: Glacial Acetic Acid ($H\,C_2\,H_3\,O_2$).
- SPHERES OF ACTION: Mind, G.I.T., Uro-genital tract, Blood Vascular system.
- SUMMARY OF INDICATIONS: Trauma–Shock and haemorrhag–Post operative shock–Post Partum Collapse.

THERAPEUTIC PICTURE OF DRUG

C_{N-1} ➲ Suitable for pale, lean persons with lax, flabby muscles.

C_{N-2} ➲ Face is pale and waxy (ferr-met.)

M_{D-1} ➲ Great Prostration after trauma (Sulph-acid.), Surgery, shock, haemorrhage, Post–delivery shock and after anaesthesia.

M_{D-2} ➲ Very dull and low-Spirited; irritable.

M_{D-3} ➲ Alternate stupor and delirium.

M_{D-4} ➲ Grieves much, sighs often.

M_{D-5} ➲ Horrible attacks of anxiety with difficult breathing.

M_{D-6} ➲ Vertigo with feebleness and fainting.

DS_1 ➲ Contents of stomach feel as if in a ferment.

DS_2 ➲ Violent burning Pain in stomach and in chest, followed by coldness of skin and cold sweat on fore head: burning worse lying on back.

DS_3 ➲ Diarrhoea liquid or undigested, with swelling of legs and feet(Phthisis).

DS_4 ➲ Diarrhoea in the later stages of abdominal typhus.

RS_1 ➲ Hoarseness, with laryngeal irritation.

RS_2 ➲ Croup, especially when the face is bright red.

RS_3 ➲ Croup like sound; a hollow sound with each inhalation.

RS_4 ➲ Inhalaion of vapour of cider vinegar has been successfully used in croup and malignant diphtheria.

FGS_1 ➲ Metrorrhagia, after parturition, with great thirst.

FGS_2 ➲ Excessive catamenia.

FGS_3 ➲ Sour belching and vomiting during pregnancy.

FGS_4 ➲ Breasts Painfully enlarged (mastitis), distended with milk.

FGS_5 ➲ Milk impoverished, bluish, transparent, sour.

MGS_1 ➲ Very weakening, nightly emissions.

F_{R1} ➲ Hectic fevers, with cough, dyspnoea, night- sweats, diarrhoea. Oedema and emaciation.

F_{R2} ➲ Febrile heat, with a dry skin; in bilious, putrid and typhoid fevers. Typus with delirium.

F_{R3} ➲ Profuse sweating; night sweats.; and no thirst during fever.

PG_1 ➲ Thirst: intense, burning, insatiable, even after drinking large quantities of fluids in diabetes mellitus; chronic diarrhoea and oedema, but no thirst during fever.

PG_2 ➲ Cannot sleep lying on the back; a sensation of Sinking in the abdomen causing dyspnoea; rests better when lying on the belly (Amm-Carb.)

PG_3 ➲ Drenching night sweats.

Modalities

Aggravation

➲ Lying on back.

➲ Fumes of Charcoal & gas.

➲ Anaesthetic vapors.

Amelioration

➲ Lying on belly.

Relations

➲ COMPARE:	Apis; Ars; Carbol-ac; Lac-defl; Lact-ac
➲ COMPLEMENTARY:	China
➲ FOLLOWS WELL:	After China In haemorrhagic, After digitalis in dropsy.
➲ ANTIDOTES:	Aco; Nat-m; Nux-vom; Sep; Tabac.
➲ INIMICALS:	Bor; Caust; Sars; Ran-b.

Aconitum napellus

- PROVED BY: Hahnemann.
- DURATION: 1 hour to several weeks.
- COMMON NAME: Monkshood (Wolfbane).
- FAMILY/KINGDOM: Ranunculaceae.
- RELATION COLD/HEAT: Warm blooded.
- MIASM: Psora.
- DIATHESIS: Not define.
- TEMPERAMENT: Sanguine.
- SOURCE: Tincture of whole plant with root when begining to flower.
- SPHERES OF ACTION: Cerebro-spinal N.S., brain, serous and mucous membrane.
- SUMMARY OF INDICATIONS: Fear of death–acute inflammations–Pain–fever–Preoperative medication before surgery (to allay anxiety).

THERAPEUTIC PICTURE OF DRUG

C_{N-1} ➲ Generally indicated in acute or recent cases occuring in young Persons.

C_{N-2} ➲ Especially girls of a full, plethoric habit who lead sedentary life.

C_{N-3} ➲ Persons easily affected by atmospheric changes.

C_{N-4} ➲ Adapted to Persons, dark hairs and eyes, rigid muscular fibre.

M_{D-1} ➲ Great fear and anxiety of mind with worry accompany every ailment, however trivial.

M_{D-2} ➲ Music is unbearable; makes her sad (Ambr.).

M_{D-3} ➲ Delirium is characterised by unhappiness, worry, fear, raving, but the patient is rarely unconscious.

M_{D-4} ➲ Fears death but believes that he will soon die; Predicts the day.

M_{D-5} ➲ Fears the future, a crowd, crossing the street.

M_{D-6} ➲ Fears of death during Pregnancy.

M_{D-7} ➲ Anxiety, Restless, Agonized tossing about.

M_{D-8} ➲ Over sensitive can not light or noise.

M_{D-9} ➲ Magination acute, clairvoyance.

M_{D-10} ➲ Thinks his thoughts come from the stomach that parts of her body are abnormally thick.

H_{D1} ➲ Burning, throbbing headache; sensation as if there is a tight band around the head.

NS_1 ➲ Puerperal convulsions, from fright; great cerebral excitement; hot, dry skin, thirst, restlessness and fear of death.

RS_1 ➲ Laryngitis, with inflammatory fever; also with suffocating spasms.

RS_2 ➲ Croup: awaking in first sleep; child in agony impatient, tosses about; dry short cough.

RS_3 ➲ Chough and loud breathing during expiration; every expiration ending with a hoarse, hacking cough; after exposure to dry,cold wind.

RS_4 ➲ Cough; dry and painful; shout, dry, hacking, excited by tickling in the larynx; spasmodic. Rough, croaking. With danger of suffocation; dry, hard, ringing.

FGS_1 ➲ Menses too abundant and too Protracted.

FGS_2 ➲ Amenorrhoea in plethoric young girls; after fright, to prevent Suppresion of menses.

FGS_3 ➲ Stitching Pains move to right of fundus uteri; sharp shooting pains, abdomen exceedingly sensitive.

FGS_4 ➲ Uterine haemorrhage; active, much excitability, giddy, cannot sit up; fear of death.

FGS_5 ➲ Childbed fever, after suppression of lochia, mammae lax, no milk; dry, hot skin; hard, frequent pulse, or tensive, contractedl; fearful; wild staring, glittering eyes; dry tongue, great thirst; inflated abdomen, sensitive to the slightest touch.

MGS_1 ➲ Sexual desire increased; fits of lasciviousness.

MGS_2 ➲ Bruised pain in the testicles.

MGS_3 ➲ Testes feel swollen and hard.

F_{R1} ➲ Fevers of sudden onset; hot, dry skin; often one cheek is red and the other is pale.

F_{R2} ➲ Cold stage is most marked.

F_{R3} ➲ Cold at the beginning violent, more in the evening after lying down, often with hot cheek and contracted Pupils.

F_{R4} ➲ Cold, if uncovered or touched.

F_{R5} ➲ Dry heat, with thirst, short breathing, quick, hard, full pulse.

F_{R6} ➲ Most valuable febrifuge with mental anxiety, restlessness etc.

F_{R7} ➲ Shivering ascends from feet to chest.

$F_{R\,8}$ ➲ Covered or affected parts sweat Profusely; likes to be uncovered.
$F_{R\,9}$ ➲ Profuse hot sweat during sleep.
$F_{R\,10}$ ➲ Bad effects from suppressed sweat.
$F_{R\,11}$ ➲ Sweat drenching, on parts lain on; relieving all symptoms.
PG_1 ➲ Unquenchable thirst for large quantities of water.
PG_2 ➲ Disorders from fright and of sudden onset with acute symptoms.
PG_3 ➲ Pain followed by numbness and tingling.

Modalities

Aggravation

- ➲ Music, Evening & Night.
- ➲ Lying on affected side,worm room.
- ➲ Tobacco smoke, dry, cold wind.

Amelioration

- ➲ Open air

Relations

➲ COMPARE:	Acon; Ars; Rhus-t.
➲ COMPLEMENTARY:	Sulph; Arn; Coff.
➲ FOLLOWS WELL:	Arn; Ars; Bell; Bry; Cact; Canth; Cocc; Hep; Ip; Kali-br; Merc; Puls. Sep.
➲ ANTIDOTES:	Acet-ac; Bell; Wine; Nux-v; Sulph.

Actea racemosa (Cimicifuga racemosa)

- ➲ PROVED BY: Jeanes.
- ➲ DURATION: 08–12 days.
- ➲ COMMON NAME: Black Kohosh.
- ➲ FAMILY/KINGDOM: Ranunculaceae.
- ➲ RELATION COLD/HEAT: Chilly.
- ➲ MIASM: Psora.
- ➲ DIATHESIS: Rheumatic & Gouty.
- ➲ TEMPERAMENT: Hysterical.
- ➲ SOURCE: Tincture of the root. Trituration of the resinoid, macrotyn.
- ➲ SPHERES OF ACTION: N.S., female generative organs esp. upon the uterus, ovaries & Joints.
- ➲ SUMMARY OF INDICATIONS: Threatened abortion–difficult labour–Puerperal disorders.

THERAPEUTIC PICTURE OF DRUG

M_{D-1} ➲ Puerperal mania. Tries to injure her self. Suicide (constantly thinks about).

M_{D-2} ➲ Sensation as if a heavy black cloud has settled all over (her) the patient.

M_{D-3} ➲ Great depression, with dreams of impending evil.

M_{D-4} ➲ Fears riding in a closed carriage, of being obliged to jump out.

M_{D-5} ➲ Incessant talking.

M_{D-6} ➲ Visions of rats, mice, etc.

M_{D-7} ➲ Mania following disappearance of neuralgia.

SO_1 ➲ Aching or sharp, darting, shooting pains in orbits of eyes.

NS_1 ➲ Great debility between the menses.

NS_2 ➲ Alternate tonic and clonic spasms.

NS_3 ➲ Hysteric spasms.

- NS_4 ➲ Epilepsy, periodical convulsions, with uterine diseases.
- CVS_1 ➲ Heart disorders from uterine of ovarian affections; palpitation following the least motion.
- FGS_1 ➲ Increase of mental symptoms during menses.
- FGS_2 ➲ Menses Profuse, early; dark, coagulated; scanty, irregular, delayed.
- FGS_3 ➲ Hysterical or epileptical spasms at time of menses.
- FGS_4 ➲ Pains in uterine region shoot side to side.
- FGS_5 ➲ Pains in ovarian region shoot upward.
- FGS_6 ➲ Bearing down in uterine region and small of back; limb feel heavy, torpid.
- FGS_7 ➲ Rheumatic dysmenorrhoea.
- FGS_8 ➲ Leucorrhoea, with sensation of weight in the uterus.
- FGS_9 ➲ During Pregnancy; nausea; false labour–like pains; sharp pains across abdomen; sleeplessness.
- FGS_{10} ➲ During parturition 'shivers,' first stage; pains too strong; spasmodic cardiac neuralgia; lochia suppressed (by cold or emotions); puerperal mania.
- FGS_{11} ➲ Tendency to abort at third month (sab.)
- FGS_{12} ➲ When given during last month of pregnancy it shortens labour, if symptoms correspond (caul-thal., Puls-nig.).
- FGS_{13} ➲ Infra-mammary Pains, worst on left side.
- FGS_{14} ➲ Burning in the mammae.
- LS_1 ➲ Rheumatic pains in muscles of neck and back.
- LS_2 ➲ Pain in the muscles, worse from motion.
- LS_3 ➲ Hand tremble, especially when writing.
- LS_4 ➲ Rheumatism affection the belly of the muscles; Cramping, stitching pains.

Modalities

Aggravation

- ➲ During menstrual period and climacteric.
- ➲ From cold, damp air.
- ➲ Sitting and Alcohol.
- ➲ More profuse the flow, the greater the suffering.

Amelioration

- ➲ In open air, eating.
- ➲ Continued motion.
- ➲ Pressure & warm covering.

Relations

- ➲ ANTIDOTES: Acon; Bapt; Bry; Gels; Puls; Cham; Camph; Bell.
- ➲ SIMILAR: Caul & Puls. in uterine and rheumatic affection; to Agar; Lil-t; Sep.

Aesculus Hippocastanum

- PROVED BY: Dr. Cooly.
- DURATION: 30 days.
- COMMON NAME: Horse Chestnut.
- FAMILY/KINGDOM: Sapindaceae.
- SOURCE: Tincture of fruit with capsul.
- TEMPERAMENT: Irritable.
- SPHERES OF ACTION: Uterus, Lumbo-sacral articulation, venous esp. portal system, liver.
- SUMMARY OF INDICATIONS: Haemorrhoids (with accompanying bad temper)-low backache.

THERAPEUTIC PICTURE OF DRUG

C_{N-1} ➲ Persons having haemorrhoidal tendencies.

C_{N-2} ➲ Who suffer with gastric, bilious, catarrhal troubles.

C_{N-3} ➲ Plethoric Persons with vascular fullness which affects the extremities and the whole body.

M_{D-1} ➲ Depressed; gloomy; low-spirited; irritable.

M_{D-2} ➲ Losses temper easily, regains it slowly.

M_{D-3} ➲ Unable to fix his attention.

DS_1 ➲ Follicular pharyngitis.

DS_2 ➲ Pricking in fauces; Pressure as if something had lodged there.

DS_3 ➲ Dryness, burning and constriction in fauces.

DS_4 ➲ Frequent neuralgic pain in the fauces.

DS_5 ➲ Soreness, burning, itching, fullness and urging at the anus.

DS_6 ➲ Dryness, heat and constriction of the rectum; rectum feels as if full of small sticks; knife- like pain in anus.

DS_7 ➲ Haemorrhoids blind, purple, Painful sensation of burning; seldom bleed. Aching and lameness, or shooting in back.

DS_8 ➲ Stool large, dry, hard and knotty; difficult, dark; mushy, light brown, first part hard, black, the last of about natural consistency, but white as milk.

DS_9 ➲ Stools followed by fullness of the rectum and intense pain of the anal orifice for several hours; (Aloe; Ign., Mur-ac., sulph.) feels like a bunch of small sticks in the rectum.

FGS_1 ➲ Inflamed cervix uteri, retroversion, prolapsus, inlargement and induration, when characterised by great tenderness, heat and throbbing.

FGS_2 ➲ Old cases of leucorrhoea, with lumbo-sacral backache, of a dark yellow colour, thick and sticky, worse after menstrual period, increased by walking, corrodes the labia, with aching in the sacrum and knees.

FGS_3 ➲ Uterine soreness with throbbing in hypogastrium.

FGS_4 ➲ Back 'gives out' during pregnancy, prolapsus, leucorrhoea; when walking or stooping; must sit or lie down.

B_{K-1} ➲ Severe dull backache in the lumbo-sacral region, more or less constant affecting the sacrum and hips as well.

B_{K-2} ➲ Lameness and weariness, in back of neck.

B_{K-3} ➲ Sacrum and hips; worse stooping forward and when walking.

PG_1 ➲ Fullness in various parts.

PG_2 ➲ Venous congestion, especially portal and haemorrhoidal.

Modalities

Aggravation

- ➲ Motion.
- ➲ In morning on awaking.
- ➲ Backache & soreness by walking and stooping.

Amelioration

- ➲ From rest.
- ➲ Cool open air.

Relations

- ➲ COMPARE: Aesc-gl; Alo; Collins; Merc; Nux-vom; Pod; Sul.
- ➲ ANTIDOTES: Nux-vom.
- ➲ SIMILAR: Aloe; Ign; Nux; Sulph; Mur-ac; in haemorrhoids.

Aethusa Cynapium

- PROVED BY: Nenning.
- DURATION: 20-30 days.
- COMMON NAME: Fool's Parsley.
- FAMILY/KINGDOM: Umbelliferae.
- RELATION COLD/HEAT: Hot.
- MIASM: Psora, Syphilis & Psycosis.
- TEMPERAMENT: Idiotic, confused and unable to think.
- SOURCE: Tincture of whole flowering plant.
- SPHERES OF ACTION: Nervous system, glandular system, mucous membrane and skin.
- SUMMARY OF INDICATIONS: Nauses and vomiting of infants and children-convulsions, epilepsy-disorders of dentition.

THERAPEUTIC PICTURE OF DRUG

C_{N-1} ➲ Especially useful for children during the period of dentition.

C_{N-2} ➲ Features expressive of Pain and anxiety.

C_{N-3} ➲ Herpetic eruption on end of the nose.

C_{N-4} ➲ Sunkenness in the face with marked linea nasalis.

M_{D-1} ➲ Epileptic spasms, with clenched thumbs, red face, eyes turned downwards, Pupils fixed and dilated; foam at the mouth, jaws locked.

M_{D-2} ➲ Incapacity of mind to think, confused, idiocy.

M_{D-3} ➲ Gread sadness when alone; hallucinations.

M_{D-4} ➲ Delirium: sees cats and dogs; tries to jump out of window.

M_{D-5} ➲ Anxiety and restlessness, afterwards headache and colic.

M_{D-6} ➲ Irritability, especially in the afternoon and in the open air.

DS_1 ➲ Can not tolerate milk in any form.

DS_2 ➲ Violent sudden vomiting: of frothy white substance; of yellow fluid, followed by curdled milk and cheesy matter.

DS_3 ➲ Vomiting of greenish phlegm, similar to stools.

DS_4 ➲ Nursing child: the child is forcibly ejected soon after been taken; then weakness causes drowsiness.

DS_5 ➲ Regurgitation of food on hour or so after eating.

PG_1 ➲ Complete absence of thirst (Apis; Puls;)

PG_2 ➲ Physically the child is so weak that he is unable to stand or hold up the head.

Modalities

Aggravation

- After eating or drinking.
- After vomiting.
- After stool.
- After spasms.

Amelioration

- Opening air.
- Company.

Relations

- COMPLEMENTARY: Calc.
- ANTIDOTES: Vegetables (raw); acids.
- SIMILAR: Ant-c; Ars; Calc-OS; Sonic.

Agaricus muscarius = Amanita

- PROVED BY: Schbeter and stapf.
- DURATION: 40 days.
- COMMON NAME: Toad stool (fly fungus).
- FAMILY/KINGDOM: Plants.
- RELATION COLD/HEAT: Chilly.
- MIASM: Psora and syphilis.
- TEMPERAMENT: Nervous.
- SOURCE: Tincture of fresh fungus.
- SPHERES OF ACTION: Nerves, mind,mucous membrane, brain, circulation and skin.
- SUMMARY OF INDICATIONS: Alcoholism–chorea, epilepsy–disorders due to exposure to cold and inclement weathe.

THERAPEUTIC PICTURE OF DRUG

C_{N-1} ➲ Persons with light hair, skin and muscles lax.

C_{N-2} ➲ It is best adapted to old persons with weak.indolent circulation

M_{D-1} ➲ Delirium characterized by singing, shouting, and muttering; rhymes and prophesies.

M_{D-2} ➲ Begins with a Paroxysm of yawning.

M_{D-3} ➲ Loquacity; aversion to work; Indifference; and fearless.

M_{D-4} ➲ Very much out of humor.

NS_1 ➲ Involuntary movements while awake, which Cease during sleep; chorea, varying from simple group of muscles, to dancing and trembling of the whole body; twitching of the muscles of the face (Mygale lasiodora).

NS_2 ➲ Epilepsy caused by suppressed eruptions (Psor., Sulph.).

NS_3 ➲ Strange, rare, Peculiar: Sensation as if Pierced by needles.

NS_4 ➲ Uncertainty in walking, stumbling gait.

FGS_1 ➲ Leucorrhoea, with much itching internally and externally.

FGS_2 ➲ Sexual excitement; Nipples itch & burn.

FGS_3 ➲ Awafully bearing down Pain almost intolerable.

FGS_4 ➲ Itching and irritation of the Parts with strong desire for an embrace.

FGS_5 ➲ During menses: headache, toothache. Pain and itching in left arm; itching; Palpitation; Salivation.

MGS_1 ➲ Great desire for an embrance, the Penis being relaxed.

MGS_2 ➲ Voluptuous itching of the genitals.

MGS_3 ➲ After coitus: great debility; profuse night-sweats; burning, itching of the skin.

B_{K-1} ➲ Pain in lumbar region and sacrum; a sort of crick in the back; extends along to the nape of the neck.

B_{K-2} ➲ Spine sensitive to touch; worse mornings.

B_{K-3} ➲ Every motion, every turn of body, causes pain in spine.

$S_{N\ 1}$ ➲ Chilblains, that itch and burn intolerably.

S_{N-1} ➲ Chilblains, that itch and burn intolerably.

S_{N-2} ➲ Burning–itching, redness and swelling, as from frostbites.

S_{N-3} ➲ Military eruptions close and white, with intolerable burning, itching.

S_{N-4} ➲ Itching stitches in various parts.

S_{N-5} ➲ Violent itching between thumb and forefinger, left hand.

PG_1 ➲ Hang over headaches; ill effects following excess of food and alcohal (Lab–inf;Nux–vom; Rann- bul.].

PG_2 ➲ Complaints appear diagonally; (Upper left and lower right side: Ant–tart,stra; upper right, lower left: - Ambra–grisea, Medorrh,Phos,Sul-acid.).

PG_3 ➲ Nervous prostration after sexual debauches.

PG_4 ➲ Exceedingly sensitive to cold air.

Modalities

Aggravation

- ➲ After eating, cold air, after coitus.
- ➲ Mental work, ice cold weather
- ➲ Before a thunder-storm.

Amelioration

- ➲ Moving about slowly.
- ➲ In open air.
- ➲ Warm application.

Relations

- ➲ FOLLOWS WELL: Bell; Op; Puls; Sil; Rhust.
- ➲ ANTIDOTES: Col-corb; Puls; Wine.

Agnus castus

- ➲ PROVED BY: Hahnemann.
- ➲ DURATION: 8-14 days.
- ➲ COMMON NAME: Chaste tree.
- ➲ FAMILY/KINGDOM: Verbenaceac.
- ➲ RELATION COLD/HEAT: Chilly.
- ➲ SOURCE: Tincture of ripe berries.
- ➲ SPHERES OF ACTION: Sexual organs of female & Male, mind and nerves.
- ➲ SUMMARY OF INDICATIONS: Leucorrhoea–deficient lactation–disorders of memory–endogenous depression.

THERAPEUTIC PICTURE OF DRUG

C_{N-1} ➲ Persons to suppress the sexual desire.

C_{N-2} ➲ For the lymphatic constitution.

M_{D-1} ➲ Extreme absence of mind; unable to recollect things;finds it difficult to read or keep up the train of thought.

M_{D-2} ➲ Despairing, sadness; low-spirited; fears of approaching death; keeps repeating that she will soon die.

M_{D-3} ➲ Premature old age; melancholy, apathy, mental distraction, self contempt; arising in young persons from abuse of sexual powers.

FGS_1 ➲ Transparent leucorrhoea; Parts very relaxed.

FGS_2 ➲ Leucorrhoea spotting linen yellow.

FGS_3 ➲ Sterility, with suppressed menses, and want of sexual desire.

FGS_4 ➲ Milk scanty or entirely suppressed. (Asaf, Lac-c.Lac-.d.).

FGS_5 ➲ Deficient secretion of milk in lying–in women.

FGS_6 ➲ Swelling and inflammation of the uterus.

FGS_7 ➲ Retained placenta Pain as if dislocated in joint.

FGS_8 ➲ Suppressed menses with abdominal Pain.

MGS_1 ➲ Sexual desire lessened, almost lost; impotence with spermatorrhoea.

MGS_2 ➲ Feeble erections, no sexual desire.

MGS_3 ➲ Penis so relaxed that voluptuous fancies excite no erections.

MGS_4 ➲ Impotence, with gleet, especially with those who have frequently had gonorrhoea.

MGS_5 ➲ Gleet, with want of sexual desire or erections.

PG_1 ➲ Hysteria with maniacal lasciviousness.

PG_2 ➲ Complains of imaginary odours,as of rotten herrings faecal matter and other offensive smell.

PG_3 ➲ Prevents excoriation, from walking.

PG_4 ➲ Splenomegaly, spleen is swollen and sore.

PG_5 ➲ Nausea with sensation as if intestines were pressed downwards; wants to support bowels (ascites).

Modalities

Aggravation

➲ Sexual excess.

Amelioration

➲ By pressure.

Relations

➲ COMPARE: Nux-v; Chel; Carb.

➲ FOLLOWS WELL: Lyc; Selen; Sulph; Ign.

➲ ANTIDOTES: Camph; Nux; Nat-Mur.

Aletris farinosa

- ➲ COMMON NAME: Star grass (Belzing grass).
- ➲ FAMILY/KINGDOM: Haemodoraceae.
- ➲ SOURCE: Tincture of root.
- ➲ SPHERES OF ACTION: Mucous membrane, Uteres, Ovary.

THERAPEUTIC PICTURE OF DRUG

C_{N-1} ➲ An anaemic relaxed condition.

C_{N-2} ➲ Chlorotic girl.

M_{D-1} ➲ Confused feelings.

M_{D-2} ➲ Can not concentrate mind.

M_{D-3} ➲ Power & energy weakend.

DS_1 ➲ Much forthy saliva.

FGS_1 ➲ Permature and profouse menses; with labor–like pains.

FGS_2 ➲ Uterus seems heavy.

FGS_3 ➲ Leucorrhoea due to weakness & Anemia.

FGS_4 ➲ Habitual tendency to abortion.

FGS_5 ➲ The patient is Tired all the time and suffer from prolapsus, Leucorrhoea, Rectal distress etc.

FGS_6 ➲ Obstinate vomiting of pregnancy.

FGS_7 ➲ Retarted and Scanty flow.

FGS_8 ➲ Prolapse with pain in right inguinal region.

FGS_9 ➲ Muscular pain during pregnancy.

Modalities

Aggravation

- ➲ Bending forward.
- ➲ By food.

Amelioration

- ➲ Open air, Rubbing.

Relations

- ➲ COMPARE: Helonias, dioica; China, Sabin.

Allium cepa

- ➲ PROVED BY: Hering.
- ➲ DURATION: 1 day.
- ➲ COMMON NAME: Onion.
- ➲ FAMILY/KINGDOM: Liliaceae.
- ➲ RELATION COLD/HEAT: Hot.
- ➲ MIASM: Psora.
- ➲ SOURCE: Tincture of the onion or of while fresh plant gathered from July to August.
- ➲ SPHERES OF ACTION: Conjunctiva, mucous membrane of nose, respiratory tract, intestine, nerves and veins.
- ➲ SUMMARY OF INDICATIONS: Frontal headaches- common cold- Pharyngitis- laryngitis- infantile colic (Infantile gastro-enteristis).

THERAPEUTIC PICTURE OF DRUG

Note: This remedy helps at the commencement of a cold. The patients looks as if he or she had been Peeling onions. There is frequent sneezing and the eyes are tearing; a watery discharge irritates the nose. The person may also have laryngitis, with a raw, painful sensation extending into the chest.

M_{D-1} ➲ Very melancholy.

M_{D-2} ➲ Fear pains will become unbearable.

M_{D-3} ➲ Often very anxious, with catarrh, dullness of intellect.

H_{D-1} ➲ Catarrhal headache, mostly in the forehead region; worse in a warm room, toward evening.

H_{D-2} ➲ Thread like Pains in the face.

H_{D-3} ➲ Headache ceases during menses; returnes when flow disappears.

SO_1 ➲ Excessive non-excoriating lachrymation.

SO_2 ➲ Itching, biting, burning in the eyes.

- SO_3 ➲ Dulness of the eyes, with aversion to light, and coryza.
- NS_1 ➲ Neuralgic Pains, like a fine thread, following amputations or injuries to nerves.
- NS_2 ➲ Traumatic chronic neuritis; neuralgia of stump after amputation burning and stinging pains.
- RS_1 ➲ Catarrhal laryngitis, with severe cough which compels the patient to grasp the larynx; seems as if the cough would tear a larynx.
- RS_2 ➲ Coryza: is spring coryza after exposure to dump north western wind; discharges burn and corrode the nose and upper lip.
- RS_3 ➲ Coryza; Profuse, watery and acrid nasal discharge with Profuse, bland lachrymation.
- RS_4 ➲ Cough when exposure to the cold air. Grasps the throat when coughing; patient feels as if the cough would spilt or tear the chest.
- PG_1 ➲ Spring coryza, after dump northeasterly winds.
- PG_2 ➲ Indicated in infants with colicky pains in the abdomen.
- PG_3 ➲ Symptoms-usually commence on the left side and extend towards the right.

Modalities

Aggravation

- ➲ Evening.
- ➲ Warm room.

Amelioration

- ➲ Open air.
- ➲ Cold room.

Relations

- ➲ COMPLEMENTARY: Phos; Puls; Sars; Thuj.
- ➲ FOLLOWS WELL: Calc., Sil.
- ➲ ANTIDOTES: Arn. Cham. Verat; Thuja Nux-x.
- ➲ INIMICALS: All-s.

Allium sativum

- ➲ COMMON NAME: Garlic.
- ➲ FAMILY/KINGDOM: Liliaceae.
- ➲ RELATION COLD/HEAT: Hot.
- ➲ MIASM: Psora & Syphilis.
- ➲ DIATHESIS: Haemorrhagic.
- ➲ SOURCE: Tincture of fresh bulb.
- ➲ SPHERES OF ACTION: Has vaso-dilatory Properties.

THERAPEUTIC PICTURE OF DRUG

C_{N-1} ➲ Tubercular constitution.

C_{N-2} ➲ Lean, thin, emaciated.

M_{D-1} ➲ Anxiety and impatient.

M_{D-2} ➲ Fears he won't recover; that he won't be able to bear any medicine.

M_{D-3} ➲ Fears he won't Poisoned.

DS_1 ➲ Voracious appetite.

DS_2 ➲ Burnig eructations (dyspepsia) and least change in diet caused trouble.

DS_3 ➲ Tongue Pale, red papillae.

DS_4 ➲ Sweetish Saliva after meals and at night. Sensation of a hair on the tongue or in the throat.

RS_1 ➲ Constont rattling of mucus in the branchi

FGS_1 ➲ Menses to early; headache and dizziness lessen as the flow becomes established.

FGS_2 ➲ During menses extensive excoriations of skin of internal Portions of thigh.

FGS_3 ➲ Bright red spots, with itching and smarting on the inside of the labia majora and at entrance of vagina.

FGS $_4$ ➲ Eruption of red blotches between the breasts and around the nipples.

LS $_1$ ➲ Pain in hip, pain in psoas and iliac muscles.

Modalities

Aggravation

➲ Least motion, movement. ➲ Open air.

Amelioration

➲ Sitting bent, onset of menses.

Relations

- ➲ COMPARE: Capsium; kal-nit; Senega.
- ➲ COMPLEMENTARY: Ars.
- ➲ ANTIDOTES: Lycopodium.
- ➲ INIMICALS: Aloe; All-c, Silic.

Aloe socotrina

- PROVED BY: Helbig.
- DURATION: 20-30 days.
- COMMON NAME: Socotrine Aloes.
- FAMILY/KINGDOM: Liliaceae.
- RELATION COLD/HEAT: Hot.
- MIASM: Psora.
- TEMPERAMENT: Bilious.
- SOURCE: Trituration or Solution in sprit of the gum.
- SPHERES OF ACTION: .Nervous System, Portal system liver, intestine, blood and skin.
- SUMMARY OF INDICATIONS: Chronic and acute diarrhoea- haemorrhoid-constipation.

THERAPEUTIC PICTURE OF DRUG

C_{N-1} ➲ Old people (especially women) of relaxed, Phlegmatic habits.

C_{N-2} ➲ Extreme Prostration with Perspiration.

C_{N-3} ➲ Indolent weary Persons leading sedentary life, averse to either Physical and mental labour.

M_{D-1} ➲ Lassitude, alternating with great mental activity.

M_{D-2} ➲ Great disinclination to mental labor; it fatigues him; general languor.

M_{D-3} ➲ He is dissatisfied and angry about himself; more so when he is constipated or when he suffers from Pain; better in the open air.

H_{D-1} ➲ Headache alternate with lumbago, with intestinal and uterine affections.

H_{D-2} ➲ Headache above forehead, with heaviness in eyes, must close them partially.

H_{D-3} ➲ Headache after stool.

H_{D-4} ➲ Headache better from cold application, pressive pain: worse from heat.

DS_1 ➲ Diarrhoea: has to hurry to toilet immediately after eating or drinking; lax sphincter ani; driving patient out of bed early in the morning.

DS_2 ➲ Diarrhoea; in hot, damp weather; evening, night and morning; from vinegar; from cold, damp room; when walking or standing; when passing urine.

DS_3 ➲ Abdominal muscles Pain (colic) when touched, when pressing at stool, or on rising from a recumbent position.

DS_4 ➲ Discharge of much flatulency, burning, smelling offensive, relieving the pain in the abdomen; after each meal, in the evening and morning, before stool.

DS_5 ➲ Urgency as with diarrhoea, only hot flatus passes, with great relief.

DS_6 ➲ Urging wakens at night, drives out of bed at 6 A.M.

DS_7 ➲ Gurgling of flatus in descending colon; worse after eating.

DS_8 ➲ During stool: tenesmus and much flatus.

DS_9 ➲ Before stool: rumbling, violent sudden urging, heariness in rectum.

DS_{10} ➲ After stool: faintness.

DS_{11} ➲ Haemorrhoids: blue, like a bunch of grapes. Thrombosis of the haemorroids. Constipation, with pressure on the lower abdomen.

DS_{12} ➲ Itching and burning in the anus; Preventing sleep.

DS_{13} ➲ Weakness or loss of power of sphincter ani.

Modalities

Aggravation

- Early morning.
- Hot, dry weather.
- Standing or walking.
- Sedentary.
- After eating or drinking.

Amelioration

- Cold water.
- Cold weather.
- Discharge of flatus and stool.

Relations

- COMPLEMENTARY: Sulph.
- FOLLOWS WELL: Kali-bi; Sep., Sulph; Sul-ac.
- ANTIDOTES: Camph; Lyc; Nux-v.
- INIMICALS: All-s.

Alumina

- PROVED BY: Hahnemann.
- DURATION: 40-60days.
- COMMON NAME: Pure clay [Argilla =oxide of aluminium].
- FAMILY/KINGDOM: Minerals.
- RELATION COLD/HEAT: Very chilly.
- MIASM: Psora.
- DIATHESIS: Scrofulous.
- TEMPERAMENT: Hypochondriac.
- SOURCE: Trituration of $Al_2O_3.3H_2O$.
- SPHERES OF ACTION: Mucous membrane, fibrous tissue, motor nerves, female sexual organs. and skin.
- SUMMARY OF INDICATIONS: Constipation (obstinate)–leucorrhoea.

THERAPEUTIC PICTURE OF DRUG

C_{N-1} ➲ Persons is spare, dry, thin, having dark complexion.

C_{N-2} ➲ Persons of sedentary habits who suffer from chronic ailments. Constitutions deficient in animal heat.

M_{D-1} ➲ Variable mood.

M_{D-2} ➲ Suicidal tendency on seeing a knife or blood.

M_{D-3} ➲ Time passes too slowly; an hour seems half as a day. (canni.)

M_{D-4} ➲ Low spirited; fears loss of reason.

M_{D-5} ➲ Confused about their personal identity.

M_{D-6} ➲ Mild, cheerful disposition; hypochondriacs.

M_{D-7} ➲ Dispoisition to be angry-unfitness for Labours.

M_{D-8} ➲ Better as day advances.

DS_1 ➲ Inactivity of rectum, even soft stool requires great straining (Anac;Plat; sil: verat.).

DS_2 ➲ Constipation: no desire for and inability to defaecate, until there is large accumulation (Melilotus alba); severe straining, must grasp the seat of the closet tightly; stool hard, knotty.

DS_3 ➲ Constipation of sucklings.

DS_4 ➲ Diarrhoea; with urging in rectum; when she urinates.

DS_5 ➲ Clots of blood pass from the anus.

DS_6 ➲ Haemorrhoids worse in evenings, better after night's rest.

DS_7 ➲ Itching and burning at the anus; fistula ani.

DS_8 ➲ Eructations: sour; bitter, after Potatoes; worse evening.

FGS_1 ➲ Leucorrhoea: acrid and profuse, running down to the heels (syph.).; worse during day time; better cold bathing.

FGS_2 ➲ Corrosive leucorrhoea, with smarting in the genital parts.

FGS_3 ➲ Leucorrhoea before or after the menses, and often with trembling fatigue, and colic.

FGS_4 ➲ Leucorrhoea flesh coloured, or aquous, and causing stiffness of the linen; transparent mucous before and after menstruation.

FGS_5 ➲ Menstruation scantly, too early, and of short duration; blood pale.

FGS_6 ➲ Menses too copious,with inflation of the abdomen.

FGS_7 ➲ During the period of menstruation, sleep agitated, with many dreams.

FGS_8 ➲ Before and during menstruation, colics, headaches, and other painful affections.

FGS_9 ➲ After menses: exhausted physically and mentally, scarcely able to speak (carb-an.Cocc)

S_{N-1} ➲ Dry, tettery, itching eruption, worse in winter.

PG_1 ➲ Inability to walk, except with the eyes open, and in the day time: tottering and falling when closing eyes (Arg-n.,Gels.).

Modalities

Aggravation

- During day time.
- from wine.
- After coitus.
- Walking.
- At new moon and full moon.

Amelioration

- Mild summer weather.
- Open air.
- from warm drinks.
- By cold bathing.

Relations

- COMPARE: Aluminium.
- COMPLEMENTARY: Bryonia; Ferr.
- FOLLOWS WELL: Bryonia; Lach; Sulph; Arg-met.
- ANTIDOTES: Lead; Ipec; Nux-v; Camph; Cham.
- SIMILAR: Arg-nit.

Ambra grisea

- ➲ COMMON NAME: Ambergris.
- ➲ DURATION: 40 days.
- ➲ RELATION COLD/HEAT: Worse to hot and better to cold.
- ➲ FAMILY/KINGDOM: A Nosode.
- ➲ MIASM: Psora and syphilis.
- ➲ SOURCE: A morbid secretion of the whale.
- ➲ TEMPERAMENT: Nervous, bilious.
- ➲ SPHERES OF ACTION: Nervous system, GIT, respiratory tract and female genital organs.
- ➲ SUMMARY OF INDICATIONS: Anxiety neurosis–frequent colds-bronchitis.

THERAPEUTIC PICTURE OF DRUG

C_{N-1} ➲ It is suited to old people & children, especially young girls who are excitable, nervous and physically weak.

C_{N-2} ➲ Thin scrawny womens (Sec: Cor.).

C_{N-3} ➲ Nervous and emaciated persons.

M_{D-1} ➲ Desire to be alone.

M_{D-2} ➲ Music causes: weeping.

M_{D-3} ➲ Great sadness, sits for days weeping.

M_{D-4} ➲ Great Restlessness, memory impaired.

M_{D-5} ➲ Despair, loathing of life.

M_{D-6} ➲ After business embarrassments, unable to sleep, must get up (Cimic; sep.).

SO_1 ➲ Ranula with foetid breath.

DS_1 ➲ Distension of stomach after midnight.

DS_2 ➲ The presence of others, even the nurse, is unbearable during stool; frequent, in effectual desire, which makes her anxious.

FGS_1 ➲ Menses too early; and too profuse.

FGS_2 ➲ Discharge of blood between the periods, at every little accident a long walk, after every hard stool, etc.

FGS_3 ➲ Leucorrhoea preceded by shootings pains in the vagina.

FGS_4 ➲ Running of white–bluish matter from the vagina.

FGS_5 ➲ Leucorrhoea: Thick, bluish–white mucus, especially or only at night [Caust; Merc; Nit- ac.].

FGS_6 ➲ Burning, Pain of excoriation, and itching, in the sexual parts.

FGS_7 ➲ Violent itching, with swelling of the external parts.

FGS_8 ➲ During menstruation,Increased swelling of varicose veins, with Pressure in the legs.

PG_1 ➲ The pelvic organs are painfully influenced.

Modalities

Aggravation

- ➲ Warm drinks.
- ➲ Warm room.
- ➲ Music.

Amelioration

- ➲ After eating.
- ➲ Cold air.
- ➲ Cold food and drinks.
- ➲ Rising from bed.

Relations

- ➲ COMPARE: Moschus; Pso.
- ➲ FOLLOWS WELL: Lyc; Puls; Sep; Sulph.
- ➲ ANTIDOTES: Camph-office; Coff; Nux-v.
- ➲ SIMILAR: Cimic; Asaf; Coca; Ign; Mosch; Phos; Valer.

Ammonium carbonicum

- PROVED BY: Hahnemann.
- DURATION: 40 days.
- COMMON NAME: Smelling Salts.
- FAMILY/KINGDOM: Minerals.
- RELATION COLD/HEAT: Very Chilly.
- MIASM: Psora.
- DIATHESIS: Haemorrhagic.
- SOURCE: Sesqui carbonate of Ammonia $2[(NH_4)_2CO_3]CO_2$. Solution in distilled water.
- SPHERES OF ACTION: Female genital organs, Nerves, GIT. blood, cardio-vascular system.
- SUMMARY OF INDICATIONS: Emphysema-obesity.

THERAPEUTIC PICTURE OF DRUG

C_{N-1} ➲ Stout, fleshy and delicate women who lead sedentary life with a "Smelling-bottle" always in the hand. Readily catch cold in winter.

M_{D-1} ➲ Sadness, with disposition to weep, apprehensions and anguish, which often disappear towards the evening.

M_{D-2} ➲ Talking and hearing others talk, affects greatly.

M_{D-3} ➲ Ill-humour in the morning, and when it is bad weather,

M_{D-4} ➲ Morose and passionate humour.

M_{D-5} ➲ Great absence of mind and weakness of memory.

SO_1 ➲ Nose bleed: when washing the face (Arn; mag-c).

SO_2 ➲ Stopping of nose, mostly at night; must breath through the mouth.

RS_1 ➲ One of the choice remedies in emphysema. Epistaxis.

RS_2 ➲ Dyspnoea with palpitation, worse with the least exertion such as ascending a few steps; worse in a worm room.

RS_3 ➲ Cough; at night, about midnight, violent, about 3 or 4 A.M.

FGS$_1$ ➲ Swelling, itching, and burning in the external genital parts of the female.

FGS$_2$ ➲ Aversion to the other sex.

FGS$_3$ ➲ Excoriation of the skin in the parts, and in the anus.

FGS$_4$ ➲ Leucorrhoea watery, burning from the uterus; acrid, profuse from the vagina; excoriation of vulva.

FGS$_5$ ➲ Menses too frequent, profuse, early (menorrhagia), Copious, clotted, black.

FGS$_6$ ➲ Great weakness during the menstrual flow; haemorrhoids< during.

FGS$_7$ ➲ Before and during the catamenia, colic and pain in the loins.

FGS$_8$ ➲ during the catamenia, toothache, pressure on the matrix, cutting, acute drawings in the back and in the genital parts,, desire to lie down, paleness of the face, shivering, coryza, and sadness.

FGS$_9$ ➲ Cholera- like symptoms at the commencement of menstruation (Bov;verat.).

Modalities

Aggravation

- ➲ Cold, wet weather.
- ➲ Wet poultices.
- ➲ From washing or bathing.
- ➲ During menstruation.

Amelioration

- ➲ Lying on abdomen (acet-ac.).
- ➲ On Painful side (Puls; nig; Bry;). In dry weather.

Relations

➲ COMPARE:	Ant-t; ars; phos; Lach; Puls.;rhus.
➲ FOLLOWS WELL:	Bell; Calc; Lyc; Phos; Puls; Rhus-t. sep; sulph.
➲ ANTIDOTES:	Arn; camph; hep.
➲ INIMICALS:	Lachesis.

Ammonicum Muriaticum

- ➲ PROVED BY: Nenning.
- ➲ DURATION: 20–30 days.
- ➲ COMMON NAME: Salt Ammoniac (NH_4Cl).
- ➲ FAMILY/KINGDOM: Minerals.
- ➲ RELATION COLD/HEAT: Chilly.
- ➲ MIASM: Psoric and syphilitic.
- ➲ SOURCE: NH_4Cl–Trituration of (NH_4Cl).
- ➲ TEMPERAMENT: Melancholic and disposition to tears.
- ➲ SPHERES OF ACTION: Mucous membrane, Liver & Female genital Organs.
- ➲ SUMMARY OF INDICATIONS: Coryza–gastroenteritis–Polyneuropathy.

THERAPEUTIC PICTURE OF DRUG

C_{N-1} ➲ Especially adapted to those persons who are fat and sluggish.

C_{N-2} ➲ Persons which have body large and fat, but legs too thin.

C_{N-3} ➲ Womens having large buttocks.

M_{D-1} ➲ Melancholy, apprehension; from internal grief.

M_{D-2} ➲ Full of grief, but cannot weep.

M_{D-3} ➲ Morose, apathetic humour, with repugnance to conversation.

M_{D-4} ➲ Mild cheerful disposition; hypochondriacs.

M_{D-5} ➲ Time passes too slowly; an hour seems half a day(Canni.).

M_{D-6} ➲ He is ill-humoured with irritability and disposition to be angry.

M_{D-7} ➲ He has antipathy to certain persons which is very peculiar to herself.

DS_1 ➲ Stitching or tearing pain in Perineum, when walking.

DS_2 ➲ Burning in the rectum during, and for house after, stool.

DS_3 ➲ Diarrhoea, with soreness of anus, sore pustules near it.

DS_4 ➲ Diarrhoea after eating, with pain in abdomen, back, small of back and limbs; much flatus.

DS_5 ➲ Green, slimy, diarrhoeic stools, in the mornings.

DS_6 ➲ Haemorrhoids, sore and smarting.

DS_7 ➲ Harmorrhoids after suppressed leucorrhoea.

DS_8 ➲ Hard, crumbling stools require great effort in expulsion.

RS_1 ➲ Acrid coryza, corroding the lip (All-c).

FGS_1 ➲ Leucorrhoea; like white of egg. preceded by griping pain about the navel;brown, Slimy,painless, after, every urination.

FGS_2 ➲ Menses too early, too free, clark, clotted; flow more at night (menorrhagia).

FGS_3 ➲ During the menses, vomiting and diarrhoea, drawing in the feet, or discharge of blood on going to stool.

FGS_4 ➲ During menses, neuralgic pains in the feet.

FGS_5 ➲ During menses, diarrhoea; greenish mucoid stools, and pain around the navel.

FGS_6 ➲ During pregnancy pain as if sprained, in the left side of abdomen.

PG_1 ➲ Offensive sweat of the feet (Alum;Graph;Psor;Sani;Silic.).

PG_2 ➲ Sensation of coldness in the back and between the scapulae (Lach-tinc.).

PG_3 ➲ Hard, crumbling stools require great effort in expulsion; crumble from the verge ofanus (Mag-m.) vary in colour, no two stools alike(puls.).

Modalities

Aggravation

➲ Head and chest symptoms.

➲ Abdominal symptoms in the afternoon.

Amelioration

➲ Open air.

Relations

➲ COMPARE:	Calc; Seneg; caust.
➲ FOLLOWS WELL:	Ant-c; merc; Nux-v.
	Phos; puls; Rhus-t.
➲ ANTIDOTES:	Coff; Nux-vom; Caust.

Anacardium orientale

- PROVED BY: Stapf.
- DURATION: 30–40 days.
- COMMON NAME: Marking Nut.
- FAMILY/KINGDOM: Anacardiaceae.
- RELATION COLD/HEAT: Neither chilly not hot.
- MIASM: Psora and Syphilis.
- TEMPERAMENT: Highly irritable.
- SPHERES OF ACTION: Mind, nerves, stomach, rectum and skin.

THERAPEUTIC PICTURE OF DRUG

C_{N-1} ➲ Pale face with blue ring around the eyes.

M_{D-1} ➲ Hypochondriacal sadness, and melancholy ideas.

M_{D-2} ➲ Weakness of mind and of memory.

M_{D-3} ➲ Sudden loss of memory.

M_{D-4} ➲ Fixed ideas. Hallucinations; thinks he is possessed by two people or wills.

M_{D-5} ➲ Disposition to laugh at serious things and to maintain a serious demeanour when anything laughable occurs.

M_{D-6} ➲ Lack of confidence in himself or others.

M_{D-7} ➲ Irresistible desire to curse and swear.

H_{D-1} ➲ Headache worse during mental work, with sensation of heat in the head; better during a meal, worse after.

H_{D-2} ➲ Headache, worse during motion and work.

H_{D-3} ➲ Nervous and gastric headache of sedentary persons.

H_{D-4} ➲ Headache with giddiness and vertigo, aggravated by movement.

DS_1 ➲ Symptoms disappear during dinner; begin a new after two hours.

DS_2 ➲ Eructations: empty, frequent fluid, causing choking; with spasmodic pain in stomach.

DS_3 ➲ First, sensation of fasting in pit of stomach, then pressure in stomach.

DS_4 ➲ Weak digestion, with fullness and distention of abdomen.

DS_5 ➲ Great and urgent desire for stool, but with the effort the desire passes away, without an evacuation; the rectum seems powerless, with sensation as if plugged up.

DS_6 ➲ Inactivity of rectum, even soft stool passed with difficulty.

FGS_1 ➲ Frequent but scanty menses, Sometimes with spasmodic pains in abdomen.

FGS_2 ➲ Weakness of all senses during pregnancy.

FGS_3 ➲ Headache may also appear during menses; headache-relieved entirely when eating.

PG_1 ➲ Weakness of the all senses.

Modalities

Aggravation

- ➲ On application of hot water.
- ➲ During motion.
- ➲ Mental work and empty stomach.

Amelioration

- ➲ From eating.
- ➲ When lying down on side.
- ➲ From rubbing.

Relations

➲ COMPARE:	Rhus-t.
➲ FOLLOWS WELL:	Lyc; Plat; Puls.
➲ ANTIDOTES:	Coff; clematis erecta, cro-tig., Jug; Ran-bulb.

Antimonium crudum

- PROVED BY: CASPARI.
- DURATION: 40 days.
- COMMON NAME: Black sulphide of antimony [Sb_2S_3].
- FAMILY/KINGDOM: Minerals.
- RELATION COLD/HEAT: Affected by elxtremes of heat & cold.
- MIASM: Psora and Sycosis.
- TEMPERAMENT: Irritable.
- SOURCE: Solution & Trituration of Sb_2S_3.
- SPHERES OF ACTION: On mucous membrane, skin, mind, stomach and intestine.
- SUMMARY OF INDICATIONS: Chronic colitis–Chronic gastritis–mental depression.

THERAPEUTIC PICTURE OF DRUG

C_{N-1} ➲ Young People & children, who are inclined to grow fat-extremes of life.

C_{N-2} ➲ Having tendency to thick unhealthy skin.

M_{D-1} ➲ Child is fretful and peevish, does not wish to be touched or looked at.

M_{D-2} ➲ Child delirious, drowsy, with nausea, hot and red face; pulse irregular; feverish heat; cries when washed in cold water; better washed in warm water.

M_{D-3} ➲ Dull intellect, imbecility.

M_{D-4} ➲ Disgust of life, with an inclination to blow one's brains out, or to drown oneself.

M_{D-5} ➲ Sentimental mood in moonlight, particularly ecstatic love.

M_{D-6} ➲ Great sadness and woeful mood.

M_{D-7} ➲ Anxious reflection in relation to his present and future.

DS_1 ➲ Thick milky–while coating on the tongue.

DS_2 ➲ Stomach weak, easily disturbed digestion.

- DS_3 ➲ Gastric catarrh; nausea and vomiting; cough; bowels loose or stools in lumps, caused by: over eating, sour wine, hot weather, bathing; during measles; metastasis of gout orrheumatism.
- DS_4 ➲ Alternate diarrhoea and constipation, with old people.
- DS_5 ➲ Diarrhoea, worse from vinegar and other acids; sour wine; overheating; after cold bath; night and early morning.
- DS_6 ➲ Difficult, hard stool, feces too large, costive, with incarcerated flatus.
- DS_7 ➲ Copious harmorrhage from bowels, with solid feces; haemorrhoidal.
- DS_8 ➲ Mucous Piles, pricking, burning; continuous mucous discharge, staining yellow, sometimes ichor oozes out.
- RS_1 ➲ Great weakness, or entire loss of voice, chiefly on becoming warm.
- RS_2 ➲ Cough: in the hot sun; on coming into warm room from cold; whooping-cough after measles.
- RS_3 ➲ Looking into the fire increases cough.
- FGS_1 ➲ Menses suppressed from cold bathing,with feeling of pressure in pelvis and tenderness in ovarian region.
- FGS_2 ➲ Toothache, before menses.
- FGS_3 ➲ Leucorrhoea watery, acrid lumpy–Exited, part & itch.
- FGS_4 ➲ Haemorrhoidal affections during pregnancy; nausea and vomiting.
- S_{N-1} ➲ Eruption like boils and blisters.
- S_{N-2} ➲ Measle–like eruption; smooth warts; horny excrescences.
- PG_1 ➲ Disposition to start even at slight noises.
- PG_2 ➲ The symptoms are aggravated in the heat of the sun.
- PG_3 ➲ Great sensibility to cold.
- PG_4 ➲ Emaciation, or great obesity.

Modalities

Aggravation

- ➲ After eating, cold bath.
- ➲ After heat of sun or fire.
- ➲ Extremes of cold & heat.

Amelioration

- ➲ In open air.
- ➲ During rest.
- ➲ After a worm bath.

Relations

- ➲ COMPLEMENTARY: Squilla & sulphur.
- ➲ FOLLOWS WELL: Calc; Lach; Merc; Puls; Sep; Sulph.
- ➲ ANTIDOTES: Calc; Hep; Merc.

Antimonium tartaricum

- PROVED BY: Stapf.
- DURATION: 20-30 days.
- COMMON NAME: Tartar Emetic.
  Tartrate of Antimony and Potash = [2k(sbO) $C_4H_4O_6H_2O_2$).
- FAMILY/KINGDOM: Minerals.
- RELATION COLD/HEAT: Complaints are caused by wet weather and over covering.
- MIASM: Psora and sycosis.
- DIATHESIS: Scrofulous.
- SOURCE: Trituration and solutions of 2k(sbO) $C_4H_4O_6H_2O_2$.
- SPHERES OF ACTION: Respiratory organs, salivary glands, mucous membranes, brain, nerve and skin.
- SUMMARY OF INDICATIONS: Bronchitis-emphysema- Pneumonia-asphyxia neonatorum.

THERAPEUTIC PICTURE OF DRUG

Note: This remedy will benefit the patient who suffers from bronchitis and has a wheezing cough with mucus in the chest, which makes a rattling of bubbling sound, as if the patient is drowing in his own secretions. The patient is Pale, has a cold sweat, and looks seriously ill; lack of energy.

C_{N-1} ➲ Hydrogenoid constitution of Grauvogl, torpid, Phlegmatic persons.

C_{N-2} ➲ Child at birth is Pale.

M_{D-1} ➲ The child will not allow itself to be touched without whining and crying.

M_{D-2} ➲ Bad humor.

M_{D-3} ➲ Excessively peevish and quarrelsome.

M_{D-4} ➲ Frightened at every trifle.

RS_1 ➲ Rattling of mucus when coughing or breathing.

RS_2 ➲ Bronchinal catarrh: Rattling, originating in upper bronchia can be heart at great distance, short cough with a shrill sound.

- RS_3 ➲ Suffocated and oppressed about 2 A.M., must sit up to get air; after cough and expectoration she become better.
- RS_4 ➲ Respiration with great rattling of mucus.
- RS_5 ➲ Cough, with heat and moisture of the hands, and perspiration on the head, chiefly on the forehead.
- RS_6 ➲ Cough, if children get angry, also after eating; child vomits foods and mucus.
- RS_7 ➲ Child breathless and pale when born, gasping; asphyxia neonatorum.
- RS_8 ➲ Cough compels the patient to sit up, is moist and rattling, but no expectoration.
- RS_9 ➲ Cough grows less frequent, patient shows sign of " Carbonized blood".
- DS_1 ➲ Tongue moist, clean or loaded with a brown coating.
- DS_2 ➲ Tongue: red dry in middle; red in streaks, thick, white, pasty coat, thick white fur.
- DS_3 ➲ Nausea: causing anxiety; with slight pressure in out of stomach, followed by headache in forehead; and incessant vomiting whole night, with diarrhoea.
- DS_4 ➲ Vomiting is followed with great languor, drowsiness, loothing, desire for cooling things.
- S_{N-1} ➲ Face: Pale, Sunken; Pole, Puffed, with coma; bluish.
- S_{N-2} ➲ Pustular eruption leaves bluish-red marks on face, also similar eruption on genitals and thighs, painful.
- PG_1 ➲ Tearing Pain in while side of face, even head and neck of the side.
- PG_2 ➲ In same forms of Pneumonia so great is the Prostration that the patient is constantly slipping down in bed.
- PG_3 ➲ Great debility, weakness and excessive lassitude; feels best when sitting still doing nothing.

Modalities

Aggravation

- ➲ Damp, cold weather.
- ➲ Evening.
- ➲ Warmth of room, lying down.
- ➲ All sour foods, milk and milk produce.

Amelioration

- ➲ Open air, cold.
- ➲ Sitting erect.
- ➲ Belching.
- ➲ Expectoration.
- ➲ Lying on the right side.

Relations

- ➲ FOLLOWS WELL: Bar-c; Camph; Cina; Ip; Kali-bi; Pulsi Sep; Sulph.
- ➲ ANTIDOTES: Asaf; Chin; Cocc; Laur; OP; Rush-tax.
- ➲ SIMILAR: Lyc; Verat; Ip.

Apis mellifeca

- ➲ PROVED BY: BRAUNS.
- ➲ FAMILY/KINGDOM: Animals.
- ➲ COMMON NAME: Honey Bee [Apium virus].
- ➲ MIASM: Psora.
- ➲ RELATION COLD/HEAT: Hot.
- ➲ TEMPERAMENT: Irritable.
- ➲ DIATHESIS: Scrofulous.
- ➲ SOURCE: Derived from poison of Honey Bee.
- ➲ SPHERES OF ACTION: Cellular tissues, Brain, glands, skin, urinary System, heart and serous membrane.
- ➲ SUMMARY OF INDICATIONS: Insect bites–Urticaria–Kidney & bladder disorders–Oedema and ascites.

THERAPEUTIC PICTURE OF DRUG

C_{N-1} ➲ Strumous constitution and bag like swelling under the lower eyelids.

C_{N-2} ➲ Pale, waxy, oedematous face.

C_{N-3} ➲ Gland enlarge indurated scirrhous or open cancer.

M_{D-1} ➲ Great tearfulness, cannot help crying.

M_{D-2} ➲ In women: jealousy; mania from sexual irritation.

M_{D-3} ➲ Depression, feels as if about to die.

M_{D-4} ➲ Sopor interrupted by Piercing shrieks.

M_{D-5} ➲ Indifference (dullness of head), sudden shrill screams.

SO_1 ➲ Eyes: Burning, stinging, shooting pains.

SO_2 ➲ Oedematous with bag-like swelling under the eye; non-inflammatory oedema; feels stiff.

SO_3 ➲ Scalding tears, profuse; great sensitiveness to light.

DS_1 ➲ Walls of abdomen tense; sensitiveness of ileo-coecal region.

DS_2 ➲ Diarrhoea: watery; yellow, with griping; watery and foul-smelling; watery, copious, black; greenish-yellow mucus, worse morning.

DS_3 ➲ Stool with every motion of body, as if anus were constantly open.

DS_4 ➲ Haemorrhage from bowels, with burning pains, excoriation of open anus, constant tenesmus.

FGS_1 ➲ Oedma of labia,Relieved by cold water.

FGS_2 ➲ Soreness & stinging pain, Ovaritis, worse in right side.

FGS_3 ➲ Metrorrhagia profuse with heavy abdomen stinging pain.

FGS_4 ➲ Ovarian tumors, metritis with stinging pain.

FGS_5 ➲ Enlargement and induration of the mammae, with stinging, burning pains; Suppuration, with great tenderness; Erysipelatous inflammation of the mammae; discharge bloody milk.

US_1 ➲ Incontinence of urine,with great irritation of the parts.

LS_1 ➲ Oedema of the hands.

LS_2 ➲ Panaritium, with burning, stinging and throbbing; very sensitive to touch; especially in "runround", after abuse of sulphur.

LS_3 ➲ Legs and feet waxy, pale, sollen, oedematous.

PG_1 ➲ Extreme Sensitiveness to touch.

PG_2 ➲ Sudden "Putting up" of whole body.

PG_3 ➲ Complete anasarca, no thirst, pale, waxy, almost transparent.

PG_4 ➲ Burning, stinging pains, like be-strings, occurring occasionally.

Modalities

Aggravation

- After sleeping.
- Warmed &Heated especially closed rooms are intolerable.
- From getting wet.

Amelioration

- Open air.
- Cold water & cold bathing.
- Walking are changing position.
- When sitting erect (All).

Relations

- COMPARE: Acet-acid; Anac; Bell.
- COMPLEMENTARY: Nat-m.
- FOLLOWS WELL: Ars; Graph; iod; Lyc; Puls; Sulph.
- ANTIDOTES: Ip; Lach; Lac-ac.
- INIMICALS: Phos; Rhus-t.

Apocynum cannabinum

- PROVED BY: FREITAG.
- DURATION: 20 Days.
- COMMON NAME: Indian Hemp.
- FAMILY/KINGDOM: Apocynaceae.
- RELATION COLD/HEAT: Cold.
- MIASM: Mixed.
- SOURCE: The whole fresh plant, root included, should be used for making the tincture or infusion.
- SPHERES OF ACTION: Urinary Organs, Heart, Uterus and digestive tract.
- SUMMARY OF INDICATIONS: Disorders with inflammation of serous membranes-Oedema, ascites-acute hydrocephalus.

THERAPEUTIC PICTURE OF DRUG

M_{D-1} ➲ Bewildered; low-spirited.

M_{D-2} ➲ Nervousness, Confused, Dizziness.

M_{D-3} ➲ Sluggish memory.

FGS_1 ➲ Amenorrhoea in young girls bloating or dropsical extension of abdomen and extremities.

FGS_2 ➲ Metrorrhagia with continued or paroxysmal flow and fluid or clotted blood, nausea, vomiting, palpitation, pulse quick, feeble when moved.

FGS_3 ➲ Vital depress, on, fainting when rising from pillow.

FGS_4 ➲ Haemorrhages (Menorrhagia) at change of life (Menopause).

LS_1 ➲ Constant and voluntary motion of one arm and one leg.

PG_1 ➲ Excertions diminished, especially urine and sweat.

PG_2 ➲ Dropsy of serous membranes.

Modalities

Aggravation

- Cold weather.
- Cold drinks.
- Uncovering.

Amelioration

- Hot applications.

Relations

- COMPARE: Apoc-andr; Alstonia const; Strophanth; Acet-ac; Apis.

Argentum metallicum

- PROVED BY: Hahnemann.
- DURATION: 30 Days.
- COMMON NAME: Pure Silver.
- FAMILY/KINGDOM: Minerals.
- RELATION COLD/HEAT: Chilly.
- MIASM: Syphilis.
- SOURCE: Silver leaf and precipitated silver.
- TEMPERAMENT: Irritable.
- SPHERES OF ACTION: Mucous membrane of female genital organs,nose, ears, bone & joints.
- SUMMARY OF INDICATIONS: Laryngitis and pharyngitis (aphonia & dysphonia).

THERAPEUTIC PICTURE OF DRUG

C_{N-1} ➲ Tall, thin, irritable persons, with constitutional effects of onanism and abuse of mercury.

M_{D-1} ➲ Delirious rage (Mania; after epilepsy).

M_{D-2} ➲ Hurried feeling; time passes slowly; melancholy.

M_{D-3} ➲ Restless, which forces one to walk quickly.

M_{D-4} ➲ ill-humour and aversion to talking.

M_{D-5} ➲ When pleased, excessively merry, but cries a long time about a trifle.

RS_1 ➲ Rowness and soreness in upper part of larynx, when coughing, not when swallowing.

RS_2 ➲ Hoarseness; especially of Professional singers, speakers, etc.

RS_3 ➲ Cannot speak a loud word; constant tickling in the throat, provoking cough.

RS_4 ➲ Over the bifurcation of the trachea, a raw spot; hoarse-ness; worse when using the voice.

FGS_1 ➲ Ovary feels too large. Bearing down pain. Prolapse of uterus.

FGS_2 ➲ Eroded spongy cervix. Leucorrhoea foul, excoriating.

FGS_3 ➲ Palliative in scirrhus of uterus pain in the left ovary and back climacteric haemorrhage.

FGS_4 ➲ Uterine disease with pain in joints and limbs.

FGS_5 ➲ Palpitation, at night; during pregnancy.

FGS_6 ➲Greate weakness of the breast.

MGS_1 ➲ Seminal emissions almost every night, without ejection, with atrophy of Penis; after onanism.

MGS_2 ➲ Crushed pain in the testicles; clothing increases the pain on walking; also evening in bed.

MGS_3 ➲ Scrotum and feet oedematous.

PG_1 ➲ Sore feeling throughout the abdomen; worse by jarring.

PG_2 ➲ Arg.met. acts more on the left side than the right.

PG_3 ➲ Affects the cartilages, tarsal, ears,nose, Eustachian; the structures entering into joints.

Modalities

Aggravation

- ➲ Riding in a carriage.
- ➲ When touched or pressed upon.

Amelioration

- ➲ Open air.

Relations

- ➲ FOLLOWS WELL: Calc; Puls; Sep.
- ➲ ANTIDOTES: Merc; Puls.

Argentum nitricum

- ➲ PROVED BY: J.O. Mueller.
- ➲ DURATION: 30 Days.
- ➲ COMMON NAME: Silver nitrate [Lunar caustic] = [Ag NO_3].
- ➲ FAMILY/KINGDOM: Mineral.
- ➲ RELATION COLD/HEAT: Hot.
- ➲ MIASM: Psora, Syphilic and Sycotic.
- ➲ DIATHESIS: Neurosycotic.
- ➲ TEMPERAMENT: Bilious.
- ➲ SOURCE: Trituration and solution of [Ag NO_3].
- ➲ SPHERES OF ACTION: Brain, Spinal cord, Nerves blood, Mucous membrane.
- ➲ SUMMARY OF INDICATIONS: ophthalmia neonatorum–gastroenteritis–diarrhoea–impontence.

THERAPEUTIC PICTURE OF DRUG

C_{N-1} ➲ Adoped to hysterical nervous persons with vivid imagination, having carbo-nitrogenoid or hydrogenoid constitution.

C_{N-2} ➲ Cachectic, scrawny, withered, dried, up, old looking young persons, having history of unusal or long continued mental exertion.

M_{D-1} ➲ Mental anxiety.

M_{D-2} ➲ Very impulsive; always in a hurry but accomplishes nothing; in continual; he walks fast.

M_{D-3} ➲ Hurries restlessly to fulfills engagements, fears to be late when there is plenty of time.

M_{D-4} ➲ Melancholic; does not undertake anything lest he should not succeed.

M_{D-5} ➲ Impulse to throw herself from the window.

M_{D-6} ➲ Frequent errors of perception; mistakes distances; fears house-corners.

M_{D-7} ➲ Time seems to pass very slowly.

M_{D-8} ➲ Apprehension when ready to go to church or opera, bringing on diarrhoea.

M_{D-9} ➲ Easily angered or excited, anger brings on symptoms, cough, pain.

M_{D-10} ➲ Profound melancholy; imagines if left alone will die; apprehends incurable disease of brain.

M_{D-11} ➲ Night nervousness, with heat and fullness in the head.

M_{D-12} ➲ Nervous, faintish and tremulous sensation.

M_{D-13} ➲ Awful faces appear on shotting eyes.

M_{D-14} ➲ Mental operation sluggish; thought requires effort.

M_{D-15} ➲ Complete loss of conciousness.

M_{D-16} ➲ Memory impaired, can not find the right word.

M_{D-17} ➲ Building castles in the air by day; monstrous visions by night.

SO_1 ➲ Cornea opaque; Ulceration of the cornea in newborn infants; Profuse Purulent discharge from the lids.

SO_2 ➲ Ciliary blepharitis from being over a fire; better from cold air and cold applications.

NS_1 ➲ Puerperal convulsions; just after attack lies quiet, but become very restless before another.

DS_1 ➲ Belching accompanies most gastric ailments.

DS_2 ➲ Belching after every meal; stomach as if it would burst with wind; belching difficult, finally air rushes out with great violence.

DS_3 ➲ After ice cream, gastralgia, pain radiating in all directions, worse after food.

DS_4 ➲ Green stool spoor, large Puplis.

DS_5 ➲ Masses of epithelium connected by muco-lymph, looking red of green and shreddy, with severe bearing down in hypogastrium; advanced dysentery, with suspected ulceration.

DS_6 ➲ Diarrhoea as soon as he drinks.

DS_7 ➲ Child is very fond of sugar, but diarrhoea results from eating it.

DS_8 ➲ Diarrhoea: green mucus, like chopped spinach in flakes.

FGS_1 ➲ Prolapsus with ulceration of as or cervix; with copious yellow, corroding leucorrhoea and frequent bleeding from points of ulceration.

FGS_2 ➲ All Symptoms worse before and during menses.

FGS_3 ➲ Coition painfull, followed by bleeding from the vagina.

FGS_4 ➲ Metrorrhagia, with nervous erethism at change of life; also in young widows and those who have born no children; returning in attacks, region of ovaries painful, with pains radiating to sacrum and thighs.

FGS_5 ➲ Menses irregular; scanty with asthma.

FGS_6 ➲ During pregnancy, stomach as if it would burst with wind; head feels expanded.

MGS_1 ➲ Impotence erection fails when coition is attempted.

MGS_2 ➲ Ulcer on the Prepuce small, covered with Pus; later spreading, bowl-shaped, with a tallow-like coating.

PG_1 ➲ Chilly when uncovered, get feels smothered if wrapped up; craves fresh air.

Modalities

Aggravation

➲ Cold food; cold air.

➲ Eating sugar; ice cream.

➲ Unusual mental exertion.

Amelioration

➲ Open air; eructation, pressure.

➲ Craves the wind blowing in her face.

➲ Bathing with cold water.

Relations

➲ FOLLOWS WELL: Calc; Kali-c; Lyc; Merc;Puls; Sep; Sil.

➲ ANTIDOTES: Ars;Iod; Nat-mur; Phos; Rhust-t; Sulph.

➲ SIMILAR: Aur; Cupr; Lach; Nat-m; Nit-ac.

Arnica montana

- ➲ PROVED BY: Hahnemann.
- ➲ DURATION: 6–10 days.
- ➲ COMMON NAME: Leopard's bane.
- ➲ FAMILY/KINGDOM: Compositeae.
- ➲ RELATION COLD/HEAT: Chilly.
- ➲ MIASM: Psora.
- ➲ SOURCE: Tincture of whole fresh plant- Tincture of root.
- ➲ TEMPERAMENT: Nervous.
- ➲ SPHERES OF ACTION: Blood & blood vessels, Particularly on capillaries.
- ➲ SUMMARY OF INDICATIONS: Injuries–Postperotive–injury of perineum at childbirth.

THERAPEUTIC PICTURE OF DRUG

Note: The remedy of choice for the effects of trauma, over-exertion of injuries from a blunt instrument.

C_{N-1} ➲ The person who needs Arnica feels bruised and sore.

C_{N-2} ➲ Bruising injuries to all soft tissues, such as injuries from blows, falls or blunt object.

C_{N-3} ➲ Nervous, sanguine, Plethoric. women, liely expression and very red face.

C_{N-4} ➲ Who are disposed to cerebral congestion.

M_{D-1} ➲ Fears touch, or the approach of anyone.

M_{D-2} ➲ Unconsciousness: when spoken to answers correctly, and completely, but unconsciousness and delirium at once return.

M_{D-3} ➲ Indifference; inability to Perform continuous active work; morose delirious.

M_{D-4} ➲ Nervous can not bear pain;the whole body is oversensitive, Says that nothing is the matter with him. wants to be left alone.

M_{D-5} ➲ Agrophobia (fear of space). After mental strain or shock.

SO_1 ➲ Eye injuries, "a black eye", retinal haemorrhage.

CVS_1 ➲ Fatty degeneration of heart.

CVS_2 ➲ "Strain of the heart" from violent running.

CVS_3 ➲ Pressure under the sternum, anguish, collapse; small, irregular pulse, dyspnoea; angina pectoris.

RS_1 ➲ Hemorrhage after mechanical injuries; slight spitting of black, thick, viscid blood, or bright red, frothy blood, mixed with mucus and coagula.

RS_2 ➲ Pleurisy after mechanical injuries; must continually change position, bed feels so hard.

RS_3 ➲ Pneumothorax from external injuries.

FGS_1 ➲ Soreness of Parts ofter labour; Prevents Post–Partum haemorrhage and puerperal complications.

FGS_2 ➲ Retension or in continence of urine after labour.

FGS_3 ➲ discharge of blood from the uterus, between the periods, with nausea.

FGS_4 ➲ Vomiting of Pregnancy.

FGS_5 ➲ Threatened abortion from fall.

FGS_6 ➲ Feeling as if foetus were lying cross wise.

FGS_7 ➲ Excoriation and ulceration of the breasts.

FGS_8 ➲ Erysipelatous inflammation of the mammae and nipples.

F_{R-1} ➲ Fevers: intermittent; typhoid; traumatic.

F_{R-2} ➲ Pulse very variable, mostly hard, full and quick.

F_{R-3} ➲ Chillness, internally with external heat, with heat and redness of one cheek.

F_{R-4} ➲ Head alone, or face alone, hot, rest of body cool.

F_{R-5} ➲ Fever, with much thirst, even before the shiverings.

F_{R-6} ➲ Heat in the evening or at night, with shivering on raising the bed-clothers, even slightly, and frequently with pain in the back and in the limbs.

PG_1 ➲ Promotes healing of all injuries.

PG_2 ➲ Soreness of muscles from over-exertion.

PG_3 ➲ Bleeding caused by injury.

PG_4 ➲ Helpful even in every old injuries, especially of the soft tissues.

PG_5 ➲ Denies he or she is ill or that there is anything wrong, although the patient is acutely ill.

PG_6 ➲ Mechanical injuries; concussion of brain while there are unconsciousness, pallor, or drowsiness, weak, intermitting pulse, cold surface, and other indications of depressed vitality from shock.

PG_7 ➲ Sprains with much swelling, bluish redness, intense soreness.

PG_8 ➲ Contusions without laceration.

PG_9 ➲ Compound fractures, and their profuse suppuration.

PG_{10} ➲ Heat of upper Part of body; coldness of lower.

PG_{11} ➲ Every thing on which he lies seems too hard.

PG_{12} ➲ Gout & Rheumatism, with great fear of being touched by person coming near him.

Modalities

Aggravation

- ➲ At rest and Heat.
- ➲ When lying down.
- ➲ Form wine.

Amelioration

- ➲ From contact.
- ➲ Motion.

Relations

- ➲ COMPLEMENTARY: Acon.
- ➲ FOLLOWS WELL: Acon; Ars; Bell; Bry; Cact; Calc; Cham; Chin; Con; Hep; Iod; Ip; Nux-v; Phos; Puls; Rhus-t; Sulph; Sul-ac.
- ➲ ANTIDOTES: Ars; Camph; Chin; Ign.

Arsenicum album

- ➲ PROVED BY: Hahnemann.
- ➲ DURATION: 60-90 days.
- ➲ COMMON NAME: white oxide of metallic Arsenic[As_2O_3].
- ➲ FAMILY/KINGDOM: Minerals.
- ➲ RELATION COLD/HEAT: Chilly.
- ➲ MIASM: Psora, syphilis and sycosis.
- ➲ DIATHESIS: Scrofulous.
- ➲ TEMPERAMENT: Fastidious.
- ➲ SOURCE: solution and trituration of $As_2\,O_3$.
- ➲ SPHERES OF ACTION: Mind, nerves, mucous membrane, joints, peritoneum, liver, blood, lungs, skin, stomach.
- ➲ SUMMARY OF INDICATIONS: Anxiety–overwork–gastrointestinal disorders–bronchil asthima–coryza–skin disorders–(esp. when there is hyperpigmentation).

THERAPEUTIC PICTURE OF DRUG

C_{N-1} ➲ The patient is lean, thin, debilitated.

C_{N-2} ➲ Having Hippocratic face, dirty and waxy look of the skin.

C_{N-3} ➲ Patient is anxious, fear full and restless.

M_{D-1} ➲ Fear of death and patient thinks it is pointless to take any treatment.

M_{D-2} ➲ Anxious, mentally and physically (change places), restless and fearful, irritable, weak and exhausted. Desire fresh air.

M_{D-3} ➲ Weak and exhausted.

M_{D-4} ➲ Desires fresh are but is sensitive to the cold.

M_{D-5} ➲ Fear of death when alone, or on going to bed.

M_{D-6} ➲ Determined to commit suicide, he suffers so.

M_{D-7} ➲ Intense anxiety and with restlessness, worse after midnight; driving out of bed.

M_{D-8} ➲ Great anxiety, with contriction of chest and dyspnoea.

M_{D-9} ➲ Vexations, with anxiety, restlessness and chilliness.

M_{D-10} ➲ Great fear, restlessness, trembling, cold sweat, prostation.

SO_1 ➲ Later stages of a head cold with sneezing: red nose, eyes and profuse watery discharge.

DS_1 ➲ Violent vomiting of food and gastric fluids; vomit usually scanty.

DS_2 ➲ Pressure in the region of the stomach; weight, as of a stone.

DS_3 ➲ Intense heat and burning in stomach and pit of stomach.

DS_4 ➲ Great anxiety about the epigastric region.

DS_5 ➲ Violent pains in abdomen, with great anguish, has no rest anywhere, rolls about on floor and despairs of life.

DS_6 ➲ Diarrhoea after chillings stomach by taking cold substances. Diarrhoea; slimy, green mucus; of pieces of mucus, with tenesmus and cutting pain in anus.

DS_7 ➲ Diarrheoa worse after midnight, also in morning after rising.

DS_8 ➲ Haemorrhoids: with stitching Pain when walking or sitting, not when at stool; with burning Pain, relieved by heat.Haemorrhages from bowels, dark, offensive.

RS_1 ➲ Bronchial asthma, worse after midnight: fears suffocation while lying down.

FGS_1 ➲ Venereal disease in women.

FGS_2 ➲ Burning in ovarian region,. Ovarian pain as if from red hot wires, worse least exertion, causes great fatigue. better in worm room.

FGS_3 ➲ Catamenia Suppressed,with pains in the sacrum and in the shoulders.

FGS_4 ➲ Stitching pains in the pelvis extending down the thighs.

S_{N-1} ➲ Scaly eruptions as in Psoriasis.

F_{R-1} ➲ Intermittent fever: Quotidian, tertian, quartum, double tertian; anticipates every 14 days, every year; remittent and relapsing typhoid and malarial fevers due to abuse of quinine derivatives.

F_{R-2} ➲ Afternoon Parorcysmus (1-2 a.m. and 12-2 p.m.).

F_{R-3} ➲ Chill without thirst, followed by heat with much thirst and no sweat.

F_{R-4} ➲ Blue nails and lips during chill.

F_{R-5} ➲ Internal burning, dry heat; inclination to uncover.

F_{R-6} ➲ Dry heat, evening and night, with thirst and frequent drinking of but a small quantity at a time.

F_{R-7} ➲ Sweats on going to sleep; goes of after sweating a little.

PG_1 ➲ Great prostration, with rapid sinking of the vital forces; fainting.

PG_2 ➲ Burning pains; the affected parts burn like fire.

PG_3 ➲ Can not bear the smell or sight of food.

PG_4 ➲ Great thirst for cold water; drinks often, but little at a time.

PG_5 ➲ Sleepiness but unable to sleep; restlessness.

Modalities

Aggravation

- ➲ After midnight (1to 2AM.orPM).
- ➲ From cold; cold drink or food.
- ➲ Sight of food. smell of food.
- ➲ When lying on affected side or wit the head low.

Amelioration

- ➲ From heat in general.
- ➲ Head elevated.
- ➲ Warm food and warm drinks.

Relations

➲ COMPLEMENTARY:	All-s; Carb–v; Nat-s; Phos; thuj.
➲ FOLLOWS WELL:	Apis; Aran; Bell;Cact; chel; Chin; cic; Ferr; Fl-ac; Hep; Ip; Iod;Kali-bi;Lyc; Merc; Sulph; Verat.
➲ ANTIDOTES:	Camph; chin; chinin–s; Ferr; Graph; Hep; Iod; Ip; Nux-m; Nux-v; Samb; Sulph; Tab; Verat.

Asterias rubens

- ➲ COMMON NAME: Red star fish.
- ➲ FAMILY/KINGDOM: Animal-Radiata.
- ➲ RELATION COLD/HEAT: Cold.
- ➲ MIASM: .sycotic.
- ➲ SOURCE: Tincture of fish.
- ➲ TEMPERAMENT: Irritable.
- ➲ SPHERES OF ACTION: uterus, mucus membrane, nerves, female organs & rectum.
- ➲ SUMMARY OF INDICATIONS: stroke–carcinoma of the breast–nymphomania muscular dystrophy–epilepsy.

THERAPEUTIC PICTURE OF DRUG

C_{N-1} ➲ Apoplexy; face red, pulse rapid and full.

C_{N-2} ➲ Lymphatic constitution, flabby, with red face.

M_{D-1} ➲ Nervous disturbances, Neuralgias, Chorea and Hysteria.

M_{D-2} ➲ Can not bear contradiction.

M_{D-3} ➲ Heat in head, as if surrounded by hot air.

FGS_1 ➲ Breasts swell and pain, worse left side.

FGS_2 ➲ Colic and other sufferings cease with appearance of flow.

FGS_3 ➲ Excitement of sexual instinct with nervous agitaion.

FGS_4 ➲ Nodes and indurations of mammary gland dull aching, neuralgic pain in this region (con).

FGS_5 ➲ Has been used for cancer of Breast, and has an unquestioned influence over cancerous disease.

FGS_6 ➲ Sexual desire increased in women.

LS_1 ➲ Pain radiates to the left arm and fingers, worse motion.

B_{K1} ➲ Ulceration with sharp pains, piercing the scapulas.

PG_1 ➲ Gait unsteady: incoordination of the muscles.

Modalities

Aggravation

- Coffee, Night.
- Cold damp Weather.
- Left side, By motion.

Amelioration

- Open air.

Relations

- COMPLEMENTARY: Con; Carb–v; Ars.
- ANTIDOTES: Plb; Zinc.
- INIMICALS: Nux-v; Coff.

Aurum metallicum

- PROVED BY: Hahnemann.
- DURATION: 50–60 Days.
- COMMON NAME: Metallic gold.
- FAMILY/KINGDOM: Minerals.
- RELATION COLD/HEAT: Chilly.
- MIASM: Syphilis.
- DIATHESIS: Scrofulous.
- TEMPERAMENT: Melancholic & irritable.
- SOURCE: Trituration of Metallic gold.
- SPHERES OF ACTION: Mind, Nerves, genito-Urinary organs, glands, bones, cardio-vas. system.
- SUMMARY OF INDICATIONS: Mental depression with suicidal tendencies-anxiety syndromes-headaches-behaviour disorders-osteomyelities.

THERAPEUTIC PICTURE OF DRUG

C_{N-1} ➲ Sanguine, ruddy people,with black hair and eyes;

C_{N-2} ➲ Lively, restless, anxious about the future.

C_{N-3} ➲ Old people; weak vision; corpulent; tried of life due to their missdeeds, having no desire to live and low-spirited, lifeless pining boys.

C_{N-4} ➲ Constitution broken down by bad effects of mercury & syphilis.

M_{D-1} ➲ Melancholy, disposed to weep; imagines he is unfit for this word, that he can never succeed.

M_{D-2} ➲ Great anguish, which even induces a disposition to suicide.

M_{D-3} ➲ Weakness of the memory.

M_{D-4} ➲ Uneasy, hurried, desire for mental and bodily activity; cannot do things fast enough.

M_{D-5} ➲ Apprehensiveness, full of fear; a mere noise at the door makes him anxious.

CVS_1 ➲ Strong beating of heart, with anxiety and congestion to the head, after metrorrhagia; also exertion.

CVS_2 ➲ Palpitation with irregular, intermittent pulse; short breathing.

CVS_3 ➲ Weak pulse, cardiac asthma, mental depression; great debility.

FGS_1 ➲ Prolapsed and indurated uterus; from over reaching or straining. from hypertrophy.

FGS_2 ➲ Menstrual and uterine affections, with great melancholy; < at menstrual period.

FGS_3 ➲ Great sensitiveness of the vagina.

FGS_4 ➲ Pain in the abdomen, as if the catamenia were coming.

FGS_5 ➲ Uterine affections with depression and tendency to suicide.

FGS_6 ➲ Drawing pain in pubes; right inguinal region sore to touch.

FGS_7 ➲ Before menses: swelling of axillary glands.

FGS_8 ➲ During menses: colic; prolapse of rectum.

FGS_9 ➲ During pregnancy; suicidal melancholia; jaundice.

FGS_{10} ➲ Foul breath; in girls at puberty.

PG_1 ➲ Falling of the head hair (alopecia).

PG_2 ➲ Bone disorders, necrosis of bones, osteomyelites, bone pains.

Modalities

Aggravation

- ➲ In cold air; when getting cold;–While lying down.
- ➲ Mental exertion.
- ➲ Many complaints come on only in winter.

Amelioration

- ➲ In warm air,;when growing warm in the morning.
- ➲ During summer.

Relations

➲ FOLLOWS WELL:	Acon; Bell; Calc; Chin; lyc; Merc; Nit–ac; Puls; Rhus-t; Sep; Sulph.
➲ ANTIDOTES:	Cocc; Coff; Cupr; Sol-n; Spig.
➲ SIMILAR:	Asaf; Calc-os; Plat; Sep; Tarent.

Badiaga

➲ COMMON NAME: Fresh water sponge.

➲ FAMILY/KINGDOM: Animals.

➲ RELATION COLD/HEAT: Cold.

➲ MIASM: Syphilis.

➲ SOURCE: Trituration of the dried sponge gathered in autumn.

THERAPEUTIC PICTURE OF DRUG

M_{D-1} ➲ After pleasurable emotions, palpitation.

M_{D-2} ➲ Mind generally clear, active in spite of headache.

FGS_1 ➲ Metrorrhagia, worse at night, with feeling of enlargement of head.

FGS_2 ➲ Cancer of breast.

FGS_3 ➲ A lady has for months off and an a severe pain in right eye ball, which extended to fore head over this eye, then to temple, always < in afternoon.

PG_1 ➲ Soreness of muscles and integuments.

Modalities

Aggravation

➲ By cold.

➲ At night.

Amelioration

➲ By heat.

Relations

➲ COMPARE:	Spongia; Seneg; Kali-c.
➲ COMPLEMENTARY:	Sul; Iod; Merc.
➲ FOLLOWS WELL:	Lach.

Baptisia tinctoria

- PROVED BY: W.H.BURT.
- DURATION: 6-8 days.
- COMMON NAME: Wild Indigo.
- FAMILY/KINGDOM: Leguminasae.
- RELATION COLD/HEAT: Chilly.
- MIASM: Psora.
- SOURCE: Trncture of fresh root and its bark.
- TEMPERAMENT: Lymphatic.
- SPHERES OF ACTION: Blood, mind, nerves. And mucous membrane of digestive tract.
- SUMMARY OF INDICATIONS: Mantal apathy–pharyngitis-polymyositis.

THERAPEUTIC PICTURE OF DRUG

C_{N-1} ➲ Face flushed, dusky, dark-red, with a stupid, be–sotted drunken expression.

C_{N-2} ➲ Ulcerated mouth, with offensive smell and offensive breath.

M_{D-1} ➲ Indisposed to think, want of power; mind seems weak, confused, as if drunk.

M_{D-2} ➲ Cannot confine his mind, a sort of wild, wandering feeling, Gloomy, unhappy state of mind.

M_{D-3} ➲ Stupor; falls asleep while being spoken to, or answering; heavy sleep till aroused; awakes only to again fall asleep in the midst of his answer, which he vainly endeavors to finish.

M_{D-4} ➲ Mind wanders as soon as the eyes are closed.

M_{D-5} ➲ Mentally restless but too lifeless to move.

M_{D-6} ➲ Can not go to sleep because she can not get herself together; head or body feels scattere about the bed tosses about to get the pieces together; thought she was as three persons, could not keep them covered.

DS_1 ➲ Painless pharyngitis.

DS_2 ➲ Tongue: at first coated white with red papillae; dry and yellow–brown in center.

DS_3 ➲ Fetid, exhausting diarrhoea, causing excoriation.

DS_4 ➲ Offensive diarrhoea day and night; child can swallow nothing but milk.

DS_5 ➲ Dysentery; rigors, Pains in the limbs, and small of the back; stools small, all blood, not very dark, but thick; tenesmus; great Prostration, brown tongue, low fever; in the autumn, or in hot weather.

FGS_1 ➲ Menses too early and too profuse (menorrhagia).

FGS_2 ➲ Excites abortion.

FGS_3 ➲ Lochia acrid, fetid.

FGS_4 ➲ Puerperal fever.

FGS_5 ➲ Stomatitis materna.

FGS_6 ➲ Threatened miscarriage from mental depression, shock, night watching.

F_{R-1} ➲ Typhoid and cerebral forms of fever.

F_{R-2} ➲ Beginning of typhus when the so-called nervous symptoms Predominate; causes sweat to break our and relieve; typhus; critical sweat on forehead and face.

F_{R-3} ➲ On awaking at 3 A.M., flashes of heat, feeling as if sweat would break out.

F_{R-4} ➲ Fever originating from confinement on shiphoard, with out good care or food.

F_{R-5} ➲ Fetid sweat; frequent sweating; also worse from small of back in all directons.

PG_1 ➲ All excretions very offensive.

PG_2 ➲ Can swallow only liquids, solid food gags.

PG_3 ➲ Muscular pains; parts rested upon feel sore.

Modalities

Aggravation

- ➲ Humid heat.
- ➲ Fog.
- ➲ Indoors.

Relations

- ➲ FOLLOWS WELL: Crot; Ham; Nit–ac; Pyrog; Ter.
- ➲ ANTIDOTES: Nux-Vom.
- ➲ SIMILAR: Arn; Ars; Bry; Gel.

Baryta carbonica

- PROVED BY: Hanemann.
- DURATION: 40 days.
- COMMON NAME: BariumCarbonate[$BaCO_3$].
- FAMILY/KINGDOM: Minerals.
- RELATION COLD/HEAT: Chilly.
- MIASM: Psora.
- DIATHESIS: Tubercular and Scrofulous.
- TEMPERAMNT: Melancholic.
- SOURCE: Trituration of[$BaCO_3$].
- SPHERES OF ACTION: Glands, throat,heart, blood vessels and Nerve.
- SUMMARY OF INDICATIONS: Amnesia- geriatric disorders-dworfism-mental deficiency in female child.

THERAPEUTIC PICTURE OF DRUG

C_{N-1} ➲ Children present a picture of typical cretinism, having short stature, swollen abdomen, Puffy face, in larged glands, thick lips and idiotic appearance.

C_{N-2} ➲ Dwarfish in Appearance, mentally deficient and physically weak and short.

C_{N-3} ➲ Old people weak & fatty but childish in behavior.

M_{D-1} ➲ Memory deficient, forgetful, inattentive, Child can not learn on account of a poor memory.

M_{D-2} ➲ Threatened idiocy.

M_{D-3} ➲ Idiotic &foolish,with loss of memory or deficient Intelligence.

M_{D-4} ➲ Loss of confidence in him self; Disponding; pusillanimous.

M_{D-5} ➲ Child does not want to play, but sits in the corner doing nothing.

M_{D-6} ➲ Great mental and bodily weakness, childishness; old people.

M_{D-7} ➲ Sadness, dejection of spirits, grief over trifles.

M_{D-8} ➲ Thinks his legs are cut off an he is walking on his knees.

M_{D-9} ➲ Thinking's of one's complaint's makes them worse.

- FGS_1 ➲ Before menses, pain in stomach and small of back.
- FGS_2 ➲ Menses scanty.
- FGS_3 ➲ Dwarfish, Hysterical women and old maids with scanty menses, deficient heat, always cold and chilly.
- FGS_4 ➲ Female child both physically and mentally weak.
- MGS_1 ➲ Excoriation between the scrotum and thigh.
- MGS_2 ➲ Sweat about the scrotum.
- MGS_3 ➲ Diminished sexual ability.
- MGS_4 ➲ Hypertrophy or induration of Prostate and testes.
- PG_1 ➲ Great sensitiveness to cold.
- PG_2 ➲ Deficient heat, always, cold and chilly.
- PG_3 ➲ Old, cachetic people; scrofulous, especially when fat.; or those who suffer from gouty complaints.
- PG_4 ➲ Emaciation or bloating of the body and of the face, with inflation of the abdomen.
- PG_5 ➲ Great tendency to catch cold, which commonly occasions inflammation in the throat.
- PG_6 ➲ Great uneasiness and over excitability of the all senses.
- PG_7 ➲ Swelling and induration of the gland.
- PG_8 ➲ Paralysis and Palsy of aged Persons.
- PG_9 ➲ Acute drawing Pains in limbs, with shuddering.

Modalities

Aggravation

- ➲ When thinking of his disease.
- ➲ Washing affected parts.
- ➲ Lying on painful side.

Amelioration

- ➲ Walking in open air.

Relations

➲ COMPARE:	Digitalis; Astrag; Radium.
➲ COMPLEMENTARY:	Dulc; Silica; Psor.
➲ FOLLOWS WELL:	Lyco; Ac-nit; Sulph; Tuberc.
➲ ANTIDOTES:	Ant-t; Bell; Zinc.
➲ INIMICALS:	After Calc.
➲ SIMILAR:	Alum; Calc-I; Dulc; Iod.

Belladonna

- PROVED BY: Hahnemann.
- DURATION: 1–7 Days.
- COMMON NAME: Deadly night shade.
- FAMILY/KINGDOM: Solanaceae.
- RELATION COLD/HEAT: Chilly.
- MIASM: Psora.
- DIATHESIS: Tubercular.
- TEMPERAMENT: Bilious, Lymphatic.
- SOURCE: Tincture of whole plant when beginning to flower.
- SPHERES OF ACTION: Cerebrum, mucous membrane,Brain and its membranes, heart lungs, Skin etc.
- SUMMARY OF INDICATIONS: Fever-headache-influenza-ear disorders-conjuctivitis-" blood boils"-rhinitis-sore throat-inflamed tonsils-Sunstrok.

THERAPEUTIC PICTURE OF DRUG

C_{N-1} ➲ Children & women with light hair & blue eyes; sensitive, Nervous, threatened with convulsions; tubercular patients.

C_{N-2} ➲ Bilious, plethoric person with red face and to a condition in them of local plethora.

C_{N-3} ➲ Lymphatic constitution with fine complexion and delicate skin

M_{D-1} ➲ Dotage, delirium, and mania, with groaning, disposition to dance, to laugh, to sing, and to whistle; mania with groans, or with involuntary laugher; nocturnal delirium; delirium with murmuring; delirium during which are seen wolves, dogs, fires; delirium by fits, and sometimes with fixedness of look.

M_{D-2} ➲ Lamentations, groans, cries and tears.

M_{D-3} ➲ Ill-humour, disposition irritable and sensitive, with an inclination to be angry and to give offence.

M_{D-4} ➲ Timidit, disposition fearful, mistrustful and suspicious; apprehension and inclination to run away.

M_{D-5} ➲ Furry and rage, with desire to strike, to spite, to bite and to tear everything, and sometimes with growling and barking like a dog.

M_{D-6} ➲ Complete loss of reason, stupidity, inadvertence, and distraction, inaptitude for thought, and great weakness of memory.

H_{D-1} ➲ Rush of blood to head and face.

H_{D-2} ➲ Headache, congestive, with red face, throbbing of brain & carotids.

H_{D-3} ➲ Headache as if a stone were pressing the forehead.

H_{D-4} ➲ Violent throbbing in brain from behind forward and towards both sides; the throbbing ends on the surface in Painful shootings.

H_{D-5} ➲ Boring, tearing, cutting, shooting Pains in various Parts of head, generally worse on right side and in forehead, less in occiput.

H_{D-6} ➲ Headache from the head of the sun.

DS_1 ➲ During the Pain, the transverse colon Protrudes like a pad all the way across the abdomen.

DS_2 ➲ Great pain in right ileo-coecal region, cannot bear the slightest touch, not even the bed-cover.

FGS_1 ➲ Dryness and heat of vagina.

FGS_2 ➲ Sensitive forcing downwards, as if all the viscera would protuded at genitals.

FGS_3 ➲ Dragging around loin, pain in sacrum.

FGS_4 ➲ Menses increased,bright red, too early,too profuse.

FGS_5 ➲ Haemorrhage hot.

FGS_6 ➲ Cutting pain from hip to hip.

FGS_7 ➲ Menses and lochia very offensive & hot.

FGS_8 ➲ Mastitis pain, throbbing, redness, streaks radiate from nipple

FGS_9 ➲ Breast feel heavy, are hard & red.

FGS_{10} ➲ Tumors of breast, pain worse lying down.

FGS_{11} ➲ Diminished lochia.

S_{N-1} ➲ Heat over whole body, with bluish redness of whole surface.

S_{N-2} ➲ Skin imparts a burning sensation to the examining hand.

S_{N-3} ➲ Skin scarlet and smooth.

F_{R-1} ➲ Burning, pungent, steaming heat.

F_{R-2} ➲ Feet icy cold.

F_{R-3} ➲ A high feverish state, with comparative absence of toxemia.

F_{R-4} ➲ Superficial blood vessels, distended.

F_{R-5} ➲ Perspiration dry, only on the head.

F_{R-6} ➲ No thirst with fever.

F_{R-7} ➲ Heat predominating; averse to uncovering.

F_{R-8} ➲ Heat of forehead with cold cheeks; of head, with redness of face and delirium.
F_{R-9} ➲ Internal heat, with anxiety and restlessness.
PG_1 ➲ Quick sensation and motion.
PG_2 ➲ Patient is sleepy but unable to sleep. Restless sleep with muscular twitching.
PG_3 ➲ Sunstroke or heatstroke with a pounding pulse.
PG_4 ➲ Throbbing pains, worse during motion or jarring.
PG_5 ➲ Vomiting due to fright or nervousness. Hallucinations.

Modalities

Aggravation

- From touch, motion, noise.
- Draft of air, After 3 A.M.
- Night, After midnight, summer sun.

Amelioration

- Rest.
- Standing or sitting erect.
- Worm Room.

Relations

➲ COMPLEMENTARY:	Calcarea.
➲ FOLLOWS WELL:	Cham; Carb-v; Sil; Sep; Sulph.
➲ ANTIDOTES:	Aco; Camph; Coff; Hep; Puls.
➲ INIMICALS:	Dulc; Ac-acet.
➲ SIMILAR:	Acon; Bry; Gels; Hyos; Meli; Op.

Berberis vulgaris

- ➲ COMMON NAME: Barberry.
- ➲ DURATION: 20-30 days.
- ➲ SOURCE: Tincure of the bark of the root.
- ➲ FAMILY/KINGDOM: Berberidaceae.
- ➲ SPHERES OF ACTION: Kidney, Urinary bladder, liver, & gall bladder.
- ➲ SUMMARY OF INDICATIONS: Rheumaticand other locomotor disorders–Polyneuropathy–Urinary disorders- renal colic.

THERAPEUTIC PICTURE OF DRUG

C_{N-1} ➲ Face looks pale, earthy complexion, sunken cheeks.

C_{N-2} ➲ Hollow eyes with blue circles around them.

M_{D-1} ➲ Careless, calm, apathetic humour.

M_{D-2} ➲ ill-humour, disgust to life.

M_{D-3} ➲ Melancholy, inclination to weep dislike to conversation.

M_{D-4} ➲ Anxiety, great fear and disposition to take fright.

M_{D-5} ➲ In the twilight, all subjects seem larger than they really are.

M_{D-6} ➲ Intellectual labours are performed with difficulty and prone. fatiguing, esp. in the morning.

DS_1 ➲ Colic from gall-stones.

DS_2 ➲ Colic like pains, especially about the navel.

DS_3 ➲ Hard stool, like sheep's dung passed after much straining.

DS_4 ➲ Soreness in the anus, with burning; pain when touched, and great sensitiveness when sitting.

DS_5 ➲ Fistula in ano, with itching there; short cough and chest complaints.

FGS_1 ➲ Tardy enjoyment in women, during coition, and often accompanied with incisive or shooting pains.

FGS_2 ➲ Sensation of burning and excoriation in the vagina, extending to the labia.

FGS_3 ➲ Menses, consisting of gray mucus or brown blood.

FGS_4 ➲ Leucorrhoea, grayish mucus, with painful urinary symptoms.

FGS_5 ➲ Neuralgia of ovaries and vagina.

FGS_6 ➲ During the catamenia, pains in the genital parts and in the loins, or violent pains in the head,with sensation of fainting.

FGS_7 ➲ Catamenia insufficient, with acute drowing pains in the whole body,painful inflation of the abdomen, pain in the loins, shooting s in the chest, dejected aspect, with violent pains in the head; or with ill–humour, disgust of life, dejection, smarting pains in the vagina, sensation of burning and excoriation in the anus, and pains in the arms, as far as the shoulders and the nape of the neck.

MGS_1 ➲ Sensation of weakness and unexcitablely in the parts, especially after urination.

MGS_2 ➲ Neuralgia of testes and cords; parts swollen, tender.

US_1 ➲ Burning and soreness in region of kidneys.

US_2 ➲ Stitching, cutting pain from left kidney following course. of ureter in to bladder and urethra.

US_3 ➲ Sharp pain in right kidney, near the spine, thence downwards into the bladder.

US_4 ➲ Tearing, pulsating pain in right kidney.

US_5 ➲ Pressure and contraction in the vesical region when pressed upon, with burning in the urethra.

US_6 ➲ Cutting or burning in the urethra, worse when not urinating, frequently more on one side.

US_7 ➲ Urine: increased and clear, with small slimy sediment, at the beginning and during the exacerbation of complaints.

US_8 ➲ Urine: with pain in lumbar and renal region; dark or bright yellow, or red, with sediment; blood red, speedily becoming, or turbid, depositing thick mucus and bright red mealy sediment.

PG_1 ➲ Rheumatic and gouty disorders, with diseases of the urinary organs.

PG_2 ➲ The renal or vesical symptoms predominate.

PG_3 ➲ Bubbling sensation in kidneys.

Modalities

Aggravation

➲ Motion. ➲ Walking or carriage.

➲ Any sudden jarring movement.

Amelioration

➲ With rest.

Relations

➲ ANTIDOTES: Bell; Camph.

➲ SIMILAR: Canth; Lyc; Sars; Tab.

Bismuth

- ➲ PROVED BY: Hahnemann.
- ➲ DURATION: 20-50 days.
- ➲ COMMON NAME: Hydrated Oxide of Bismuth ($Bi_2O_3OH_2$).
- ➲ MIASM: Psora and syphilis.
- ➲ SOURCE: Trituration of $Bi_2O_3OH_2$.
- ➲ SPHERES OF ACTION: GIT, mind and nervous system.
- ➲ SUMMARY OF INDICATIONS: Anxiety- headaches- restlessness—gastra-enteritis.

THERAPEUTIC PICTURE OF DRUG

CN_1 ➲ Face: earth complexion, blue around the eyes; features changed, as if he had been very sick.

M_{D-1} ➲ Solitude is unbearable; desire for company.

M_{D-2} ➲ Complains about his condition.

M_{D-3} ➲ Unstable minded; begins now this again that, holds but a short time to any one thing.

M_{D-4} ➲ Anguish; the Patient sits, then walk, then lies down, never rests too long in one place.

DS_1 ➲ Toothache relived by taking cold water in the mouth worse when it become warm.

DS_2 ➲ Tongue coated while and has a sweet, metallic taste.

DS_3 ➲ Nausea at the stomach after eating or nursing.

DS_4 ➲ Vomiting of bile without effort.

DS_5 ➲ Vomiting: convulsive gagging and in expressible pain in the stomach; after operations on the abdomen.

DS_6 ➲ Vomits: only at intervals of days when food has filled the stomach; then vomits enormous quantities, lasting all days; all fluids.

DS_7 ➲ Pressure as from a load in one spot.

DS_8 ➲ Crampy, spasmodic pains in stomach; burning alternating with pressure; Pressure in spire, must bend backwards.

DS_9 ➲ Stools: Papecent, foul; watery, cadaverous, smelling.

PG_1 ➲ Thirst for cold drinks. Eructations after drinking.

PG_2 ➲ Cholera morbits and summer complaint.

PG_3 ➲ Symptoms of inflammation of the alimentary canal. Headache alternates with gastritis.

Modalities

Aggravation

➲ After eating.

➲ With motion.

Amelioration

➲ With cold.

➲ With cold drink.

Relations

➲ FOLLOWS WELL: Bell; Calc; Puls; Sep.

➲ ANTIDOTES: Calc; Caps; Coff; Nux-v.

Borax veneta

- ➲ PROVED BY: Hahnemann.
- ➲ DURATION: 30 days.
- ➲ COMMON NAME: Biborate of soda [$Na_2B_4O_7$].
- ➲ FAMILY/KINGDOM: Minerals.
- ➲ RELATION COLD/HEAT: Hot.
- ➲ MIASM: Psora.
- ➲ SOURCE: Trituration and solution of[$Na_2B_4O_7$].
- ➲ SPHERES OF ACTION: GIT, female genital organs-especially vagina,vulva, skin and blood.
- ➲ SUMMURY OF INDICATIONS: Female trouble–blepharitis- Great anxiety.

THERAPEUTIC PICTURE OF DRUG

CN_1 ➲ Borax is especially suited to women & children with pale earthy face.

CN_2 ➲ Red nose of young women.

CN_3 ➲ Lax skin and muscles.

CN_4 ➲ Tangled and frowsy hair.

M_{D-1} ➲ Dread of down word motion in nearly all complaints.

M_{D-2} ➲ Great anxiety,esp. when riding in a carriage or descending a mountain.

M_{D-3} ➲ Children wake suddenly, screaming and grasping the side of the cradle without an apparent cause.

M_{D-4} ➲ Easily frightened and startled with least noise. Before stool irritable, cheerful and happy after.

M_{D-5} ➲ Fear of being infected by some contagious disease.

M_{D-6} ➲ Excessively nervous; easily frightened.

M_{D-7} ➲ Sensitive to sudden noise eg. unusual sharp sound, a cough, sneeze, a cry, etc.

SO_1 ➲ Inflammation of the left eye at inner canthus, with nightly agglutination.

SO_2 ➲ Inflammation of right eye at external canthus, with irregularity of the lashes; nightly agglutination.

SO_3 ➲ Itching in the nose, with tingling.

SO_4 ➲ Nostrils ulcerated, with swelling and pan, as of excoriation at the point of the nose.

SO_5 ➲ Red and shining swelling of the nose, with throbbing and tensive sensation.

DS_1 ➲ Aphthae in the mouth and on the tongue, which bleed easily.

DS_2 ➲ Spasmodic stiffness and torpor of the tongue.

DS_3 ➲ Skin of the palat hard and wrinkled.

FGS_1 ➲ Leucorrhoea: Profuse, albuminous,starchy, with sensation as if warm water were flowing down; for two weeks between the catamenia.

FGS_2 ➲ Menses: too soon, Profuse with gripping pain nausea and pain in the stomach extending to the lumbosacral region.

FGS_3 ➲ Membranous dysmenorrhoea when there is violent, labour-like pain before and during the flow, as if the uterus would expel itself through the vagina.

FGS_4 ➲ Favors easy conception.

FGS_5 ➲ Sensation of distention in clitoris with sticking.

FGS_6 ➲ Pruritus pudendai and eczema of the vulva.

FGS_7 ➲ During the catamenia, Pulsative pains in the head, buzzing in the ears, nausea, with pain in the stomach and in the loins, or shootings and aching in the groin.

FGS_8 ➲ Labour pains: spasmodic: more in stomach than in uterus.

FGS_9 ➲ Pain in the breasts when suckling.

S_{N-1} ➲ Acne, in plethoric young females.

PG_1 ➲ Hair becomes frowsy and tangled.

Modalities

Aggravation

- ➲ Down ward motion.
- ➲ From sudden slight noise.
- ➲ Smoking, warm weather.
- ➲ Before urinating.

Amelioration

- ➲ Pressure.
- ➲ Holding painful side with hand.
- ➲ Evening, cold weather.

Relations

➲ FOLLOWS WELL:	Cala; Nux-vom.
➲ ANTIDOTES:	Cham; Coff.
➲ INIMICALS:	Acet-ac; wine.

Bovista lycoperdon

- ➲ PROVED BY: Hartlaub.
- ➲ DURATION: 7-14 days.
- ➲ COMMON NAME: Puff ball.
- ➲ FAMILY/KINGDOM: Fungi.
- ➲ RELATION COLD/HEAT: Chilly.
- ➲ MIASM: Sycosis.
- ➲ TEMPERAMENT: Nervous.
- ➲ SOURCE: Trituration of puff ball.
- ➲ SPHERES OF ACTION: Female uro-genital systems, Abdomen Blood & skin.
- ➲ SUMMURY OF INDICATIONS: Stammering–haemorrhages–epistaxis-Pruitus–acne–menstrual disorders Gariatric diarrhoea.

THERAPEUTIC PICTURE OF DRUG

CN_1 ➲ Adapted to old maids who suffer from tettery type of eruptions.
M_{D-1} ➲ Dejection and sadness, when a lone.
M_{D-2} ➲ Placid melancholy, with inquietude and somber thoughts.
M_{D-3} ➲ Sad depressed, and desponding.
M_{D-4} ➲ Weakness of memory and Absence of mind.
FGS_1 ➲ Menses flow only at night, not in day time.
FGS_2 ➲ Diarrhoea before and during menses.
FGS_3 ➲ Menses too early and profuse worse at night.
FGS_4 ➲ Leucorrhoea acrid, thick, tough, greenish, follows menses.
FGS_5 ➲ Cannot bear tight clothing around waist.
FGS_6 ➲ Traces of menses between menstruation.
FGS_7 ➲ Soreness of pubes during menses.
FGS_8 ➲ Metrorrhagia, para ovarian cysts.

PG_1 ➲ Usually deep impression on finger from using blunt instruments, Scissors, knife.

PG_2 ➲ Discharge from nose and all mucous membranes very tough, stringy,tenacious.

PG_3 ➲ Great lassitude and want of strength, esp. in joints.

PG_4 ➲ Ebullition of the blood, with much thirst.

Modalities

Aggravation

- Cold food.
- Morning, At fullmoon.
- From wine, from Coffee.

Amelioration

- Hot food.

Relations

➲ COMPARE:	Calc; Cicuta; Rhus-t; Sepia.
➲ FOLLOWS WELL:	Alum; Rhus; Sep; Verat.
➲ ANTIDOTES:	Camph.
➲ INIMICALS:	Coff.

Bromium

- ➲ DURATION: 20-30 days.
- ➲ COMMON NAME: Bromine [Br].
- ➲ FAMILY/KINGDOM: Minerals .
- ➲ RELATION COLD/HEAT: Chilly.
- ➲ MIASM: Psora, Syphilis and sycosis.
- ➲ DIATHESIS: Scrofulous.
- ➲ SOURCE: Solution in distilled water of Br.
- ➲ SPHERES OF ACTION: Glands of body, female genital organs, Respiratory tract and heart.
- ➲ SUMMARY OF INDICATIONS: Bronchial asthma and other respiratory– goitre.

THERAPEUTIC PICTURE OF DRUG

Note: The chief distinction between bromium and iodum is that the former cures the blue-eyed and the latter the dark–eyed patients–HERING

C_{N-1} ➲ It acts best on womens with light blue eyes flaxen hair, light eye brows.

C_{N-2} ➲ Fair delicate skin.

C_{N-3} ➲ Blonde, red cheeked, Scrofulous.

M_{D-1} ➲ Cheerful, desire for mental labour.

M_{D-2} ➲ Low–spirited and out of humour.

M_{D-3} ➲ Crying and lamentation, with hoarse voice.

M_{D-4} ➲ Anxiety; originating in body (heart, lungs), Patient expect to see things jump around the floor.

M_{D-5} ➲ In evening when alone, feels as if he should see something if he should turn round; as if some one were behind him.

RS_1 ➲ Membranous and diphtheritic crup;much rattling of mucus during cough.

RS_2 ➲ Cold sensation in larynx, with cold feeling when inspiring, after breakfast; better after shaving.

RS_3 ➲ Deep, forcible inspiration, is necessary, from time to time.

RS_4 ➲ Difficultly of breathing; cannot inspire deep enough.

RS_5 ➲ Cough, with sudden Paroxysms of suffocation, on swallowing; respiration very short; obliged to catch for breath.

RS_6 ➲ Whooping-cough, with croupish hoarseness of the cough.

RS_7 ➲ Affections being in bronchi and ascend to larynx.

RS_8 ➲ Sensation of weakness and exhaustion in the chest.

RS_9 ➲ Sensation as if the air passages were full of smoke.

FGS_1 ➲ During menses pain in abdomen and small of back.

FGS_2 ➲ Menses too early and too profuse. of bright red blood: flow passive. with much exhaustion; or membranous shreds may pass off.

FGS_3 ➲ Membranous dysmenorrhoea.

FGS_4 ➲ Physometra; loud emission of flatus from the vagina.

FGS_5 ➲ Tumor in breasts, with stitching pains; worse left. side.

FGS_6 ➲ Stitching pains from the breast to the axillae. can not bear pressure (scirrhus).

FGS_7 ➲ Sharp shooting pains in the left breast, worse, pressure.

FGS_8 ➲ Violent contractive spasm before or during menses, lasting hours, leaving the abdomen sore,.

PG_1 ➲ Stony, hard, scrofulous or tuberculous swelling of gland.

PG_2 ➲ Sensation of cobwebs on the face.

PG_3 ➲ For goitre after iodum has failed to cure.

PG_4 ➲ Excessive languor and debility (worse after breakfast).

PG_5 ➲ Tremulousness all over.

PG_6 ➲ Shivering with yawning and stretching; repeated every other day, as a chilliness and cold feet.

PG_7 ➲ Great weakness and lassitude after all the symptoms passed off; in diphtheria.

Modalities

Aggravation

- ➲ From evening until mid night.
- ➲ When sitting in worm room.
- ➲ Worm,damp weather.
- ➲ When at rest.
- ➲ Lying left side.

Amelioration

- ➲ From any motion.
- ➲ Exercise.

Relations

- ➲ FOLLOWS WELL: Arg-n; Kali-c.
- ➲ ANTIDOTES: Am-c; Mag-c; Op.

Bryonia alba

- ➲ PROVED BY: Hahnemann.
- ➲ DURATION: 7-21 days.
- ➲ COMMON NAME: Wild hop.
- ➲ FAMILY/KINGDOM: Cucurbitaceae.
- ➲ RELATION COLD/HEAT: Hot.
- ➲ MIASM: Psora.
- ➲ DIATHESIS: Rheumatic and gouty.
- ➲ TEMPERAMENT: Irritable.
- ➲ SOURCE: Tincture of root produce before flowering.
- ➲ SPHERES OF ACTION: Serous membrane, fibrous tissue, brain, liver respiratory system.
- ➲ SUMMARY OF INDICATIONS: Gout–rheumatism- degenerative joint disorders–fevers–constipation.

THERAPEUTIC PICTURE OF DRUG

Note: Bryonia is called the "grumpy bear" remedy, because the person who needs this remedy is irritable and wishes to be left all alone. Whatever the disorder-fever, headache, sore throat or gastritis the patient feels worse with the slightest movement and is very thirsty.

C_{N-1} ➲ Dark or black hair, dark complexion,firm muscular fibre dry, nervous,slender people.

C_{N-1} ➲ Persons.of a gouty & Rheumatic diathesis, prove to so–called bilious attacks.

M_{D-1} ➲ Irritable mood, wishes to be alone-very irritable; inclined to fright, fear and vexation.

M_{D-2} ➲ Anxiety and inquietude, with fear of the future.

M_{D-3} ➲ Patient desire to go home.

M_{D-4} ➲ Great depression and very morose mood, without cause.

M_{D-5} ➲ Irritable mood, wishes to be alone, very irritable; inclined to fright, fear and vexation.

M_{D-6} ➲ After having been angry he is chilly; has a red face and heat in the head.
M_{D-7} ➲ Irascibility and pation.
M_{D-8} ➲ Delirium (at night) and ravings about the transactions of the day.
H_{D-1} ➲ Headache commence in morning not on waking, but when first opening eyes.
H_{D-2} ➲ Tearing across the forehead, then the cervical muscles, then in right arm.
H_{D-3} ➲ Headache as though the head would burst, commencing in morning and gradually increasing till evening.
H_{D-4} ➲ Pain sharp with the slightest cough.
DS_1 ➲ Pressure, as if from a stone in the stomach, esp. after a meal, or on walking sometimes accompanied by ill-homour.
DS_2 ➲ Pain, as of excoriation, in the pit of the stomach, sensible to the touch, or on coughing.
DS_3 ➲ Constipation: faeces too large, with difficult evacuation.
DS_4 ➲ Stool too large in size; too hard and dry.
DS_5 ➲ Faeces scanty, but hard, and as if burnt.
DS_6 ➲ Diarrhoea: bilious, acrid stools, with soreness of anus
DS_7 ➲ Diarrhoea like dirty water with whitish granulated sediment of undigested food.
DS_8 ➲ Diarrhoea: mostly at night or after eating; after eating fruit or sour-krout; morning, after getting up, preceded by cutting pains in bowels; burning, worse in warm weather.
DS_9 ➲ Alternation of diarrhoea and constipation.
RS_1 ➲ Dry, violent, spasmodic cough with stitching pain in the chest.
RS_2 ➲ Cough is worse at night, after eating and drinking, taking a deep breath and when entering a warm room.
RS_3 ➲ Nausea excites cough, and coughing often excites vomiting.
RS_4 ➲ Cough, with constant crawling, upwards, in the throat, followed by expectoration of mucus.
FGS_1 ➲ Menses too early, too profuse,worse from motion, with tearing pain in legs.
FGS_2 ➲ Stitching pains in ovaries on taking a deep inspiration, very sensitive to touch.
FGS_3 ➲ Pain in right ovary as if torn, extending to thigh.
FGS_4 ➲ Milk fever.
FGS_5 ➲ Pain in breasts at menstrual period.
FGS_6 ➲ Breasts hot and painful hard.
FGS_7 ➲ Abscess of mammae.
FGS_8 ➲ Frequent bleeding of nose at appearance of menses.
FGS_9 ➲ Intermenstrual pain, with great abdominal and pelvic soreness.

FGS_{10} ➲ Mammae heavy,of a stony hardness, pale but hard hot, & painful, must support the breast.

F_{R-1} ➲ Pulse full, hard, tense, and quick.

F_{R-2} ➲ Chills with external coldness, dry cough, stitches.

F_{R-3} ➲ Sour sweat after slight exertion and internal heat.

F_{R-4} ➲ Easy, profuse perspiration.

F_{R-5} ➲ Rheumatic fever and typhoid marked by gastro-hepatic complications.

F_{R-6} ➲ Wants to drink much water during chill and fever.

PG_1 ➲ Excessive dryness of mucous membrane of entire body, with great thirst.

PG_2 ➲ Thirsty, but drinking makes headache worse. Thirst for large quantities of cold drinks at long intervals.

PG_3 ➲ Dryness from mouth to anus.

PG_4 ➲ Rheumatism with red, swollen, hot shiny joint. Rest touch and pressure relieve the pain.

PG_5 ➲ Stitching pains, better with firm pressure, worse on motion.

PG_6 ➲ Patient can not sit up from nausea and faintness.

PG_7 ➲ Children dislike to be carried, or to be raised.

PG_8 ➲ Symptoms progress slowly, usually worse on the right side.

Modalities

Aggravation

- ➲ Motion, exertion, touch.
- ➲ Can not sit up, warmth.
- ➲ From any motion.
- ➲ Suppressed discharge of any kind.

Amelioration

- ➲ Lying especially on painful side.
- ➲ Pressure, rest, cold, eating cold things.
- ➲ Absolute rest, either mental and physical.

Relations

- ➲ COMPLEMENTARY: Alumina and Rhus-tox.
- ➲ FOLLOWS WELL: Acon; Nux; Op; sul.
- ➲ ANTIDOTES: Alum; Coff; Ign;Mrc; Nux.
- ➲ SIMILAR: Bell; Hep; Ran-b.

Bufo rana

- ➲ PROVED BY: Dr. Carl Heneke.
- ➲ FAMILY/KINGDOM: Bufonnidae.
- ➲ COMMON NAME: Poison of the toad.
- ➲ SOURCE: Solution in rectified sprit of the poison expressed from the cutaneous glands.
- ➲ SPHERES OF ACTION: Nervous system, skin and female genital symptoms.

THERAPEUTIC PICTURE OF DRUG

C_{N-1} ➲ Feeble minded female child who are prematurely senile.

C_{N-2} ➲ The female has great sensitiveness to cold.

M_{D-1} ➲ Weak memory; idiotic.

M_{D-2} ➲ Desire for solitude.

M_{D-3} ➲ Inclination to be angry; to bite.

FGS_1 ➲ Menses too early and too profuse (menorrhagia),clots. and bloody discharge at other times (Metrorrhagia)

FGS_2 ➲ Watery leucorrhoea.

FGS_3 ➲ Burning in the ovaries and uterus.

FGS_4 ➲ Ulceration of the cervix.

FGS_5 ➲ Offensive bloody discharge.

FGS_6 ➲ Epileptic attacks with menses.

FGS_7 ➲ Headache with or before menses.

FGS_8 ➲ Cancer of breast & especially useful when the milk is mixed with blood.

FGS_9 ➲ Burning in ovaries and uterus.

FGS_{10} ➲ Tumors and polypi of the womb.

PG_1 ➲ Cord–like swelling from groin to knee (milk–leg =Phlegmasia albadollens.)

PG_2 ➲ Lymphangitis of septic origin.

PG_3 ➲ Veins swollen.

Modalities

Aggravation

- At night.
- During sleep.
- In warm room.

Amelioration

- From bathing and cold air.
- From putting feet in hot water.

Relations

- COMPLEMENTARY: Salamandra.
- ANTIDOTES: Lach; Senega.

Cactus grandiflorus
II
Selenicereus spinulosus

- PROVED BY: Rubini.
- DURATION: 7–10 days.
- COMMON NAME: Night blooming cereus.
- FAMILY/KINGDOM: Cactaceae.
- MIASM: Psora.
- TEMPERAMET: Sanguine.
- SOURCE: Tincture of youngest and tenderest stems and flowers.
- SPHERES OF ACTION: Heart, blood vessels, Uterus, ovary etc.
- SUMMARY OF INDICATIONS: Headaches and neuralgia constricting in motion- menopausal– headaches–heart disorders.

THERAPEUTIC PICTURE OF DRUG

C_{N-1} ➲ Sanguineous congestions in person of plethoric habit,often resulting in haemorrhage; sanguineous apoplexy

M_{D-1} ➲ Fear of death, believes the disease incurable.

M_{D-2} ➲ Melancholy, taciturn, sad, ill humored, screams with pain. anxiety.

H_{D-1} ➲ Heavy pressing in the head as if a great weight lay on the vertex; better from pressure; worse from noise (even talking) and light.

H_{D-2} ➲ Vertigo from sanguineous congestions to head.

HD_3 ➲ Throbbing pain with sensation of weigh and violent neuralgias in right side of head; periodic.

CVS_1 ➲ Sensation of constriction in heart, as if an iron hand prevented its normal movements.

CVS_2 ➲ Pricking pains impeding breathing and movements of the body; oppression; cannot lie on the left side; blue face; pulse quick, throbbing, tense and hard.

CVS_3 ➲ Palpitation with vertigo, loss of consciousness, dyspnoea; worse walking, at night, lying on the left side, at the approach of the menses and from any exertion.

CVS_4 ➲ Irregularity of the heart's action, at times frequent, at others slow; great irritation of the cardiac nerves; enlarged left ventricle.

CVS_5 ➲ Endocardial murmurs; excessive impulse; increased precardial dullness; enlarged ventricle.

CVS_6 ➲ Heart disease with oedema of left hand only.

FGS_1 ➲ Constriction in uterine region and ovaries.

FGS_2 ➲ Dysmenorrhoea,pulsating pain in uterus and ovaries.

FGS_3 ➲ Viginismus.

FGS_4 ➲ Menses early, dark, pitch–like.Cease on lying down, with heart symptoms

F_{R-1} ➲ Chilliness, with chattering of the teeth.

F_{R-2} ➲ Chilliness not relieved by covering; 11 am and 11 pm.

F_{R-3} ➲ Burning heat, with shortness of breath.

F_{R-4} ➲ Intermittent fever (quotidian) recurring every day at the same hour (for many successive days)

F_{R-5} ➲ Scorching heat at night, with headache, following a chill and terminating in perspiration.

F_{R-6} ➲ Coldness in back and icy cold hands.

F_{R-7} ➲ Heat after chill, with dyspnoea, headache and thirst; with insensibility till midnight, then shortness of breath and inability to remain lying, followed by profuse sweat, with great thirst.

PG_1 ➲ Whole body feels as if caged, each wire being twisted tighter and tighter.

PG_2 ➲ Haemorrhages: from nose; lungs; rectum; bladder; stomach.

PG_3 ➲ Sensation of constriction: in throat; chest; heart; bladder; rectum.

PG_4 ➲ General weakness and prostration of strength.

PG_5 ➲ Congestions.

Modalities

Aggravation

- ➲ About noon, lying on left side.
- ➲ Walking.
- ➲ Going up stairs.
- ➲ 11 A.M. & 11 P.M.

Amelioration

- Open air.
- From rest.
- When sitting.

Relations

- COMPARE: Acon; Gels; Lacs; Naja; Spig.
- FOLLOWS WELL: Dig; Eupat; Lach; Nux; Sulph.
- ANTIDOTES: Camph; Chin.

Caladium seguinum

- PROVED BY: E.W. Berridge.
- DURATION: 30–40 days.
- COMMON NAME: American Arum.
- FAMILY/KINGDOM: Araceal.
- SOURCE: Ticture of whole fresh plant.
- SUMMARY OF INDICATIONS: Pruritus valvae–Chronic gastritis.

THERAPEUTIC PICTURE OF DRUG

M_{D-1} ➲ Mind depressed.

M_{D-2} ➲ Lascivious ideas.

M_{D-3} ➲ Restless, Cannot control himself after smoking.

M_{D-4} ➲ Unconciousness or coma.

FGS_1 ➲ Pruritus of vulva and vagina; induces onanism; during pregnancy; with mucous discharge.

FGS_2 ➲ Voluptuousness.

FGS_3 ➲ Cramp pains in uterus at night.

FGS_4 ➲ Pulsating pain in uterus and ovaries.

FGS_5 ➲ Constriction in uterine region, around pelvis.

FGS_6 ➲ Constriction of vagina prevent coition (vaginismus).

FGS_7 ➲ Very painful menstruation, extorting loud cries.

MGS_1 ➲ Sexual desire with relaxed penis, or painful erections without desire.

MGS_2 ➲ Impotence with mental depression.

MGS_3 ➲ Glans; very red, covered with fine red points; dry with desire to rub it.

MGS_4 ➲ Prepuce much swollen at the margin, sore and painful.

MGS_5 ➲ Pimples on the mons veneris.

PG_1 ➲ Weariness over the whole body.

PG_2 ➲ Attack like fainting after writing and thinking, when lying down, or when rising.

PG_3 ➲ Sighing respiration; dryness of parts which are usually moist.

PG_4 ➲ Sweet sweat attracts the flies.

PG_5 ➲ Aversion to motion, dread to move.

Modalities

Aggravation

- Motion.
- From warmth.

Amelioration

- From sweat.
- After short sleep, cold water.

Relations

- COMPARE: Capsic; Caust; Phos; Selen; Lyco.
- COMPLEMENTARY: Nit-ac.
- FOLLOWS WELL: Acon; Pulsa; Sepia.
- ANTIDOTES: Mer-car; Hyos; Carb-v.
- INIMICALS: Arum-triph.

Calcarea carbonica or Calcarea ostreaum

- PROVED BY: Hahnemann.
- DURATION: 60 days.
- COMMON NAME: Carbonate of lime = $CaCO_3$.
- FAMILY/KINGDOM: Minerals.
- RELATION COLD/HEAT: Chilly.
- MIASM: Anti-psoric and Antisycotic remedies.
- DIATHESIS: Scrofulous, rachitic & tubercular.
- TEMPERAMENT: Leucophlegmatic.
- SOURCE: Trituration of the middle layer of oster shell.
- SPHERES OF ACTION: Female genital organs, bones, glands, blood, skin, mind etc.
- SUMMARY OF INDICATIONS: Rickets-constipation-Menstrual disorders.

THERAPEUTIC PICTURE OF DRUG

C_{N-1} ➲ Children who grow fat, chalky look with red face, large belly like an inverted saucer.

C_{N-2} ➲ Children with large head, open fontanelles and sutures, flabby muscles, plale skin, soft bones.

C_{N-3} ➲ Who sweat easily, specially on back side of the head and neck and swollen glands.

C_{N-4} ➲ Girls who are fleshy, plethoric and grow too rapidly.

C_{N-5} ➲ It is suited to fair, fatty and flabby patient who becomes easily fatigued and tired on walking.

C_{N-6} ➲ Patient with much sweating, cold extremities and sour smell of the body.

C_{N-7} ➲ There is tendency to obesity in youth and slow in movement.

M_{D-1} ➲ Fears she will lose her reason or that people will observe her mental confusion.

M_{D-2} ➲ Anxiety with palpitations.

M_{D-3} ➲ Obstinancy; slight mental effort produces a hot head.

M_{D-4} ➲ Averse to work exertion.

DS_1 ➲ Teath particularly sensitive to cold air.

DS_2 ➲ Difficult dentition.

DS_3 ➲ Toothache: after drinking cold liquids, or excited by draught or cold; drawing, shooting or boring; during and after menstruation; during pregnancy; worse from worm or cold drinks.

DS_4 ➲ Eructations: tasting of the food eaten; bitter; sour; of tasteless fluid; of food; burning.

DS_5 ➲ Vomit: sour, of bitter slime; of what has been eaten; black; bloody; of milk in thick curds during dentition.

DS_6 ➲ Pit of stomach swollen like a saucer turned bottom up; painful to pressure.

DS_7 ➲ Stools: frequent; first hard, then pasty, then liquid; thin, offensive, like bad eggs; yellowish, grey, or clay-like, fecal; whitish, watery worse in the after part of the day, often of sour smell; undigested, hard

DS_8 ➲ Stools look like lumps of chalk, in children during dentition.

FGS_1 ➲ Menstruation too early, too profuse too long lasting; with subsequent amenorrhoea and chlorosis with menses scanty or suppressed.

FGS_2 ➲ Women: menses too early, too profuse; feet habitually cold and damp, as if they had on colddamp stockings; continually cold in bed.

FGS_3 ➲ Theleast mental excitement cause profuse return of menstrual flow.

FGS_4 ➲ Itching or pressing in the vagina.

FGS_5 ➲ Shootings in the orifice of the matrix and pressive pain in the vagina.

FGS_6 ➲ Prolapsus Uteri, with pressure on the parts.

FGS_7 ➲ Itching in the womb.

FGS_8 ➲ Inflammation and swelling of the womb, with redness, Purulent discharge and burning pain.

FGS_9 ➲ Varices in the labia majora.

FGS_{10} ➲ Leucorrhoea, with burning itching or else like milk, flowing by fits, and during the emission of urine.

FGS_{11} ➲ Burning and itching of parts before and after menstruation; in little girls.

FGS_{12} ➲ Increase sexual desire (Nymphomania)

FGS_{13} ➲ Before the catamenia, mammae swollen and painful, fatigue headache, disposition to be frightened colic and shivering.

FGS_{14} ➲ During the catamenia, congestion in the head, with internal heat or cuttings in the abdomen, and cramp-like pain in the lumbar region or else vertigo, headache, toothache, nausea, colic and other sufferings.

FGS_{15} ➲ Pain, as of excoriation and ulceration in the nipples.

FGS_{16} ➲ Inflammation swelling of the mammae and of the nipples.

FGS_{17} ➲ Swelling of the glands of the breast.

FGS_{18} ➲ Breasts painful and tender before menses.

FGS_{19} ➲ Milk too abundant, or suppressed.

PG_1 ➲ Head sweats profusely while sleeping, wetting pillow for around.

PG_2 ➲ Feels better in every way when constipated stools may have to be removed mechanically.

PG_3 ➲ During either sickness or convalescence, great longing for eggs; Groves for indigestible materials; aversion to meats.

PG_4 ➲ Cramps and contractions of the limbs esp. of the fingers and toes.

PG_5 ➲ Shootings and drawing pains in the limbs, chiefly at night, or in summer, and on change of weather.

PG_6 ➲ Frequently trembling of the whole body, increased in the open air.

PG_7 ➲ Curvature of bones especially of the spine and long bone; extremities deformed; bones irregularly developed.

PG_8 ➲ Hoarseness; painless, sensation, as if something were torn loose in the trachea.

PG_9 ➲ Great tendency to take cold, and great sensibility to cold and damp air.

Modalities

Aggravation

- ➲ Cold air.
- ➲ Cold weather.
- ➲ Morning.
- ➲ Wet weather.
- ➲ Washing.
- ➲ During the full moon.

Amelioration

- ➲ Dry weather, lying on painful side.
- ➲ When constipated.

Relations

➲ COMPLEMENTARY:	Bell.; Rhus-t
➲ FOLLOWS WELL:	Agar; Bell; Bism; Dros; Ip; Graph; Lyc; Nat-c; Plat; Puls; Rhus-t; Stars; Sep; Sil; Ther.
➲ ANTIDOTES:	Bryo; Camph; Chin; Iod; Nit-ac; Nit-s; Nux-v; Sep; Sulph.
➲ INIMICALS:	After kali-bi.

Calcarea phosphorica

- PROVED BY: Hering.
- DURATION: 60 days.
- COMMON NAME: Phosphate of lime [Tricalcic phosphat = Ca_3 $2PO_{4]}$.
- FAMILY/KINGDOM: Minerals.
- RELATION COLD/HEAT: Chilly.
- MIASM: Psora.
- DIATHESIS: Scrofulous and gouty.
- SOURCE: A mixture of the basic and other phosphates of lime, made by dropping dilute phosphoric acid into lime water.
- SPHERES OF ACTION: Female genital organs, teath, bone, glands and digestive system.
- SUMMARY OF INDICATIONS: Non-union of bones- gastritis with colic-deficient lactation-rheumatism-diarrhoea.

THERAPEUTIC PICTURE OF DRUG

C_{N-1} ➲ Persons who are anaemic and dark complexioned, dark hair and eyes.

C_{N-2} ➲ Thin spare subjects, instead of fat.

C_{N-3} ➲ Emaciated body, sunken flabby abdomen, soft bones bent disproportionately, enlarged head and long weak emaciated neck, unable to support head.

C_{N-4} ➲ Emaciated child; slow in learning to walk, or lose the ability; lose flesh.

M_{D-1} ➲ Great depression.

M_{D-2} ➲ Slow comprehension.

M_{D-3} ➲ Difficulty in performing intellectual operations.

M_{D-4} ➲ Always wants to go some where.

H_{D-1} ➲ Headache of school-girls; diarrhoea.

H_{D-2} ➲ Headache, worse from change of weather, extending from the forehead to nose; or from the temples to jaw, with some rheumatic teeling from the clavicles to wrists.

H_{D-3} ➲ Delayed closure, or re-opening of fontanelles.

H_{D-4} ➲ Cannot hold the head up; moves it from place to place; head totters.

DS_1 ➲ Children vomit, often and easy.

DS_2 ➲ Burning: in region of navel; in the whole abdomen, rising up into the chest or into the throat.

DS_3 ➲ Oozing of bloody fluid from navel of infants.

DS_4 ➲ Stools: green and loose, sometimes slimy, with children; soft, past with difficultly, accompanying the headache of school girls.

DS_5 ➲ Fistula in ano, alternating with chest symptoms.

DS_6 ➲ Colic and diarrhoea from: ice creams; juicy fruit or cidar; every attempt to eat; drinking cold water (colic or diarrhoea).

FGS_1 ➲ Aching in uterus; weakness and distress in uterine region; < during defication and micturition; uterine displacement.

FGS_2 ➲ Pressure upward over mons veneris, Throbbing.

FGS_3 ➲ Voluptuous feeling as if the parts were fillings up with blood; feels pulse in all the parts, with increased sexual desire.

FGS_4 ➲ Menses: too early, light, or dark (esp. with rheumatic Patients);labour-like pains.

FGS_5 ➲ Menses too early, blood bright, with girls; too late; blood dark or first bright; then dark in women.

FGS_6 ➲ Leucorrhoea, like white egg, day and night; < morning after rising of sweetish odour; increased whites with a stool of bad odour.

FGS_7 ➲ Pain in navel; sacrum; Symphysis pubis; mammae during pregnancy.

FGS_8 ➲ At puberty; acne in anaemic girls with vertex headache and flatulent dyspepsia > be eating.

PG_1 ➲ Girls at puberty tall, growing rapidly; tendency of bones to soften or spine to curve.

PG_2 ➲ Feels complaints more when thinking about them.

PG_3 ➲ spine weak, disposed to curvatures, especially to the left; unable to support body; neck weak, unable to support head.

PG_4 ➲ Non-union of bones; Promotes callous.

PG_5 ➲ Rheumatic pains of all kinds.

PG_6 ➲ Rheumatic pains in different part of the body, proceeding along the muscles in to the joints.

PG_7 ➲ Burning itching over the whole body.

PG_8 ➲ On every little cold she is much worse.

PG_9 ➲ Pains along sutures or at symphyses.

Modalities

Aggravation

- When thinking about disorder.
- Exposure to damp, cold, changeable.
- East winds (In Europe).
- Melting snow.
- Mental exertion.

Amelioration

- In summer.
- Warm, dry atmosphere.

Relations

- COMPLEMENTARY: Hep; Ruta; Sulph; Zink.
- FOLLOWS WELL: Rhus-t; Sulph.
- INIMICALS: Coft.
- SIMILAR: Carbo animalis; Cal-flu; Cal-ace; Flu-aci; Kali-pho.

Calendula officinalis

- ➲ COMMON NAME: Marigold.
- ➲ FAMILY/KINGDOM: Compositae.
- ➲ SOURCE: Tincture of the leaves and flowers.
- ➲ SPHERES OF ACTION: Muscles,Tendons, nerves, scalp and skin.
- ➲ SUMMARY OF INDICATIONS: Painful traumatic injury–surgical wounds-loss of blood and severe pain.

THERAPEUTIC PICTURE OF DRUG

Note: [Acts well in potency as well, as in tincture or lotion applied locally. Both may be administered at the same time.]

M_{D-1} ➲ Great irritability; easily frightened; hearing acute.

M_{D-2} ➲ Intense depression.

FGS_1 ➲ Warts on the os externum.

FGS_2 ➲ Menses suppressed, with cough.

FGS_3 ➲ Chronic endocervicitis.

FGS_4 ➲ Uterine hypertrophy, sensation of weight and fullness' in the pelvis; stretching and dragging in the groin; pain on sudden movement.

FGS_5 ➲ Os lower than natural (prolapsed.).

PG_1 ➲ Ulcers; irritable, inflamed, sloughing, varicose; painful as if beaten; excessive secretion of pus.

PG_2 ➲ Used in traumatic affections. This remedy is useful to secure healing of wounds by first intention and to; prevent suppuration.

PG_3 ➲ Lacerated wounds, loss of blood from wounds causing exhaustion and ulceration of skin.

PG_4 ➲ Calendula is almost specific to prevent suppuration of clean, surgical cuts or lacerated wounds. the lotion can be applied to open wounds.

PG_5 ➲ Loss of blood and severe pain.

Modalities

Aggravation

- In damp.
- Cloudy weather.
- Heavy.

Relations

- COMPARE: Ham; Hyper; Symph; Arn.
- COMPLEMENTARY: Hep.
- FOLLOWS WELL: Arn; Ars; Bry; Nit;-ac; Phos; Rhus-t.
- ANTIDOTES: Chel; Rheum.
- INIMICALS: Camph.

Camphora officinarum

- PROVED BY: Hahnemann.
- DURATION: 1 day.
- COMMON NAME: Camphor.
- FAMILY/KINGDOM Lauraceae.
- RELATION COLD/HEAT: Very chilly.
- MIASM: Psora.
- TEMPERAMENT: Irritable.
- SOURCE: A gum obtained from Laurus Camphora. Solution in rectified sprit.
- SPHERES OF ACTION: . Digestive system; cerebro-spinal nerves; urninary organs *e.g.* kidney.
- SUMMARY OF INDICATIONS: Severe gastro-enteritis (Cholera).

THERAPEUTIC PICTURE OF DRUG

C_{N-1} ➲ Especially suited to those persons who are exceedingly sensitive to cold air.

C_{N-2} ➲ Persons physically and mentally very weak.

M_{D-1} ➲ Anxiety, precordial; restless tossing about; palpitation of heart.

M_{D-2} ➲ Great anguish and discouragement.

M_{D-3} ➲ Loss of memory; Awkwardness.

M_{D-4} ➲ Delirious somnolent, with slow fever, at night.

M_{D-5} ➲ Thinking about an existing pain causes it to disappear.

DS_1 ➲ Inclination to vomit, followed by attacks of vertigo.

DS_2 ➲ Vomiting of bile or of blood.

DS_3 ➲ At the commencement of the vomiting, cold sweat, chiefly on the face.

DS_4 ➲ Absence of nausea and vomiting; body icy-cold.

DS_5 ➲ Asiatic cholera, with cramps in calves, coldness in body, anguish burning in oesophagus and stomach.

DS_6 ➲ Diarrhoea, with colicy pains, with chilliness and sensitiveness to cold air.

DS_7 ➲ Absence of discharges; body icy-cold.

S_{N-1} ➲ Skin sorely sensitive, even to the slightest touch.

S_{N-2} ➲ Blood blisters; Erysipelas; Gangrene; Hard spots.

S_{N-3} ➲ Scarlatina: with cold, blue Hippocratic face; rattling in throat; with hot breath, hot sweat on forehead, child will no be covered.

S_{N-4} ➲ Measle eruption delays; titanic rigors; skin cold, bluish; dysuria.

S_{N-5} ➲ Sudden sinking away of variola pustules.

PG_1 ➲ The symptoms often disappear as soon as attension is called to them.

PG_2 ➲ The surface of the body is cold to the touch, yet can not bear to be covered: throws off all coverings.

PG_3 ➲ Rheumatic lancinations in the muscles.

PG_4 ➲ Uneasiness, relaxation and heaviness over the whole body.

PG_5 ➲ Tetanus with loss of consciousness and vomiting.

Modalities

Aggravation

- ➲ Motion.
- ➲ Cantact or cover.
- ➲ Night.
- ➲ Cold air.

Amelioration

- ➲ When thinking of (contemptating on) the disorder.
- ➲ Warm air.
- ➲ Drinking cold water.

Relations

➲ FOLLOWS WELL:	Ant-t; Ars; Bell; Cocc; Nux-v; Rhus-t; Verat.
➲ ANTIDOTES:	Nit-s-d; Op; Phos; Dulc.
➲ INIMICALS:	After Kali-n.

Cannabis indica

- ➲ COMMON NAME: Indian Hemp.
- ➲ FAMILY/KINGDOM: Urticaceae.
- ➲ SOURCE: Tincture of young leaves and twigs.
- ➲ SUMMARY OF INDICATIONS: Amnesia-mental disorders.

THERAPEUTIC PICTURE OF DRUG

M_{D-1} ➲ Excessive loquacity; exuberance of spirits.

M_{D-2} ➲ Time seems too long; seconds seem like ages; a few rods, an immense distance.

M_{D-3} ➲ Constantly theorizing.

M_{D-4} ➲ Anxious depression. Constant fear of becoming insane.

M_{D-5} ➲ Mania, must more constantly.

M_{D-6} ➲ Very forgetful; cannot finish a sentence.

M_{D-7} ➲ Uncontrollable laughter.

M_{D-8} ➲ Delirium tremens, trembling, hallucinations; tendency to become furious; nausea; unquenchable thirst.

M_{D-9} ➲ Clairvoyance.

M_{D-10} ➲ Emotional excitement; rapid change of mood.

M_{D-11} ➲ Can not realize her identity, chronic vertigo as if flouting in air.

FGS_1 ➲ Very profuse menstruation.; Painful, dark but without clots.

FGS_2 ➲ Spasmodic uterine colic, pains returning like labor pains; great agitation and sleeplessness.

FGS_3 ➲ Threatened miscarriage in 8th month; burning on micturition with purulent discharge.

FGS_4 ➲ Dysmenorrhea with sexual desire (nymphomania)

FGS_5 ➲ Backache during menses.

PG_1 ➲ Head: sensation as if top of head were opening & shutting and as if calvarium were being lifted.

PG_1 ➲ Pain across shoulders and spine, must stoop; can not walk erect.

Modalities

Aggravation

- Morning.
- With coffee, liquor and tobacco.
- Lying on the right side.

Amelioration

- Fresh air.
- Cold water.
- Rest.

Relations

- COMPARE: Bell; Hyos; Stram.
- ANTIDOTES: Nux-vom.

Cantharis vesicatoria

- PROVED BY: Hahnemann.
- DURATION: 30-40 days.
- COMMON NAME: Spanish flies.
- FAMILY/KINGDOM: Canthariдeae.
- RELATION COLD/HEAT: Hot.
- MIASM: Psora.
- TEMPERAMENT: Irritable.
- SOURCE: Tincture of living insects.
- SPHERES OF ACTIONE: Urinary organs, Urinary bladder. Urethra,ureter, skin.
- SUMMARY OF INDICATIONS: Haemorrhages-urethritis–erysipelas-sunburn, burns and scalds–cystistis.

THERAPEUTIC PICTURE OF DRUG

M_{D-1} ➲ Furious delirium

M_{D-2} ➲ Anaxious, Restlessness ending in a rage.

M_{D-3} ➲ Acute mania, generally of a sexual type, firely sexual desire.

DS_1 ➲ Burning sensation in oesophagus, stomach and other organs; also in the soles of feet at nights.

DS_2 ➲ Passage of white, tough musus with stool, like scrapings from intestines, with streaks of blood; slimy and bloody stools.

DS_3 ➲ During stool: colic, pressing, cutting or burning pains in the anus, causing the patient to cry out.

RS_1 ➲ Burning the larynx; larynx sensitive to touch.

RS_2 ➲ Profuse catarrh of the air-passage, the mucus being tenacious, with painful hawking and nightly lancinating and dryness in the trachea.

RS_3 ➲ Exudating with in the pleura; dyspnoea, palpitation; scanty urine; tendency to syncope.

RS_4 ➲ Inflammation of serous membranes; pleurisy after Acon and Bryon.

FGS_1 ➲ Retained placenta, with painful urination.

FGS_2 ➲ Puerperal metritis, with inflammation of bladder.

FGS_3 ➲ Burning pain in ovaries, extremely sensitive.

FGS_4 ➲ Pain in os coccyx, lancinating and tearing.

MGS_1 ➲ Sexual desire greatly increased, with painful, frequent ervetations (with gonorrhoea), if long continuance, as in Priapismus; disturbing sleep at night.

MGS_2 ➲ Drawing pain in the spermatic cord, while urinating; testicles drawn up.

MGS_3 ➲ Inflammation and gangrene of the genital parts.

MGS_4 ➲ Ready emission, during amorous caresses.

MGS_5 ➲ After coition, burning pain in the urethra.

US_1 ➲ Constant urging to urinate, passing a few drops at a time mixed with blood. Intolerable urging, before, during and after urination.

US_2 ➲ Intense itching, burning, cutting pains in urethra; violent tenesmus and strangury.

US_3 ➲ Pain in the region of kidneys and urging to urinate, steadily increasing in severity.

US_4 ➲ Pain in the kidney extending in to the abdomen, the axilla, along the urethra into the bladder.

US_5 ➲ Difficult emission of urine, in a week an scattered stream.

US_6 ➲ Flow of sanguineous mucus from the bladder.

US_7 ➲ Emission of blood, drop by drop.

US_8 ➲ Inflammation and ulceration of the kidneys, of the bladder, and of the urethra.

US_9 ➲ Urine, pale yellow, or of a deep red colour.

PG_1 ➲ Pain, raw,sore, burning in every part of body, internally and externally; extreme weakness.

PG_2 ➲ Over sensitiveness of all regions of the body.

PG_3 ➲ The symptoms are renewed every seven days.

PG_4 ➲ Burning pains, as from excoriation, in all the cavities of the body.

PG_5 ➲ Ulceration and erosion of internal parts; patient lies in a stupor, with occasional twitches of the hands; symptoms of collapse.

PG_6 ➲ Haemorrhages from nose, mouth, intestines, genital and urinary organs.

PG_7 ➲ The suffering show them selves chiefly on the right side, and are mitigated in a recumbent posture.

PG_8 ➲ Disgust for everything: drink; food, tobacco- Drinking even small quantities of water increases the pain in the bladder.

Modalities

Aggravation

- From touch, urinating.
- Drinking cold water, coffee.

Amelioration

- By Rubbing.
- Lying quietly on the back.

Relations

- COMPARE: Acon; Apis; Ars; Bryo; Gels.
- COMPLEMENTARY: Camph.
- FOLLOWS WELL: Bell; Kali–Iod, Merc; Phos; Puls; Sulph.
- ANTIDOTES: Acon; Apis; Rheum; Laurl.
- INIMICALS: Coff.

Capsicum annum

- ➲ PROVED BY: Hahnemann.
- ➲ DURATION: 7 days.
- ➲ COMMON NAME: [Red pepper].
- ➲ FAMILY/KINGDOM: Solanaceae.
- ➲ RELATION COLD/HEAT: Chilly.
- ➲ MIASM: Psora.
- ➲ DIATHESIS: Phlegmatic.
- ➲ TEMPERAMENT: Nervous.
- ➲ SOURCE: Tincture of the dried pods.
- ➲ SPHERES OF ACTION: Mucous membrane *e.g.* mouth, tongue, abdomen, chest, lungs & skin.
- ➲ SUMMARY OF INDICATIONS: Obesity–tonsillitis–mastoiditis.

THERAPEUTIC PICTURE OF DRUG

C_{N-1} ➲ Especially suited to fatty persons with light hair, blue eyes, stout and plethoric.

C_{N-2} ➲ Who easily get exhausted, indolent, dread of any kind of exercise.

C_{N-3} ➲ Persons inclined to be jovial, yet angry at trifles.

C_{N-4} ➲ Children dread open air.

C_{N-5} ➲ A capsicum child is fatty, dirty, clumsy, and is always chilly.

M_{D-1} ➲ Excessive peevishness.

M_{D-2} ➲ Homesickness, with sleeplessness and disposition to suicide.

M_{D-3} ➲ Wants to be felt alone.

M_{D-4} ➲ Peppery disposition.

M_{D-5} ➲ Delirium tremens.

M_{D-6} ➲ Indolent, dreads any kinds of exercise.

M_{D-7} ➲ Children; dread open air; always chilly.

- RS_1 ➲ Burning and smarting sensation, as from cayenne pepper, in throat and other parts, not > by heat.
- RS_2 ➲ Cramp-like contraction of the throat.
- RS_3 ➲ Sore throat with painful deglution and pulling sensation in the pharynx.
- RS_4 ➲ With every explosive cough (and at no other time), there escapes a volume of pungent, fetid air.
- RS_5 ➲ Nervous, spasmodic cough.
- RS_6 ➲ Cough in sudden paroxysms, convulses whole body.
- RS_7 ➲ Tonsillitis: with burning, smarting pain; intense soreness; constriction of the throat with burning; inflamed dark red swollen.
- RS_8 ➲ Pain in ears when coughing; ears and tip of nose hot; bloody mucus from nose; eyes protrude with burning and lacrymation.
- FGS_1 ➲ Uterine haemorrhage near menopause with nausea.
- FGS_2 ➲ Sticking sensation in the left ovarian region.
- PG_1 ➲ Climacteric disturbances with burning on the tip of the tongue.
- PG_2 ➲ The burning, Spasmodic constriction and all other pains are worse between the acts of degulutition.
- PG_3 ➲ Cramps in the body, with stiffness in the arm and legs, with numbness and sensation of tingling.
- PG_4 ➲ Drawing pains in the limbs excited by movement.

Modalities

Aggravation

- ➲ Open air.
- ➲ Uncovering.
- ➲ Draughts.

Amelioration

- ➲ While eating.
- ➲ From heat.

Relations

➲ COMPARE:.	Apis; Bell; Bry; Calad; Puls.
➲ FOLLOWS WELL:	Bell; Lyc; Puls; Sil.
➲ ANTIDOTES:	Calad; Camph; Chin; Cina.

Carbo animalis

- ➲ COMMON NAME: Animal charcoal.
- ➲ DURATION: 60 days.
- ➲ RELATION COLD/HEAT: Chilly.
- ➲ MIASM: Pasora, Syphilis, Sycotic.
- ➲ SOURCE: Made from charred ax-hide. contains calc. phos.c(impure). Trituration.
- ➲ SPHERES OF ACTION: Glands, blood vessels Genito-urinary system.,respiratory skin and extremities.
- ➲ SUMMARY OF INDICATIONS: Headaches–circulatory disorders–menstrual disorders.

THERAPEUTIC PICTURE OF DRUG

C_{N-1} ➲ It is suited to old persons greatly debilitated especially when there is venous plethora and blueness of skin.

M_{D-1} ➲ Nostalgia and mournful feeling of isolation, with tears.

M_{D-2} ➲ Weeps during a meal.

M_{D-3} ➲ Fear and apprehension, esp.in the evening.

M_{D-4} ➲ Discouragement and despair.

M_{D-5} ➲ Disposition to be frightened.

M_{D-6} ➲ Fright in the dark.

M_{D-7} ➲ Alternate feeling of gaiety and gloom, or of irascibility and ill-humoured taciturnity.

M_{D-8} ➲ Confusion of ideas and dullness, esp. in the morning.

FGS_1 ➲ Premature catamenia.

FGS_2 ➲ Leucorrhoea burning, smarting, or which imparts a yellow tinge to the linen.

FGS_3 ➲ Serous and fetid lochia.

FGS_4 ➲ Menses are followed by great exhaustion, so weak, can hardly speak How only in morning.

FGS_5 ➲ Uterine hemorrhages where there is much affection of the glands.

FGS_6 ➲ Cancer of uterus, burning pain extending downs the thighs.

FGS_7 ➲ Burning in the vagina and labia.

FGS_8 ➲ Painful nodosities and indurations in the mammae.

FGS_9 ➲ Erysipelatous inflammation of the breasts.

FGS_{10} ➲ Nausea of pregnant females, coming on principally at night; faint and empty sensation in the pit of the stomach is produced by nursing.

PG_1 ➲ Hearing confused., can not tell from which direction a sound comes.

PG_2 ➲ Stitching pains remain in the chest after recovery from pleurisy.

PG_3 ➲ Aversion to open, dry, cold air.

PG_4 ➲ Easily–strained from lifting, even small weight; straining and over lifting easily produce great debility.

PG_5 ➲ Pressive pains in the joints, and the muscles of the limbs.

PG_6 ➲ Spasmodic contraction of several parts.

PG_7 ➲ Torpor of all the members, esp. of the head.

PG_8 ➲ Excessive sensitibility to the open air, and especially to the cold air of winter.

PG_9 ➲ Ebullition of the blood and tendency to become easily overheated.

Modalities

Aggravation

- ➲ Slightest touch.
- ➲ After midnight.

Relations

- ➲ COMPLEMENTARY: Calc-p; Phos.
- ➲ FOLLOWS WELL: Ars; Bell; Bry; Carb-v; Nit-ac; Phos; Puls; Sep; Sil; Sulph; Verat.
- ➲ ANTIDOTES: Camph; Nux-v; Vinum.
- ➲ INIMICALS: Carb-v.

Carbo vegetabilis

- ➲ PROVED BY: Hahnemann.
- ➲ DURATION: 60 Days.
- ➲ COMMON NAME: Vegetable Charcoal.
- ➲ FAMILY/KINGDOM: Minerals.
- ➲ RELATION COLD/HEAT: Hot.
- ➲ MIASM: Anti-psoric.
- ➲ DIATHESIS: Haemorrhagic.
- ➲ TEMPERAMENT: Sanguine.
- ➲ SOURCE: Trituration of Vegetable Charcoal.
- ➲ SPHERES OF ACTION: Nervous System, Vascular System, mucous membrane, Lungs.
- ➲ SUMMARY OF INDICATIONS: Chronic gastric disorders–alcoholism–circulatory disorders–food–poisoning–Flatulence.

THERAPEUTIC PICTURE OF DRUG

C_{N-1} ➲ Persons of advanced age; Prematurely old people

C_{N-2} ➲ Women at turn of life.

C_{N-3} ➲ Cachectic person, young or old.

C_{N-4} ➲ The face is puffy, bluish, pale & Hippocratic with cold sweat.

M_{D-1} ➲ Weakness of memory and slowness of thought.

M_{D-2} ➲ Inquietude and Anxiety esp. in the evening.

M_{D-3} ➲ Aversion to darkness, Fear of ghosts.

DS_1 ➲ Simple food disagrees (weak digestion).

DS_2 ➲ Eructation give temporary Relief.

DS_3 ➲ Sour or rancid eructations.

DS_4 ➲ Contractive cramp, also at night, extending to the chest; abdomen distended; must bend double, worse lying down; pain paroxysmal, takes away the breath

DS_5 ➲ Feels acidity in stomach while lying on the back and when walking; stomach feels very heavy and as if hanging down.

DS_6 ➲ Colic from flatulence, abdomen full to bursting pain worse about bladder, or left of epigastrium; worse from least food; better from passing flatus, or hard stool.

DS_7 ➲ Stools: burning light coloured, fetid, watery, bloody, with tenesmus; covered with filamentous yellow mucus, last part bloody; putrid, cadaverous-smelling, involuntary.

CVS_1 ➲ Blood stagnates in capillaries, cyanosis; cold face and limbs, cold sweat; complete torpor; impending paralysis of heart.

CVS_2 ➲ Palpitation: excessive for days; after eating; when sitting.

CVS_3 ➲ Pulse thread-like; weak and small; intermittent.

CVS_4 ➲ Cheyne-stokes brething in organic heart disease.

CVS_5 ➲ Haemorrhage from any mucus outlet.

CVS_6 ➲ External or internal bleeding with steady oozing.

RS_1 ➲ Rattling cough with itching in the throat. Spasmodic cough with gagging, choking and vomiting of mucus.

RS_2 ➲ Hoarseness, worse in the evenings.

RS_3 ➲ Sudden collapse from any cause. The breath is cold.

FGS_1 ➲ Premature and too copious menses, pale blood.

FGS_2 ➲ Vulva swollen, Aphthae, varices on pudenda.

FGS_3 ➲ Leucorrhoea before menses, thick, greenish, milky excoriating.

FGS_4 ➲ During menstruation, burning in hands and soles.

MGS_1 ➲ Too speedly emission in coition; followed by roaring in the head.

MGS_2 ➲ Extraordinary affluence of voluptuous thoughts.

PG_1 ➲ Desire to be constantly fanned.

PG_2 ➲ Weakness, desire for fresh, cold air. Desire to be constantly fanned.

PG_3 ➲ Limb cold, bluish skin; sweat is cold and clammy.

PG_4 ➲ Internal burning sensation and external coldness.

PG_5 ➲ For a patient who has never fully recovered from the effects of previous chronic illness, this remedy serves as a useful tonic.

PG_6 ➲ Pulsation in different parts of the body.

PG_7 ➲ Pains with anxiety, heat and complete discouragement, or with dejection after the paroxysm.

PG_8 ➲ Haemorrhage from any broken down conditions of mucous membranes.

PG_9 ➲ Bad effects from loss of vital fluid.

Modalities

Aggravation

- In evening, In open air.
- From cold, from hot food.
- Butter, coffee, milk, Alcoholic drink.

Amelioration

- From eructation.
- From fanning from a closed distance.
- By cold Application.

Relations

- COMPLEMENTARY: China; Kali-carb; Drosera.
- FOLLOWS WELL: Acid-phos; Ars; Acon; China.
- ANTIDOTES: Camphor; Ars; Coffee; Lach.
- INIMICALS: Carb-an, Keros.

Carbolicum acidum

- ➲ PROVED BY: Hahnemann.
- ➲ FAMILY/KINGDOM: Chemical .
- ➲ COMMON NAME: Glacial Carbolic Acid [C_6H_5OH] = Phenol.
- ➲ MIASM: Psora and Syphilitic.
- ➲ RELATION COLD/HEAT: Chilly.
- ➲ TEMPERAMENT: Irritable.
- ➲ SOURCE: Salution in rectified spirit .
- ➲ SPHERES OF ACTION: Nervous system, skin, All mucous membranes eg. mouth, throat, G.I.T. and urinary organs.
- ➲ SUMMARY OF INDICATIONS: Headaches–Pain syndromes–constipation.

THERAPEUTIC PICTURE OF DRUG

M_{D-1} ➲ Disinclination for mental exertion.

M_{D-2} ➲ Muddled, confused, bewildered.

H_{D-1} ➲ Dull,heavy frontal headache as if a rubber band were stretched tightly over the forehead,from temple to temple better by pressure.

H_{D-2} ➲ Headache > by green tea; while smoking; by tight band; by cold hand; by bending head forward.

DS_1 ➲ Constipation,with horribly offensive breath.

DS_2 ➲ Vomiting of drunkards.

DS_3 ➲ Excessive nausea, and inclination to vomit; while eating a little, after breakfast.

DS_4 ➲ Vomiting of: Bright's disease; sea-sickness; cancer; Pregnancy.

DS_5 ➲ Weight in epigastrium as if burdened with flatulence.

DS_6 ➲ Wants a drink of water every few minutes.

DS_7 ➲ Constant belching up of wind.

DS_8 ➲ Burning in stomach; total loss of appetite; desire for whiskey.

DS_9 ➲ Diarrhoea and dysentery; mucus stools like scrapings; stools like rice-water; thin, black, very offensive.

DS_{10} ➲ Cholera infantum, with putrid discharge like foul eggs.

FGS_1 ➲ Discharge always offensive.

FGS_2 ➲ Pustules around the vulva containing bloody pus.

FGS_3 ➲ Pain in the left ovary worse walking in open air.

FGS_4 ➲ Cervical erosions, foetid, acrid discharge.

FGS_5 ➲ leucorrhoea, acrid, copious, foetid, green.

FGS_6 ➲ Puerperal fever with offensive discharge

FGS_7 ➲ Irritating leucorrhoea, cousing, and burning.

PG_1 ➲ Agonizing backache across the loins, dragging down the thighs.

PG_2 ➲ Longing for alcohol and tobacco.

PG_3 ➲ Profound protration, collapse, surface pale and bathed in cold sweat.

PG_4 ➲ Exquisite pains come on suddenly, last a short time,disappear suddenly.

Modalities

Aggravation

➲ From cold in general.

Amelioration

➲ With green tea.

➲ While Smoking.

Relations

➲ COMPARE:	Ars; Kreos; (In burns).
➲ ANTIDOTES:	Alco; Chalky; Iod; Vin.

Caulophyllum thalictroides

- ➲ PROVED BY: Burt.
- ➲ FAMILY/KINGDOM: Berberidaceae.
- ➲ COMMON NAME: Blue cohosh.
- ➲ TEMPERAMENT: Nervous.
- ➲ RELATION COLD/HEAT: Hot.
- ➲ DIATHESIS: Rheumatic & Gourty.
- ➲ SOURCE: Tincture of root.
- ➲ SPHERES OF ACTION: Uterus, cervix, joint esp. small joints and stomach.
- ➲ SUMMARY OF INDICATIONS: Used to ensure smooth, painless child birth–rheumatoid arthritis (of women).

THERAPEUTIC PICTURE OF DRUG

C_{N-1} ➲ It is generally suited to women during pregnancy, parturition and lactation, having moth spots on the face and forehead and drooping of eyelids.

M_{D-1} ➲ Fretful, Irritable, apprehensive

FGS_1 ➲ Spasmodic rigid os, delays labor, need like pricking pain in cervix.

FGS_2 ➲ Chorea, hysteria or epilepsy at puberty, during establishment of menstrual function.

FGS_3 ➲ Sensation as if uterus was congested, with fullness and tension in hypogastric region.

FGS_4 ➲ Amenorrhoea; spasms, cramps, or great atony.

FGS_5 ➲ Painful menstruation, the flow being normal in quality.

FGS_6 ➲ Spasmodic dysmenorrhoea; spasmodic, intermittent pains in bladder, stomach, broad ligaments (grains), even chest and limbs; congestion and irritability of uterus; scanty flow.

FGS_7 ➲ Menstrual colic; uterus retroverted.

FGS_8 ➲ Irritable vagina, spasmodic, intense pains.

FGS_9 ➲ Aphthous vaginitis and spasmodic pains in the uterus.

FGS_{10} ➲ Leucorrhoea: profuse mucous; "moth spots" on the forehead; often in little girls.

FGS_{11} ➲ Threatening abortion, spasmodic bearing down pains; vascular excitement; tremulous weakness; pains severe in back and loins, but uterine contractions feeble; slight flow.

FGS_{12} ➲ Labor-pains short, irregular, spasmodic; patient very weak; no progress being made.

FGS_{13} ➲ Pains become weak, flagging from long protracted labor, causing exhaustion; thirsty, feverish.

FGS_{14} ➲ Passive haemorrhage after abortion or confinement.

FGS_{15} ➲ Protracted lochia, oozes passively from the relaxed uterine vessels, great atony.

FGS_{16} ➲ After-pains, especially after exhausting, lengthy labor; spasmodic, across the lower abdomen; extend into groins.

LS_{1} ➲ Rheumatism of women, especially of the small joints; erratic pains, changing place every few minutes; painful stiffness of the affected joints.

PG_{1} ➲ Pains are intermittent, paroxysmal, spasmodic.

Modalities

Aggravation

- ➲ In open air.
- ➲ By coffee.
- ➲ During menses.

Amelioration

- ➲ Lying on left side.
- ➲ By emission of flatus.
- ➲ Prom pressure.

Relations

➲ COMPARE:	Ambr; Ign; Mosch; Zine.
➲ ANTIDOTES:	Colch.
➲ SIMILAR:	Cimic; Bell; Puls; Sec; Vib.

Causticum

- ➲ PROVED BY: Hahnemann.
- ➲ COMMON NAME: Potassum Hydrate, [Sine kali].
- ➲ RELATION COLD/HEAT: Chilly.
- ➲ SOURCE: Obtainde by distillinbg a mixure of slaked lime and a solution of potassium.
- ➲ SPHERES OF ACTION: Mucous menbrane,nerve (Medulla oblongata and vagus), larynx, trachea, urinary bladder and flexor tendon and skin.
- ➲ SUMMARY OF INDICATIONS: Mental depression- constipation- burns and scalds–warts–Paralysis.

THERAPEUTIC PICTURE OF DRUG

C_{N-1} ➲ Person of hydrogenoid constitution.

C_{N-2} ➲ Children with dark hair and eyes, delicate, sensitive.

C_{N-3} ➲ Adapted to persons with dark hair and rigid fiber.

C_{N-4} ➲ Weakly. psoric, with excessively yellow, sallow complexion.

C_{N-5} ➲ Subject to affections of respiratory and urinary tracts.

M_{D-1} ➲ Intense sympathy for sufferings of others.

M_{D-2} ➲ Mirthfulness some times. and soon after, ill- humour.

M_{D-3} ➲ Melancholy and vexatious thoughts, day and night, with tears.

M_{D-4} ➲ Weakness of memory.

M_{D-5} ➲ Sad, hopeless;

M_{D-6} ➲ Disorders from long lasting grief and sorrow, from loss of sleep, night watching, from sudden emotions,fear, frights; joy, from anger.

NS_1 ➲ Hemiplegia after cerebral hemorrhage or softening.

NS_2 ➲ Epileptic attacks during time of puberty, also worse during new moon.

NS_3 ➲ Weakness and trembling; Faint-like sinking of strength.

NS_4 ➲ Convulsions: with screams, gnashing of the teeth, and violent movements of the limbs; with feverish heat and coldness of hand and feet.

NS_5 ➲ Chorea even at night, right side of face and tongue may be paralysed.

NS_6 ➲ Paralysis: of specific region; vocal cords, tongue, eyelids, face, extremities, bladder.

NS_7 ➲ Disturbed functional activity of brain and spinal cord, from exhausting diseases or severe mental shock resulting in paralysis.

DS_1 ➲ Chronic constipation; frequent and ineffectual efforts to evacuate, with pains, anxiety and redness of the face.

DS_2 ➲ The faeces are passed more easily, in an erect posture.

DS_3 ➲ Faeces knotty, or of a very small size, hard, tough, covered with mucus; viscid and shining, as if with fat or a bright and whitish colour.

DS_4 ➲ In the anus, appearance of haemorrhoidal tumors, which are hard, swollen, painful and which impede evacuation.

DS_5 ➲ Walking and meditation aggravate the harmorrhoidal pains, so as to render them insupportable.

DS_6 ➲ Varices of the rectum, hindering stool, large; painful; stinging; burning when touched.

DS_7 ➲ Pressure in the haemorrhoidal tumors of the rectum, so as to cause them to Protrude.

RS_1 ➲ Rawness and tickling in the throat, with dry cough and some expectoration only after long coughing.

RS_2 ➲ Hoarseness: worse morning and evening, with scraping in the throat; for several days, could not speak loud.

RS_3 ➲ Croup, especially when there is a raw sensation in the larynx..

RS_4 ➲ Cough: violent, hollow, at times dry with pain in right chest; hollow, especially night and morning, with tightly adhering mucus in the chest, and with sensation of soreness on the chest.

RS_5 ➲ Cough worse evening till midnight; from exhaling; drinking coffee; cold air; draught of air.

RS_6 ➲ Soreness in the chest; burning soreness in a stripe down under the sternum, with cough etc.

RS_7 ➲ Tightness of chest, must frequently take a deep breath.

FGS_1 ➲ Menses; too early; too feeble; only during the day; cease on lying down.

FGS_2 ➲ Catamenia retarded, but more copious, with flow of blood in large clots.

FGS_3 ➲ Excoriation between.the legs, at the vulva.

FGS_4 ➲ Profuse leucorrhoea, having the smell of the catamenia or, which flows in the night.

FGS_5 ➲ Leucorrhoea flows at night and not during the day.

FGS_6 ➲ Before the catamenia, melancholy, sacral pains and colic.

FGS_7 ➲ During the catamenia, pain in the loins, cuttings, and paleness in the face; Yellowness of the face; Vertigo.

FGS_8 ➲ Nipples excoriated, cracked,. and surrounded with tetters.

US_1 ➲ Urine: involuntary; Passage when coughing. sneezing or blowing the nose

US_2 ➲ Expelled very slowly, and sometimes retained.

US_3 ➲ Involuntary during first sleep at night (nocturnal enuresis); also from the slightest excitement.

US_4 ➲ Loss of sensibility on passing urine.

S_{N-1} ➲ Cicatrices, especially burns, scalds, freshen up, become sore again.

S_{N-2} ➲ Eruption of pimples on the tip of the nose.

S_{N-3} ➲ Injuries of the skin which had healed, become sore again.

S_{N-4} ➲ Itching: over the whole body; at various parts, especially on tip and wings of the nose; face; scrotum; back; arms; palm; dorsum of feet.

PG_1 ➲ Soreness, of scalp, throat, respiratory tract, rectum, rectum anus,Urethra. vagina, uterus,

PG_2 ➲ Contraction of the tendons, and stiffness in the flexor muscles of the limbs.

PG_3 ➲ Cramp-like contraction of several limbs.

PG_3 ➲ Jerkings and convulsive movements.

PG_4 ➲ In the evening, great dejection and oppression of the whole body.

PG_5 ➲ Paralytic weakness, with trembling and tottering of the limbs.

PG_6 ➲ Paralytic (one sided).

PG_7 ➲ Great sensibility to currents of air, and to cold.

PG_8 ➲ Aggravation of the symptoms, generally in the evening, or in the open air.

Modalities

Aggravation

- ➲ In clear, fine weather.
- ➲ Coming from the open into a warm room.
- ➲ Cold air, especially a draft of cold air.

Amelioration

- ➲ In damp, wet weather.
- ➲ Warm air.

Relations

➲ COMPLEMENTARY:	Coloc; Petros.
➲ FOLLOWS WELL:	Ant-t; Calc; Guai; Kali-I; lyc.; Nux- v; Puls; Sep; Sil; Stann; Sulph.
➲ ANTIDOTES:	Asaf; Coff; Coloc; Ntl-s-d; Nux-v.
➲ INIMICALS:	Coff; Ph-ac.

Chamomilla

- ➲ PROVED BY: Hahnemann.
- ➲ DURATION: 20-30 days.
- ➲ COMMON NAME: Matricaria Chamomilla.
- ➲ FAMILY/KINGDOM: Compsitae.
- ➲ RELATION COLD/HEAT: "<"from heat and open air relief from warm weather.
- ➲ MIASM: Psora.
- ➲ TEMPERAMENT: Nervous, Irritable.
- ➲ SOURCE: Tincture of whole fresh plant.
- ➲ SPHERES OF ACTION: Brain, mind, Intestine.
- ➲ SUMMARY OF INDICATIONS: Childhood disorders with severe irritability-acute pain syndromes.

THERAPEUTIC PICTURE OF DRUG

Note: A remedy especially indicated for children: useful during the period of dentition.

C_{N-1} ➲ Person especially children, with light brown hair, nervous.

C_{N-2} ➲ Exitable temperament.

C_{N-3} ➲ One cheek. red hot, and other pale & cold.

M_{D-1} ➲ Peevishness, ill-humour, absence of mind, taciturnity and repugnance to conversation.

M_{D-2} ➲ Desire for different things, which, when once possessed, are no longer cared for.

M_{D-3} ➲ Tendency to misapply words when speaking or writing.

M_{D-4} ➲ Disposition to weep, and to be angry, with great sensitiveness to offence.

M_{D-5} ➲ The child cries and wants to be carried on the arm.

M_{D-6} ➲ Quarrelsome and choleric humour.

M_{D-7} ➲ Mischievous disposition in children.

M_{D-8} ➲ Mental excitement with strong tendency to be frightened.

M_{D-9} ➲ Patients neither endure to be addressed by others, nor to be interrupted when conversing.

M_{D-10} ➲ Piteous moaning of child because he can not have what he wants; whining restlessness.

DS_1 ➲ Toothache: stiching;digging; gnawing; as from taking cold; during or after eating; if anything warm is taken into the mouth, especially after coffee; in open air; in the room; getting warm in bed; during menstruation; most left side and lower teeth; worse at night.

DS_2 ➲ Pain in the belly from side to side, just above the novel, corresponding to the transverse colon, commencing in the right and going over to left.

DS_3 ➲ Diarrhoea: during dentition(green mucus); in child bed, from downward motion.

DS_4 ➲ Diarrhoea: from cold, from anger, from chagrin.

DS_5 ➲ Diarrhoea: chiefly at night, with spasmodic colic.

DS_6 ➲ Stools: watery frequent, preceded by cutting, constricting belly ache, worse in epigastric region; mucus with colic and vomituritia.

DS_7 ➲ Stools: bilious, with burning in anus; painful, thin, green, consisting of feces and mucus.

DS_8 ➲ Stools: green, watery, corroding, with colic, thirst, bitter taste and bitter eructations; like chopped eggs, smelling sour; hot, smelling like rotten eggs.

FGS_1 ➲ Uterine haemorrhage. profuse discharge of clotted, dark blood with labour like pain.

FGS_2 ➲ Labour pain spasmodic, press upwards.

FGS_3 ➲ Puerperal fever Erysipelas of the mammae and soreness of the nipple.

FGS_4 ➲ Patient intolerant of pain.

FGS_5 ➲ Nipple inflamed, tender to touch.

FGS_6 ➲ Infants breasts tender.

FGS_7 ➲ Yellow acrid leucorrhoea.

FGS_8 ➲ Burning and smarting pain in vagina.

FGS_9 ➲ Milk Runs out in nurshing women.

LS_1 ➲ Violent drawing, tearing pains, from the left ischium to the or calcis and sole of the foot, with cramp-like tension of the muscles.

LS_2 ➲ Tearing pain in the feet after a severe chill; must lie down and keep quiet; pain in ankle, worse from every motion.

LS_3 ➲ Burning of the soles at night; puts the feet out of bed.

LS_4 ➲ Cracking in the joints, especially of lower limbs, with pains there in, as if bruised.

PG_1 ➲ Rheumatic, drawing pains, chiefly at night in bed, with paralytic state, and sensation of torpor in the part affected and inclination to move them continually; mitigated by external heat.

PG_2 ➲ Convulsions of children from nursing, after a fit of anger in mother.

PG_3 ➲ Children new born and during period of detition.

PG_4 ➲ Pain with thirst, heat, and redness (of one) of the cheeks, and hot sweating of the head.

PG_5 ➲ Over-excitement, and excessive sensibility of the nervous system, with great sensibility to pain, which appears insupportable and induce despair.

PG_6 ➲ Over-sensitiveness of the senses (esp. from coffee and narcotics).

PG_7 ➲ Great sensibility in open air, and principally to wind.

PG_8 ➲ Great weakness and inclination to fall, with prostration of strength to fainting as soon as the pain commences.

Modalities

Aggravation

- ➲ By heat, anger.
- ➲ Open air.
- ➲ In wind, eructation.

Amelioration

- ➲ From being carried.
- ➲ Fasting, warm wet weather.

Relations

➲ COMPARE:	Acon; Coff; Puls; Staph; Igna.
➲ COMPLEMENTARY:	Bell, Mag–c.
➲ FOLLOWS WELL:	Bell; Opium; Sil; Sulph; Nux-v.
➲ ANTIDOTES:	Camph, Nux, Puls.
➲ INIMICALS:	Zinc.

Chelidonium majus

- COMMON NAME: Celandineq.
- DURATION: 7-14 days.
- RELATION COLD/HEAT: Cold.
- FAMILY/KINGDOM: Papaveraceae.
- SOURCE: Tincture of entire fresh plant, at time of flowering.
- MIASM: Psora, syphilis andsycosis.
- TEMPERAMENT: Irritable.
- SPHERES OF ACTION: Hepato–biliary system–liver,gallbladder, bile duct etc.skin and stomach. mind, brain, mucous membrane, spleen & kidney.
- SUMMARY OF INDICATIONS: Trigeminal neuralgia–muscle sprains-Hepatic disorders.

THERAPEUTIC PICTURE OF DRUG

C_{N-1} ➲ It is adapted to persons of light complexion, blond, thin and irritable, gastric and abdominal complaints at any stage, sex and temperament.

M_{D-1} ➲ Remarkable tranquillity of mind for two or three days.

M_{D-2} ➲ Followed after a while by ill–humour.

M_{D-3} ➲ Low spirited, desponding with inclination to weep.

SO_1 ➲ Dazzling spot before the eyes, lachrymation when looking at it.

SO_2 ➲ Neuralgia of eyebrows and temples.

SO_3 ➲ Pressing pain over left eye, which seems to press down upper lid.

SO_4 ➲ Tearing pain in left eye, extending to zygoma, teeth, forehead and temple; first relieved by pressure, but soon cannot endure the slightest touch; periodic, evening in bed.

DS_1 ➲ Desire for–vary hot drinks, unless almost boiling, stomach will not retain them.

DS_2 ➲ Pain from region of liver, shooting toward the back.

DS_3 ➲ Hepatic diseases; jaundice, pain in right shoulder.

DS_4 ➲ Diarrhoea and constipation alternately.

DS_5 ➲ Stools: thin, pasty, bright yellow; pasty, light grey; pale,slimy; mucous diarrhoea, at night, constipated, like sheep's dung.

RS_1 ➲ Deep-seated pain in wholer right side of chest; Pnemonia of right lung, liver complications.

RS_2 ➲ Cough in paroxysms; throws up lumps of mucus.

RS_3 ➲ Cough after waking and on rising with sensation of dust under sternum.

RS_4 ➲ Paroxysms of cough with copious expectoration; with pain behind sternum esp. at night.

RS_5 ➲ Paroxysms of dry cough 4 P.M.

FGS_1 ➲ Menses too late and too profuse, lasting too long.

FGS_2 ➲ Pain in Right ovary.

FGS_3 ➲ Milk diminished.

B_{k-1} ➲ Constant pain, under the lower and inner angle of Right scapula.

S_{N-1} ➲ Yellow–gray colour of the skin wilted skin, of the palm of hand

S_{N-2} ➲ Red painful pimples and pustules on various parts eg. Neck, Chest and arms.

S_{N-3} ➲ Old putrid, spreading ulcer.

S_{N-4} ➲ Itching; burning like nettles, preceding eruption like measles.

Modalities

Aggravation

- ➲ Right side, Motion.
- ➲ Touch, change of weather.
- ➲ Very early in morning.

Amelioration

- ➲ After dinner.
- ➲ From Pressure.

Relations

- ➲ COMPARE: Lyco; Nux; Opium; Sulph.
- ➲ COMPLEMENTARY: Lyco; Bry.
- ➲ FOLLOWS WELL: Ars; Bry; Ipec; Nux.
- ➲ ANTIDOTES: Cham; Coff.

Cina maritima

- PROVED BY: Hahnemann.
- DURATION: 14–20 days.
- COMMON NAME: Wormseed.
- FAMILY/KINGDOM: Compositae.
- RELATION COLD/HEAT: May be any.
- MIASM: Latent psora.
- TEMPERAMENT: Irritable.
- SOURCE: Tincture of Wormseed.
- SPHERES OF ACTION: Mind, gastro–intestinal tract urinary bladder & nerves.

THERAPEUTIC PICTURE OF DRUG

C_{N-1} ➲ Especially suited to persons or children with dark Hair & complexion, pale, sickly body, whitish or bluish appearance around mouth, with dark ring around the eyes, one cheek red and other pale.

M_{D-1} ➲ Highly irritable, peevish, very cross and ill-humoured.

M_{D-2} ➲ Does not want to touch or looked at, can not bear anyone to come near him.

M_{D-3} ➲ Continual inquietude, with desire for things of all kinds, which are rejected some moment after.

M_{D-4} ➲ Disposition to be offended by trifling jests.

M_{D-5} ➲ Great anguish and anxiety on walking in the open air.

M_{D-6} ➲ Pitiful weeping when awake.

SO_1 ➲ Nose: violent sneezing, with stitches in the temples.

SO_2 ➲ Bleeding of the nose; stoppage of the nose, in the evening.

SO_3 ➲ Itching of the nose, boring in the nose, with the finger.

SO_3 ➲ Child rubs the nose on the pillow, on the shoulders of the nurse, or with the hands.

DS_1 ➲ Child, grinds the teeth at night.

DS_2 ➲ Children, suffering from worms.

DS_3 ➲ Constant pressure in the stomach at night, causing restlessness.

DS_4 ➲ Gnawing sensation in the stomach, as from hunger.

RS_1 ➲ Hoarse gagging cough, in the evening.

RS_2 ➲ Rattling cough in spells.

RS_3 ➲ Gagging cough, morning after rising; irritation renewed by inspiration.

RS_4 ➲ Violent periodically recurring paroxysms of whooping cough, excited by sensation as if down were in the throat, or by adherent mucus in larynx; after cough, gurgling sound.

FGS_1 ➲ Uterine haemorrhage before puberty.

FGS_1 ➲ Metrorrhagia-womb-trouble in general.

FGS_1 ➲ Catamenia premature, and too abundant

US_1 ➲ Urine soon becomes turbid.

US_2 ➲ Involuntary emission of urine at (night); urine milky.

US_3 ➲ Frequent want to make water, with profuse discharge and wetting the bed.

PG_1 ➲ Twisting pain about navel. white and bluish about the mouth choreic movements.

Modalities

Aggravation

- ➲ After taking sweets.
- ➲ Over eating.
- ➲ After anger.

Amelioration

- ➲ By lying on abdomen.

Relations

➲ COMPARE:	Ant-c; Ant-t; Bry; Cham; Sil; Kre; Staph-in irritability.
➲ FOLLOWS WELL:	Calc; Chin; Nux; Atann.
➲ ANTIDOTES:	Arn; Camph; Chin; Caps.

Cinchona officinalis (China)

- ➲ PROVED BY: Hahnemann.
- ➲ DURATION: 14–21 days.
- ➲ COMMON NAME: Peruvian bark–china.
- ➲ FAMILY/KINGDOM: Rubiaceae.
- ➲ RELATION COLD/HEAT: Chilly.
- ➲ MIASM: Psora.
- ➲ DIATHESIS: Haemorrhagic.
- ➲ TEMPERAMENT: Nervous.
- ➲ SOURCE: Tincture of the dried bark.
- ➲ SPHERES OF ACTION: Brain, Mind, Nervous System, Blood, liver, Spleen, G.I.T.
- ➲ SUMMARY OF INDICATIONS: Fevers, Headache, Excessive fluid loss-gastrointestinal disorders.

THERAPEUTIC PICTURE OF DRUG

C_{N-1} ➲ Pumped out Constitution (According to Dr. P.C.Paul.)

C_{N-2} ➲ Broken down from exhausting discharge & loss of vital fluid.

C_{N-3} ➲ For stout, Swarthy person, for system, once robust, which have become debilitated.

C_{N-4} ➲ Face Hippocratic, pale; eyes sunken and surrounded by blue margins; Pale, sickly expression as after excesses.

M_{D-1} ➲ Disposition to hurt other people's feelings.

M_{D-2} ➲ Cries suddenly and tossing about.

M_{D-3} ➲ Apathetic, indifferent, disobedient, taciturn, despondent.

M_{D-4} ➲ Ideas crowd in mind; prevent sleep.

H_{D-1} ➲ Headache–haemorrhage or sexual excesses.

H_{D-2} ➲ Heaviness of the head, fainting, loss of sight, ringing in ears; cold surface after haemorrhage.

H_{D-3} ➲ Intense throbbing headache; carotids throb. After loss of blood.

H_{D-4} ➲ Sensation as if head would burst, with sleeplessness; worse from motion or any jar; better in room and when opening the eyes.

H_{D-5} ➲ Headaches, worse from draught of air, in the open air, slightest touch; better from hard pressure.

H_{D-6} ➲ Headache from occiput over whole head from morning until afternoon; worse lying, must stant or walk; drives to madness.

H_{D-7} ➲ Burning in forehead, with hot sweat on it.

DS_1 ➲ Cold feeling in stomach; constant satiated feeling, yet can eat, but feels worse afterwards.

DS_2 ➲ Fullness in stomach and bowels; flatulence; belching does not relieve.

DS_3 ➲ Haematemesis, great loss of blood, weak, pale, cold hands and feet; stomach very sensitive to touch.

DS_4 ➲ Gastralgia after depletion; acidity; bloating after food or drink; satiety; relieved by motion.

DS_5 ➲ Colic better bending double and colic worse at night and after eating.

DS_6 ➲ Colic at a certain hour each afternoon; "3 months colic."

DS_7 ➲ Tympanitic abdomen, pressure as from a hard body; or, spasmodic constrictive pains from incarcerated flatulence; worse at night or after deplection; also in typhus, worse mornings.

FGS_1 ➲ Menses too early, dark clots and abdominal distention

FGS_2 ➲ Profuse menses with pain.

FGS_3 ➲ Bloody leucorrhoea.

FGS_4 ➲ Seems to take the place of the usual menstrual discharge.

FGS_5 ➲ Painful heaving in pelvis.

F_{R-1} ➲ Intermittent paroxysms return every week.

F_{R-2} ➲ All stages well marked.

F_{R-3} ➲ Chills, generally in the forenoon, commencing in the breast; thirst before chill, little and ofen.

F_{R-4} ➲ Debilitating night sweats.

F_{R-5} ➲ Free perspiration caused by every little exertion, especially on single parts.

F_{R-6} ➲ Hay fever, watery coryza, pain in the temples.

PG_1 ➲ Ailments–from loss of vital fluids, especially haemorrhages, excessive location, diarrhoea, suppuration.

PG_2 ➲ Extreme Sensitive to touch but hard pressure relieves.

PG_3 ➲ Tensive pullings, or starting and shooting tearings, esp. in the large bones of the limbs, with paralytic pains, and weakness of the parts affected.

PG_4 ➲ Pains and sufferings provoked or aggravated by touch, at night, or after a meal.

PG_5 ➲ Sensitive of torpor in different parts.

PG_6 ➲ Dropsical swelling of some parts, or of the whole body.

PG_7 ➲ Over-excitability of the whole nervous system.

PG_8 ➲ Heaviness of the whole body.

PG_9 ➲ There may be bleeding from every internal part of the body; coldness and passive haemorrhage.

Modalities

Aggravation

- ➲ From slightest touch.
- ➲ Draft of air.
- ➲ Mental emotion.
- ➲ Loss of vital fluid.

Amelioration

- ➲ Hard pressure
- ➲ Bending double

Relations

➲ COMPARE:	Chinin-s; Lyco; Carbo-v.
➲ COMPLEMENTARY:	Ferrum; Calc-phos.
➲ FOLLOWS WELL:	Calc-p in hydrocephaloid.
	Ars; Arnica; Bell; Sulph; Acid-phos.
➲ ANTIDOTES:	Apis; Lyco; Merc; Nux.
➲ INIMICALS:	After Dig and Selen.

Cinnamonum

- COMMON NAME: Cinnaman.
- FAMILY/KINGDOM: Lauraceae.

THERAPEUTIC PICTURE OF DRUG

M_{D-1} ➲ Sleepy, no desire for anything.

FGS_1 ➲ Menses early, profuse, prolonged, bright red.

FGS_2 ➲ Repeated small haemorrhages during gestation and puerperal state.

FGS_3 ➲ Menorrhagia-in females troubled with itching at nose, blood bright red < After false step or strain.

FGS_4 ➲ Uterine haemorrhages caused by overlifting, during puerperal state.

PG_1 ➲ Fingers seem swollen.

PG_2 ➲ Leading feature of cinnamon is Haemorrhage postpartum haemorrhage.

PG_3 ➲ Talking = Hysterical attacks.

Modalities

Aggravation

- By any physical exertion.
- False step or strain.
- While riding

Relations

- COMPARE: Sil; Ipec; Thrill.
- ANTIDOTES: Opium.

Cocculus indicus

- ➲ PROVED BY: Hahnemann.
- ➲ DURATION: 30 days.
- ➲ COMMON NAME: Indian Cockle.
- ➲ FAMILY/KINGDOM: Menispermaceae.
- ➲ RELATION COLD/HEAT: Agg. from sun.
- ➲ MIASM: Psora.
- ➲ TEMPERAMENT: Nervous.
- ➲ SOURCE: A tincture is prepared from the powdered seeds, which contain a crystallisable principle picrotoxine, a powerful poison.
- ➲ SPHERES OF ACTION: Cerebro-spinal system, voluntary muscular system and sensorium.
- ➲ SUMMARY OF INDICATIONS: Travel sickness–Migraine–Occipital headaches–Meniere's disease.

THERAPEUTIC PICTURE OF DRUG

C_{N-1} ➲ Especially suited for women and children with light hair and eyes, who suffer severely during menstruation and pregnancy, unmarried,and childless woman.

C_{N-2} ➲ Adopted to book worms, sensitive romantic girls with irregular menstruation, onanist & persons debilitated by sexual excesses.

M_{D-1} ➲ Capricious;heavy and stupid.

M_{D-2} ➲ Time passes too quickly; absorbed in reveries.

M_{D-3} ➲ Inclination to sing irresistible, slow in comprehension.

M_{D-4} ➲ Mind benumbed; profound sadness; can not bear contradiction,.

M_{D-5} ➲ Very anxious about the health of others.

H_{D-1} ➲ Confusion of the head, esp. after eating or drinking.

H_{D-2} ➲ Vertigo, as from intoxication, or on rising up in the bed, with inclination to vomit, which forces the patient to lie down again.

H_{D-3} ➲ Headache as if the eyes were being torn out.

H_{D-4} ➲ Pressing headache from without inwards; or as if compressed by a bandage; or as if screwed together.

H_{D-5} ➲ Pressing pain in forehead, from without inwards with nausea; aggravated by riding in a wagon; from eating; drinking and sleeping; from thinking; ameliorated during rest, in-doors.

H_{D-6} ➲ Headache in occiput and nape, sensation of opening and shutting like a door; even in spotted fever.

H_{D-7} ➲ Convulsive trembling of the head from weakness of the muscles of the neck.

FGS_1 ➲ Dysmenorrhoea, with profuse dark menses.

FGS_2 ➲ Menses too early, clotted, with spasmodic colic.

FGS_3 ➲ Painful pressing in the uterine region, followed by haemorrhoids.

FGS_4 ➲ Purulent, gushing leucorrhoea between menses; very weakening can scarcely speak.

FGS_5 ➲ So weak during menstruation, she is scarcely able to stand.

FGS_6 ➲ Premature catamenia, with cramps in the abdomen.

FGS_7 ➲ Suppression of catamenia, with spasmodic and pressive colic, flatulency, paralytic. debility, oppression, anxiety, cramps in the chest, fits of nausea, even to fainting, and convulsive movements of the limbs.

PG_1 ➲ Ill effects: from loss of sleep, mental excitement and night watching feels weak when even one hour's sleep is lost.

PG_2 ➲ Nausea or vomiting from riding in an automobile, boat or railroad car or even looking at a boat in motion; sea–sickness, car-sickness or travel sickness.

PG_3 ➲ Difficultly of speech, as from paralysis of the tongue.

PG_4 ➲ Pullings and paralytic tearings, by fits, or continuous, in the limbs and in the bones.

PG_5 ➲ Convulsive movements of the muscles in different parts.

PG_6 ➲ Weakness and loss of strength, after the least bodily fatigue, movement, or the intruption of sleep.

PG_7 ➲ The open air is insupportable, whether it be warm or cold.

Modalities

Aggravation

➲ Eating, drinking.

➲ loss of sleep.

➲ Smoking.

➲ Talking.

➲ Carriage riding.

- Motion or tossing of ship or Vehicle.
- Rising up during the pregnant state.

Relations

- COMPARE: Ign; Nux-v.
- FOLLOWS WIELL: Ars; Bell; Hep; Ign; lyc; Nux;-v; Puls; Rhul-t; Sulph.
- ANTIDOTES: Camph; Nux-v Cham; Cup-met; Ign-am.
- INIMICALS: Coff.

Coffea cruda

- ➲ PROVED BY: Hahnemann.
- ➲ DURATION: 1-7 days.
- ➲ COMMON NAME: Coffee.
- ➲ FAMILY/KINGDOM: Rubiaceae.
- ➲ RELATION COLD/HEAT: Chilly.
- ➲ MIASM: Psora.
- ➲ TEMPERAMENT: Sanguine choleric.
- ➲ SOURCE: Tincture of Raw berries.
- ➲ SPHERES OF ACTION: Cerebrospinal nervous system.
- ➲ SUMMARY OF INDICATIONS: Insomnia–anxiety–headaches.

THERAPEUTIC PICTURE OF DRUG

C_{N-1} ➲ It is suited to tall, lean, stooping persons, with dark complexion.
C_{N-2} ➲ Sanguine Choleric temperament.
M_{D-1} ➲ Unusual activity of mind & body.
M_{D-2} ➲ Over-sensitiveness; weeping mood.
M_{D-3} ➲ Sentimental ecstasy; excited imagination; increased power to think.
M_{D-4} ➲ Fright from sudden pleasant surprises.
M_{D-5} ➲ Great anguish; cannot be composed; is not able to hold the pen; trembles.
M_{D-6} ➲ Excessive weeping and lamentations over trifles.
M_{D-7} ➲ The pains seem insupportable, driving to despair.
H_{D-1} ➲ Headache; from over-mental exertion.
H_{D-2} ➲ Seems as if the brain was torn to pieces, as if a nail was driven in the head.
H_{D-3} ➲ Tight pain, worse from noise, smell, narcotics.
H_{D-4} ➲ Headache; worse in open air and sensitive hearing.
DS_1 ➲ Toothache–Intermittent, jerking, relieved by holding Ice- water in the mouth.
FGS_1 ➲ Menses too early and holding lasting.

FGS_2 ➲ Dysmenorrhoea, large clots of black blood.

FGS_3 ➲ Hypersensitive Vulva and vagina voluptuous itching.

MGS_1 ➲ Great excitement of sexual desire.

MGS_2 ➲ Flaccidity or strong irritation of the genital parts.

MGS_3 ➲ Without emission of semen, and with dry heat of the body.

PG_1 ➲ Painful sensitiveness of the parts affected.

PG_2 ➲ Great flexibility of the muscles, and activity of the whole body.

PG_3 ➲ Mental and physical excitability.

PG_4 ➲ Sleeplessness (Insomnia), from over-excitability of mind and body (sleeplessness of lying in women).

PG_5 ➲ Sleeplessness from excitement of imagination, flow of idias, and fantastic visions.

PG_6 ➲ Inclination to lie down and to shut the eyes, without being able to sleep.

PG_7 ➲ Aversion to the open air with uneasiness and aggravation of the symptoms during a walk in the open air.

Modalities

Aggravation

➲ Sudden mental emotion.

➲ Excessive, joy, cold.

➲ Open air, narcotic medicines.

Amelioration

➲ Warmth, from lying down.

➲ Holding Ice in mouth.

Relations

➲ COMPARE: Acon; Cham; Ign; Sulph.

➲ COMPLEMENTARY: Acon.

➲ FOLLOWS WIELL: Ac-flour; Acon; Aur; Bell; Lyco; Nux.

➲ ANTIDOTES: China; Merc; Puls.

➲ INIMICALS: Canth; Caust; Cocc; Ign.

Colchicum autumnale

- PROVED BY: STAPF.
- DURATION: 14–20 days.
- COMMON NAME: Meadow saffron.
- FAMILY/KINGDOM: Liliaceae.
- RELATION COLD/HEAT: Chilly.
- MIASM: Psora.
- DIATHESIS: Rheumatic and Gouty.
- TEMPERAMENT: Irritable and Melancholic.
- SOURCE: Tincture of the bulb dug in spring.
- SPHERES OF ACTION: Digestive tract, heart, pericardium, kidneys, joints.
- SUMMARY OF INDICATIONS: Rheumatic disorders- abdominal distention–nephritis.

THERAPEUTIC PICTURE OF DRUG

C_{N-1} ➲ Leucophlegmatic constitution.

C_{N-2} ➲ Adapted to the rheumatic, gouty diathesis.

C_{N-3} ➲ Persons of robust vigorous constitution.

C_{N-4} ➲ Diseases of old people.

M_{D-1} ➲ Great dejection.

M_{D-2} ➲ Ill–humour.

M_{D-3} ➲ Peevish; dissatisfied with everything.

M_{D-4} ➲ The sufferings appear insupportable.

M_{D-5} ➲ The least external impression, (bright light, strong smells bad manners) drives him to distraction.

M_{D-6} ➲ Weakness of memory.

M_{D-7} ➲ Great desire for rest and disinclination to every mental exertion; obscence of mind.

M_{D-8} ➲ Forget fullness and distraction.

DS_1 ➲ Smell painfully acute; nausea and faintness from the odour of cooking food, especially of fish, eggs or fatty meat.

DS_2 ➲ Abdomen is distended with gas, feeling as if it would burst, Burning or icy coldness in stomach and abdomen.

DS_3 ➲ Pressing, tearing, cutting or stitching pains in abdomen.

DS_4 ➲ Colic: aggravated by eating; after flatulent food; with great distention of belly; until diarrhoea sets in; better from bending double.

DS_5 ➲ Evacuations slow, difficult, scanty, with urging, even of the soft stool, with pain in the small of the back.

DS_6 ➲ Involuntary evacuation of faeces.

DS_7 ➲ Watery discharges, going off without sensation.

DS_8 ➲ Diarrhoea consisting of mucus like rice-water.

DS_9 ➲ Dysenteric diarrhoea, of white, transparent, gelatinous mucus.

DS_{10} ➲ Ineffectual pressing to stool; he feels the faeces in the rectum, but cannot expel them.

DS_{11} ➲ Discharge of much mucus from the rectum.

DS_{12} ➲ During stool sensation as if the sphincter ani were torn to pieces.

FGS_1 ➲ Pruritus of genitals.

FGS_2 ➲ Sensation of swelling in the vulva and clitoris.

FGS_3 ➲ Cold sensation in the thighs after menses.

US_1 ➲ Nephritis: oedema and ascites.

US_2 ➲ Scanty discharge of urine of a deep colour, with tenesmus, and a burning sensation.

US_3 ➲ Painful and scanty emission of urine of a bright red colour.

US_4 ➲ Urine; bloody; almost like ink; containing albumen.

US_5 ➲ Urine scanty, looking like bits of decomposed blood, with offensive smell.

PG_1 ➲ Affected parts very sensitive to contact and motion.

PG_2 ➲ Arthritic pain in joints, patient screams with pain on touching a joint or stubbing a toa.

PG_3 ➲ Tingling in many parts of the body, as if frost-bitten, when the weather changes.

PG_4 ➲ The sufferings are singularly aggravated by intellectual fatigue, by touch, by too brilliant a light, and by the smell of pork.

PG_5 ➲ Nervous fatigue and weakness from nocturnal labour.

Modalities

Aggravation

- ➲ Mental exhaustion or emotion.
- ➲ Effects of concentrated studying.

- Odour of cooking food.
- Touch.
- Night.

Amelioration

- Stooping.
- Warmth.
- Silence, lying perfectly still.

Relations

- FOLLOWS WIELL: Carb-v; Merc; Nux-v; Puls; Rhus-t.
- ANTIDOTES: Bell; Camph; Cocc; Led; Nux-v; Puls. Spi-anth; Thuj.

Collinsonia canadensis

➲ PROVED BY: Dr. Burt.

➲ DURATION: 30 days.

➲ COMMON NAME: Stone Root.

➲ FAMILY/KINGDOM: Labiatae.

➲ RELATION COLD/HEAT: Cold.

➲ DIATHESIS: Haemorrhoidal.

➲ SOURCE: Tincture of fresh Root.

➲ SUMMARY OF INDICATIONS: Haemorrhoids during pregnancy–dysenorrhoea–heart disorders.

THERAPEUTIC PICTURE OF DRUG

M_{D-1} ➲ Extremely irritable becomes angry when questioned. Mortification caused by offence.

M_{D-2} ➲ Anger, with indignation.

DS_1 ➲ Chronic, painful, bleeding piles.

DS_2 ➲ Pelvic and portal congestion resulting in dysmenorrhoea or haemorrhoids (especially in the later months of pregnancy).

DS_3 ➲ Constipation, stool light-coloured, lumpy, with hard straining.

DS_4 ➲ Chronic, painful, bleeding haemorrhoids; sensation as if sticks, sand or gravel are lodged in the rectum.

DS_5 ➲ Haemorrhoids; caused by congestive inertia of lower bowel, also for obstinate cases.

DS_6 ➲ Diarrhoea, mucous, bloody; thin, yellow matter, or watery, with violent tenesmus and sharp cutting in the bowels.

CVS_1 ➲ After heart is relieved old piles reappear, or suppressed menses return.

CVS_2 ➲ Heart disorders; tachycardia.

CVS_3 ➲ Pericardical attacks of faintness and oppression, <slightest motion.

FGS_1 ➲ Boring pain in ovary,

FGS $_2$ ➲ Must draw up double, with restlessness. Round, small, cystic tumour in ovaries or broad ligament.

FGS $_3$ ➲ Wants abdomen suppoted by pressure.

FGS $_4$ ➲ Bearing down cramps, causing her to bend double.

Modalities

Aggravation

- Slightest mental emotion.
- Excitement aggravate the symptoms.

Amelioration

- By Heat.

Relations

- COMPARE: Aesc; Aloe; Cham; Nux-v; Sulph.
- ANTIDOTES: Nux-v.

Colocynthis

- PROVED BY: Hahnemann.
- DURATION: 1-7 days.
- COMMON NAME: Squirting Cucumber.
- FAMILY/KINGDOM: Cucurbitaceae.
- DIATHESIS: Rheumatic, gouty, nervous.
- SOURCE: Tincture of pulp of fruit.
- SPHERES OF ACTION: Visceral organs female genital organs, nerves *e.g.* abdominal plexus, trigeminal and sciatic nerves.
- SUMMARY OF INDICATIONS: Abdominal disorders–lower limbs pain (Sciatica).

THERAPEUTIC PICTURE OF DRUG

M_{D-1} ➲ Greatly affected by the misfortunes of others as well as her own.

M_{D-2} ➲ Extreme irritability; nothing seems right to him; extremely impatient; every word Provokes him.

M_{D-3} ➲ Anger, with indignation; also bad effects there from, particularly vomiting and diarrhoea.

M_{D-4} ➲ Depressed, joyless; disinclined to talk, answer, to see friends.

H_{D-1} ➲ Vertigo; when quickly turning head, especially to the left.

H_{D-2} ➲ Lateral cutting headache with nausea, and vomiting (migraine).

H_{D-3} ➲ Burning pains, digging, grinding and tearing.

H_{D-4} ➲ Pain (better pressure and heat), with soreness of the scalp.

H_{D-5} ➲ Frontal headache; worse, stooping, lying on the back and moving eyelids.

DS_1 ➲ Agonizing abdominal pain causes the patient to double up; restlessness, twisting and turning to obtain relief, pain decreased by hard pressure.

DS_2 ➲ Violent cutting, tearing pains, which from different parts of chest and abdomen, concentrate in the pit of stomach, better from hard pressure and bending double; brought on by vexation and indignation.

DS_3 ➲ Cramp-like pain in both sides of abdomen, worse after pressure, or leaning with belly on a table.

DS_4 ➲ Collection of fat in abdomen since her first confinement.

DS_5 ➲ Colic so distressing that they seeks relief by pressing the corner of a table, or head of bed-post, against abdomen.

FGS_1 ➲ Cramp- like pain in left ovary; in uterus; as if parts were squeezed in a voice.

FGS_2 ➲ Ovarian cyst. Paroxysm of acute pain in abdomen, sacrum and hip > by flexing thigh on pelvis.

FGS_3 ➲ Round, small cystic tumors in the ovaries or broad ligaments.

FGS_4 ➲ Wants abdomen supported by pressure.

FGS_5 ➲ Bearing down cramps, causing her to bend double.

FGS_6 ➲ Metritis; metrorrhagia,;suppressed catamenia, with cramping pains > by bending double; of caused by indignation or chagrin.

FGS_7 ➲ Stitches in the ovaries.

FGS_8 ➲ Lochia suppressed; puerperal fever after vexation.

LS_1 ➲ Shooting pain,like lightning–shocks, down the whole limb; from the left hip to the left nee (to the popliteal fossa).

LS_2 ➲ Crampy pain in the affected hip, as though the parts were screwed in a vice; lies upon the affected side, with knee drawn up.

LS_3 ➲ Drawing twitching, with dull throbbing in region on left hip, and in right loin.

LS_4 ➲ Continuous pain in left knee-joint, impeding walking.

Modalities

Aggravation

- ➲ Anger and indignation.
- ➲ Mortification caused by humiliation.
- ➲ Cheese increases colic.

Amelioration

- ➲ From doubling up.
- ➲ Hard pressure.
- ➲ Warmth.
- ➲ Lying with head bent forwards.

Relations

➲ FOLLOWS WELL:	Bell; Bry; Caust; Cham; Merc; Nux-v; Puls; Spig; Staph.
➲ ANTIDOTES:	Camph; Coff; Opi.

Conium maculatum

- ➲ COMMON NAME: Poison Hemlock.
- ➲ DURATION: 30 days.
- ➲ RELATION COLD/HEAT: Cold.
- ➲ FAMILY/KINGDOM: Umbelliferae.
- ➲ DIATHESIS: Scrofulous.
- ➲ MIASM: Psora.
- ➲ SOURCE: Tincture of fresh plant in flower.
- ➲ TEMPERAMENT: Melancholic & Irritable
- ➲ SPHERES OF ACTION: Nerous system, female genital organs heart, Cardiovascular system, and glands.
- ➲ SUMMARY OF INDICATIONS: Geriatric and climacteric disorders of women–polyneuropathy–paraplegia.

THERAPEUTIC PICTURE OF DRUG

C_{N-1} ➲ It is mostly suited to old man and women, old bachelors, during and after climacteric age.

C_{N-2} ➲ Scrofulous people with rigid muscular fibres and light hair.

C_{N-3} ➲ Persons of lively quick sanguine disposition with marked development of glandular system.

C_{N-4} ➲ Persons having debility and diseases caused by blow or fall.

C_{N-5} ➲ Those who lead sedentary life and are easily exhausted and excited and catch cold very readily.

M_{D-1} ➲ Depressed, timid, averse to society and afraid of being alone.

M_{D-2} ➲ Excitement causes mental depression.

M_{D-3} ➲ No inclination for business or study; takes no interest in anything.

M_{D-4} ➲ Memory weak; unable to sustain any mental effort.

H_{D-1} ➲ Vertigo–especially when lying down or turning in bed or turning head to the left.

H_{D-2} ➲ Headache as if the head were too full and would burst; morning when awakening.

H_{D-3} ➲ Stitching pain from within outward, in the forehead, mornings or at noon.

H_{D-4} ➲ Sensation in right half of brain as of a large foreign body.

SO_1 ➲ Weakness of sight; also from partial paralysis of optic nerve.

SO_2 ➲ Aversion to light, without inflammation of the eyes.

SO_3 ➲ Ulcer on the cornea (right to left); great photophobia, but little injection.

SO_4 ➲ Often the students remedy for night work.

RS_1 ➲ Cough provoked by tickling and scraping in the throat.

RS_2 ➲ Dry cough, provoked by a tickling, with sanguineous expectoration, or in violent fits during the night.

RS_3 ➲ Cough, like whooping-cough, with sanguineous expectoration, or in violent fits during the night.

RS_4 ➲ Cough, caused by itching in the chest and throat, or from a small dry spot in the larynx, without expectoration at night, and difficult, bloody, purulent, offensive expectoration during the day.

FGS_1 ➲ Burning, sore, aching, sensation in the region of the uterus.

FGS_2 ➲ At every menstrual effort breasts become sore and painful.

FGS_3 ➲ Dysmenorrhoea, with shooting pain in the left chest.

FGS_4 ➲ Menses: suppressed; too late and scanty; preceded by melancholy, followed by acrid leucorrhoea.

FGS_5 ➲ Leucorrhoea: thick, milky, with contractive, labor-like colic, coming from both sides; of white, acrid mucus, causing burning.

FGS_6 ➲ Tumors in mammae, with piercing pains, worse at night, gland abnormally tender..

FGS_7 ➲ Hardness of the right mammae, with painfulness to touch, and nightly stiches in it.

FGS_8 ➲ Bad effects: of suppressed sexual desire, or suppressed menses.

MGS_1 ➲ Desire increased; power decreased.

MGS_2 ➲ Sexual nervousness, with feeble erection.

MGS_3 ➲ Testicles hard and enlarged (orchitis).

PG_1 ➲ Sweat day & night, as soon as one sleeps, or even when closing the eyes (Chin).

PG_2 ➲ Weakness of voluntary muscles. Numbers of legs.

PG_3 ➲ Swelling and induration of the glands, with tingling and shooting pains.

PG_4 ➲ Great liability to take cold.

PG_5 ➲ Great fatigue and other sufferings, from walking in the open air.

Modalities

Aggravation

- At night, lying down.
- During or rising up in the bed.
- Celibacy.

Amelioration

- In dark from letting the affected limb hang down and motion.

Relations

- COMPARE: Arnica; Rhus–t; Ruta; Calca-Carb; Psor.
- COMPLEMENTARY: Bar-m.
- FOLLOWS WELL: Arn; Ars; Bell, Calc-Carb; Calc–ars.
- ANTIDOTES: Merc. Nit-ac; Sulph.

Crocus sativa

- PROVED BY: Stapf.
- DURATION: 8 days.
- COMMON NAME: Saffron.
- FAMILY/KINGDOM: Iridaceae.
- MIASM: Syphilitic.
- DIATHESIS: Haemorrhagic.
- TEMPERAMENT: Hysterical.
- SOURCE: Tincture of dried stigmas, cooper makes a tincture of the fresh young shoots.
- SPHERES OF ACTION: Female genital organs eyes,chest,abdomen and brain.
- SUMMARY OF INDICATIONS: Extreme emotional affections–haemorrhage–menstrual headaches,

THERAPEUTIC PICTURE OF DRUG

M_{D-1} ➲ Frequent and extreme emotional changes: from the greatest hilarity to the deepest despondency.

M_{D-2} ➲ Excessively happy,affectionate,wants to kiss every body; the next moments in a violent rage.

M_{D-3} ➲ Laughter quickly followed by tears.

M_{D-4} ➲ Chorea and hysteria with great hilarity: singing and dancing alternating with melancholy and rage.

H_{D-1} ➲ Headache (in women at the climacteric.) throbbing, pulsating, increases. during the days of accustomed menstrual flow; nervous and menstrual headache before, during of after flow.

H_{D-2} ➲ Sudden broad thrust: in the right temple; extending into the brain.

SO_1 ➲ Nosebleed. black,tenacious, stringy, every drop can be turned in to a thread; with cold sweat in large drops on forehead, in children who develop too ropidly.

SO_2 ➲ Eyes feel as if in smoke.

SO_3 ➲ Pupils enlarged and react slowly.

SO_3 ➲ Ciliary neuralgia, pain from the eyes extending to the top of the head.

SO_4 ➲ Asthenopia with extreme photophobia.

SO_5 ➲ Must wipe the eyes sensation of mucus or water in them.

NS_1 ➲ Convulsion attacks, like chorea (every seven days), with laughter, dancing and leaping, alternately with violent paroxysms of whooping-cough.

NS_2 ➲ Movements, as of something alive (hopping and jumping) in various parts of the body.

NS_3 ➲ Jerking in the muscles, spasmodic contraction of single sets of muscles.

FGS_1 ➲ Sensation of some thing living and moving in the abdomen, abdomen swollen; (These symptoms, when occurring in females, as they often do at the change of life and at other times, may lead to the erroneous idea of pregnancy).

FGS_2 ➲ Urging of blood towards the genital parts as if the menses were commencing

FGS_3 ➲ Catamenia too frequent, copious and painful.

FGS_4 ➲ Metrorrhagia of black and slimy blood.

FGS_5 ➲ Flow of blood, during the new and full moon.

FGS_6 ➲ Haemorrhage from the uterus (during +the least movement); blood viscid, black, smelling badly (miscarriage third month).

FGS_7 ➲ Threatend abortion, esp. where there is a haemorrhage of dark, stringy blood.

FGS_8 ➲ Post–Partum haemorrhage.

FGS_9 ➲ Jerking pain in the interior of the left breast as if drawn towards the back by means of a thread.

FGS_{10} ➲ A bounding, feeling, as if something alive in the right breast.

PG_1 ➲ Haemorrhage from any part; blood black viscid, clotted, forming into long black strings hanging from the bleeding surface.,

PG_2 ➲ Heaviness and failing of the limbs, after light exercise.

PG_3 ➲ Striking alternation of the most opposite, physical and mental symptoms.

PG_4 ➲ Excessive general weakness, with fainting fits, during movement.

Modalities

Aggravation

- Lying down.
- Warm room.
- Fasting, before break fast.
- Hot weather.
- In morning.
- Looking fixedly at an object.

Amelioration

- In open air.

Relations

- COMPARE: Ip; Tril-p; Plat; Chin
- FOLLOWS WELL: Nux-v;Puls; Sulph.
- ANTIDOTES: Aco; Bell; Op.

Crotalus horridus

- ➲ PROVED BY: Herring.
- ➲ DURATION: 30 days.
- ➲ COMMON NAME: Poison of rattle snakes.
- ➲ FAMILY/KINGDOM: Crotalidae.
- ➲ RELATION COLD/HEAT: Hot.
- ➲ MIASM: Psora.
- ➲ DIATHESIS: Haemorrhagic.
- ➲ TEMPERAMENT: Choleric.
- ➲ SOURCE: Solution of the venom in glycerine.
- ➲ SPHERES OF ACTION: Acts upon cerebro-spinal nerve, fibrin of blood & liver.
- ➲ SUMMARY OF INDICATIONS: Haemorrhagic diathesis–jaundice (taxic hepatitis).

THERAPEUTIC PICTURE OF DRUG

C_{N-1} ➲ Strumous, debilitated broken down constitution, particularly in drunkards with tendency to carbuncles or blood boils.

M_{D-1} ➲ Weeping mood, clouded perception and memory.

M_{D-2} ➲ Impatient.

M_{D-3} ➲ Laquacious, with desire to escape, sadness.

M_{D-4} ➲ Delusion of cerebral decay.

DS_1 ➲ Tongue red and sore; yellow; stiff and numb; smoth and red; swollen and protruded.

DS_2 ➲ Great difficulty in swallowing anything solid.

DS_3 ➲ Insatiable thirst, dry tongue, fever.

DS_4 ➲ Hungry, trembling, weakness; occipital headache.

DS_5 ➲ Vomiting: and giddiness; incessant with thirst; of grass green fetid ejecta; bilious with anxiety, palpitation, weak pulse; of blood; of food, violent.

DS_6 ➲ Cannot bear clothes round stomach and below hypochondria.
DS_7 ➲ Stomach so irritable it can retain nothing.
DS_8 ➲ Swelling of the whole abdomen; yellow fever.
DS_9 ➲ Inguinal gland enlarged; sloughing, unhealthy pus.
DS_{10} ➲ Bleeding from the anus and other opening of the body.
DS_{11} ➲ Dysenteric discharges of dark, fluid blood; involuntary great debility and faintness.
CVS_1 ➲ Palpitations, especially at menstrual period.
CVS_2 ➲ Trembling feeling in the heart (apoplexy).
CVS_2 ➲ Action feeble, pulse tremulous.
FGS_1 ➲ Prolanged menses.
FGS_2 ➲ Dysmenorrhoea, pain extends down thighs, with aching in region of heart.
FGS_3 ➲ Uterine haemorrhage with faintness at stomach.
FGS_4 ➲ Puerperal fever, offensive lochia.
FGS_5 ➲ Phlegmasia alba dolens.
FGS_6 ➲ Sensation as though uterus would drop out.
FGS_7 ➲ Painfull drawing in uterine ligaments.can not keep legs still.
FGS_8 ➲ Malignant disease of uterus, great tendency to haemorrhage, blood dark, fluid, offensive.
FGS_9 ➲ Vicarious menstruation, in debilitated constitution.
S_{N-1} ➲ Yellow colour of whole body (haematic rather than hepatic jaundice).
S_{N-2} ➲ Itching stinging all over; urticaria.
S_{N-3} ➲ Suppuration, painful of old wounds.
S_{N-4} ➲ Purpura haemorrhagica; haemorrhage from every part of body.
S_{N-5} ➲ Boils, carbuncles and eruptions are surrounded by purplish, mottled skin and oedema.
S_{N-6} ➲ Anthax; sore sensation relieved by pressure.
F_{R-1} ➲ Malignant fevers of a haemorrhagic or putrescent character.
F_{R-2} ➲ Low bilious remittents.
F_{R-3} ➲ Yellow fever; bloody sweat; cerebrospinal meningitis.
F_{R-4} ➲ Surface cold, esp. extremities.
F_{R-5} ➲ Flushes of heat all over.
PG_1 ➲ Haemorrhagic diathesis, bloody sweat.
PG_2 ➲ Bad effect of vaccination.

Modalities

Aggravation

➲ Lying on right side.

- Open air, evening.
- Morning and after sleep.

Amelioration

- By rest and fanning.

Relations

- COMPARE: Lach; Pyro; Bapt.
- ANTIDOTES: Camph; Alcohol; Am-m; Lach.

Croton tiglium

- PROVED BY: Hencke.
- DURATION: 30 days.
- COMMON NAME: Croton oil seeds.
- FAMILY/KINGDOM: Euphorbiaceae.
- SOURCE: Tincture of the oil from the seeds.
- SPHERES OF ACTION: Mucous membrane of GIT and skine etc.
- SUMMARY OF INDICATIONS: In sudden evacuation of bowels–Pain in the chest (In the nursing mother).

THERAPEUTIC PICTURE OF DRUG

M_{D-1} ➲ Sadness, sometimes with dislike to labour; or else with anxiety, and displeasure concerning everythings.

M_{D-2} ➲ Frequent melancholy.

M_{D-3} ➲ Grumbling discontented humor.

M_{D-4} ➲ Dislike to labour.

M_{D-5} ➲ Nothing is desired but loitering and to avoid all serious undertakings.

M_{D-6} ➲ Disordered aspect, with eyes haggard, sparkling.

M_{D-7} ➲ Weakness of memory.

M_{D-8} ➲ Feeling as though one cannot think outside of himself, "feels all pent up" inside, and no chance for the thoughts to flow out.

DS_1 ➲ Bowels moved by spasmodic jerks, stools "coming out like a shot" as soon as women eats, drinks, or even while eating; yellow watery stool.

DS_2 ➲ Constant urging to stool followed by sudden evacuation, which is shot out of the rectum.

DS_3 ➲ Sensation in the intestines as from water before stool.

DS_4 ➲ Stools; yellow water; light brown, covered with mucus, with frequent urging; dark green, or greenish-yellow, liquid; tenacious mucus; watery mixed with whitish flakes; coming out like a shot.

DS_5 ➲ Pain in the anus, as if a plug were forcing outwards.

FGS_1 ➲ Catamenia too scanty, or altogether suppressed, with dyspnoea and palpitation of the heart, esp. on going to bed.

FGS_2 ➲ Pain and stitches through the breasts into the chest, and extending to the back, as soon as the child begins to nurse, nipple very sore.

S_{N-1} ➲ Intense itching; but scratching is painful.

S_{N-2} ➲ Pustular eruptions, especially on the face and genitals with fearful itching, followed by painful burning.

S_{N-3} ➲ Herpes zaster; stinging, smarting pains in the eruption.

S_{N-4} ➲ Vesicles; confluent oozing; vescicular erypsipelas, itching exceedingly.

S_{N-5} ➲ The patient can't bear to scratch very hard as it hurt; a very slight scratch, a mere rub suffices to allay the itching.

Modalities

Aggravation

- ➲ Diarrhoea.
- ➲ Every motion.
- ➲ After drinking.
- ➲ While eating or nursing.
- ➲ During summer.
- ➲ From fruit sweetmeats.
- ➲ The least food or drink.
- ➲ Touch.

Relations

➲ COMPARE:	Kali-br; Phos.
➲ FOLLOWS WIELL:	Rhus-t.
➲ ANTIDOTES:	Ana; Ant-t; Cle-ere; Ran-bul; Rhus-t.

Cuprum metallicum

- ➲ PROVED BY: Hahnemann.
- ➲ DURATION: 40–50 days.
- ➲ COMMON NAME: Metallic copper.
- ➲ FAMILY/KINGDOM: Minerals.
- ➲ RELATION COLD/HEAT: Agg. from cold air.
- ➲ MIASM: Anti-psoric.
- ➲ SOURCE: Cu-trituration.
- ➲ SPHERES OF ACTION: Nervous system.
- ➲ SUMMARY OF INDICATIONS: Exhaustion–cramps–Stammering–epilepsy–whooping cough.

THERAPEUTIC PICTURE OF DRUG

C_{N-1} ➲ It is suited to fair haired persons and the carbo-nitrogenoid constitution.

C_{N-2} ➲ Women who have borne many children.

M_{D-1} ➲ Mental and physical exhaustion from over–exertion of mind and loss of sleep.

M_{D-2} ➲ Attacks of unconquerable anxiety.

M_{D-3} ➲ Incoherent, delirious talk.

M_{D-4} ➲ Want of moral courage and convulsive laughter.

M_{D-5} ➲ Loss of sense and thought.

M_{D-6} ➲ Unfitness for exertion, with fear to be idle.

NS_1 ➲ Paralysis of the tongue; imperfect, stammering speech.

NS_2 ➲ Epilepsy; aura begins in knees and ascends; increases at night during sleep; about new moon at regular intervals (menses); from a fall or blow on the head; from getting wet.

NS_3 ➲ Epileptic convulsions: trembling, tottering and falling unconscious, without a scream; Preceded by drawing in the left arm.

NS_4 ➲ Eclampsia of children, during dentition.

NS_5 ➲ Child lies on belly and spasmodically thrusts breech up.

NS_6 ➲ Twitching, jerkings or startings during sleep.

NS_7 ➲ Nervous trembling, with very great acuteness and sensitiveness of the senses.

DS_1 ➲ A strong, sweetish, metallic, copper taste in the mouth and saliva.

DS_2 ➲ Constant protrusion and retraction of the tongue, like a snake.

DS_3 ➲ Hiccough preceding the spasms.

DS_4 ➲ While drinking, the fluid descends with a gurgling sound; craves cool drinks.

DS_5 ➲ Neuralgia of abdominal viscera.

DS_6 ➲ Colic, violent and intermittent; Intussusceptions.

DS_7 ➲ Cholera; with cramps in abdominal and calves.

RS_1 ➲ Spasmodic affections generally; whooping, cough where the attacks run into catalepsy; movement of the head; epilepsy.

RS_2 ➲ Dry cough, with fits of suffocation, like whooping-cough; worse 3 A.M.

RS_3 ➲ Obstinate hoarseness, with great inclination to lie down.

RS_4 ➲ Cough has a gurgling sound, better by drinking cold water.

RS_5 ➲ Spasm and constriction in the chest; spasmodic asthma, alternating with spasmodic vomiting.

RS_6 ➲ Violent asthmatic attacks come on suddenly, lasting form one to three hours, and cease suddenly.

FGS_1 ➲ Before the catamenia, ebullition of the blood, palpitation of the heart and headache.

FGS_2 ➲ Menstruation too late; protracted; complaints before.

FGS_3 ➲ Menses absent for month; violent delirium.

FGS_4 ➲ Ebullition of blood; palpitations.

FGS_5 ➲ Torpid chlorosis.

FGS_6 ➲ Before and during menses, cramps, convulsions, piercing shrieks; Spasmodic dyspnoea; violent palpitation.

FGS_7 ➲ Menses not appearing after suppression of foot-sweat.

PG_1 ➲ Pain in the extremities; cramps in the soles and soles and calves, with great weariness of limbs.

PG_2 ➲ Epileptic attacks (at night), followed by headache.

PG_3 ➲ Tonic spasms with loss of consciousness, turning of the head backwards, redness of the eyes, salivation, and frequent emition of urine.

PG_4 ➲ Great lassitude, and sinking of the whole body.

PG_5 ➲ Outward appearance of the face bluish; bluish red.

Modalities

Aggravation

- Cold air.
- Cold wind.
- At night.
- Suppressed foot sweat or exanthemata.

Amelioration

- By swallowing of cold water.
- Nausea, vomiting and cough.

Relations

- COMPARE: Ars; Verat.
- COMPLEMENTARY: Calk.
- FOLLOWS WELL: Ars; Bell; Calc; Caust; Cic; Hyos; Kali-n; Puls; Stram; verat.
- ANTIDOTES: Bell; Camph; Chin; Con; Dulc; Hep; Ip. Mere; Nux-v.

Cyclamen europaeum

- PROVED BY: Hahnemann.
- DURATION: 14-20 days.
- COMMON NAME: Sowbread.
- FAMILY/KINGDOM: Primulaceae.
- RELATION COLD/HEAT: Chilly.
- MIASM: psora and sycosis.
- TEMPERAMENT: Irritable.
- SOURCE: Tincture of the root gathered in spring.
- SPHERES OF ACTION: Cerebro–spinal system, GIT & female sexual system.
- SUMMARY OF INDICATIONS: Menstrual disorders–painful disorders of bones.

THERAPEUTIC PICTURE OF DRUG

C_{N-1} Best adapted to Blonde leuco-phlegmatic who are pale and anaemic.
M_{D-1} Irritable, peevish, morose and ill humored.
M_{D-2} There may be great sadness with weeping disposition.
SO_1 Dimness of sight, with fiery sparks before the eyes.
SO_2 Diplopia.
SO_3 Sense of smell dimished.
SO_4 Diminution of hearing, as if the ears were stopped.
DS_1 Fullness and pressure at the put of the stomach.
DS_2 Stitches in the stomach.
DS_3 Borborygmi in the abdomen, immediately after a meal.
DS_4 Pressure in rectum or anus.
DS_5 Watery diarrhoea.
FGS_1 Mental symptoms are better during profuse menstrual flow.
FGS_2 Menses profuse, black, membranous clotted too early with labor-like pains from back to pubis.

FGS_3 ➲ Menstrual irregularities with migraine and blindness or fiery spots before eyes.

FGS_4 ➲ Hiccough during pregnancy.

FGS_5 ➲ Post partum haemorrhages, with colickly bearing down pains, with relief after gush of blood.

MGS_1 ➲ Stitches in urethra.

MGS_2 ➲ Phimosis.

US_1 ➲ Urine profuse, watery and frequent.

US_2 ➲ Urine, dark red containing much sediment matter.

LS_1 ➲ Burning, sore pain in-heels.

LS_2 ➲ After waling, toes feel dead.

LS_3 ➲ Cramp-like pains in the thighs.

LS_4 ➲ Fetid sweat between the toes.

S_{N1} ➲ Itching, leaving a numb sensation.

S_{N2} ➲ Acne in young women.

PG_1 ➲ Aversion to open air.

PG_2 ➲ Pale, chloretic deranged menses, accompanied by vertigo, headache dim vision.

Modalities

Aggravation

- ➲ Open air, cold air.
- ➲ Cold bathing, By rest.
- ➲ Sitting, standing at night.
- ➲ Before menses.

Amelioration

- ➲ During menstrual flow by moving about.
- ➲ Rubbing parts.
- ➲ In warm room, indoors.

Relations

- ➲ COMPARE: China; Ferrum; Puls.
- ➲ FOLLOWS WELL: Phos; Rhus; Sep; Sulph.
- ➲ ANTIDOTES: Camphor; Coffea; Puls.

Dulcamara

- ➲ PROVED BY: Hahnemann.
- ➲ DURATION: 30 days.
- ➲ COMMON NAME: Bitter sweet.
- ➲ FAMILY/KINGDOM: Solanaceae.
- ➲ RELATION COLD/HEAT: Neither chilly not hot.
- ➲ MIASM: Sycotic & psoric.
- ➲ TEMPERAMENT: Irritable.
- ➲ SOURCE: Tincture prepared from fresh green stem & leaves. gathered just before flowering.
- ➲ SPHERES OF ACTION: All mucus membrane, skin, dura & muscles.
- ➲ SUMMARY OF INDICATIONS: Rheumatic and skin affections–cystitis.

THERAPEUTIC PICTURE OF DRUG

C_{N-1} ➲ Phlegmatic scrofulous constitution.
M_{D-1} ➲ Mental agitation.
M_{D-2} ➲ Great impatience and restlessness.
M_{D-3} ➲ Nocturnal delirium, with aggravation of pains.
H_{D-1} ➲ Ringwarm of scalp.
H_{D-2} ➲ Pressive pressure.
H_{D-3} ➲ Headache relived by conversation.
SO_1 ➲ Otalgia, at night, with nausea.
SO_2 ➲ Dry coryza.
SO_3 ➲ Stuffs up when there is a cold rain.
DS_1 ➲ Aversion of food.
DS_2 ➲ Burning thirst for cold drinks.
DS_3 ➲ Pains in the umbilical region.
DS_4 ➲ Dropsy of the abdomen.

FGS_1 ➲ Suppression of menses from cold or dampness.

FGS_2 ➲ Before appearance of menses. a rash appears on skin or Sexual excitement.

FGS_3 ➲ Dysmenorrhoea, with blotches all over mammae engorged and sore delicate, Sensitto cold.

US_1 ➲ Retention of urine, scanty and foetid urine.

US_2 ➲ Must urinate when getting chilled.

US_3 ➲ Discharge of mucus from the urethra.

LS_1 ➲ Paralysis of arms, with icy coldness, as from apoplexy.

LS_2 ➲ Perspiration on palm of hand.

LS_3 ➲ Swelling of the calf of the leg.

B_{K-1} ➲ Neck stiff, back painful, loins lame, after taking cold.

B_{K-2} ➲ Pain in small of back, as after long stooping.

S_{N-1} ➲ Dryness and heat of the skin.

S_{N-2} ➲ Pruritus always worse in cold, wet weather.

S_{N-3} ➲ Red spots, urticaria, brought on exposure, on sour stomach.

S_{N-4} ➲ Painful ulcers, discharge scanty.

S_{N-5} ➲ Skin callous.

S_{N-6} ➲ Tettery eruption, with swelling of glands.

PG_1 ➲ Every time patient takes cold or is longs exposed to cold Involuntary.

Modalities

Aggravation

➲ From cold in generals.

➲ Damp rainy weather.

➲ Cold air, suppressed eruption & sweat.

Amelioration

➲ Warmth dry weather.

➲ Warm air and walking.

Relations

➲ COMPLEMENTARY:	Bary-carb; Kali-sulph.
➲ FOLLOWS WIELL:	Bry; Calc; lyco; Rhus; Sep.
➲ ANTIDOTES:	Cup; Merc.
➲ INIMICALS:	Bell; Lach; Ac-acid.

Erigeron canadense

- PROVED BY: W.H.Burt.
- FAMILY/KINGDOM: Compositae.
- COMMON NAME: Flea-bane.
- SOURCE: Tincture from the fresh plant when in bloom.
- SPHERES OF ACTION: Female genital organs.

THERAPEUTIC PICTURE OF DRUG

H_{D-1} ➲ Congestion of head, red face, nose bleed, febrile action.

DS_1 ➲ Violent retching and burning in the stomach, with vomiting of blood.

DS_2 ➲ Dysentery, with soreness and burning in bladder.

DS_3 ➲ Dull pain in left hypogastrium and umblilicus.

FGS_1 ➲ Metrorrhagia, with violent irritation of rectum and bladder; after abortion, with diarrhoea and dysuria; with prolapsus uteri.

FGS_2 ➲ Very profuse flow of bright-red blood; every movement of patient increases the flow; pollor and weakness.

FGS_3 ➲ Leucorrhoea profuse, with spasmodic pains, and irritation of the bladder and rectum.

FGS_4 ➲ Bloody lochia rectum after the least motion; > during rest.

FGS_5 ➲ Pregnant women with "Weak uterus".

FGS_6 ➲ Chronic gonorrhoea with burning micturition; Continuous dribbling.

US_1 ➲ Urinate painful or suppressed.

US_2 ➲ Dysuria of teething children, frequent desire, crying when urinating.

Modalities

Aggravation

- Left side.

Relations

- COMPARE: Arn; Canth; Copaiv; Ham; Ipec; Sabi; Tereb.

Euphrasia-officinalis

- PROVED BY: Hahnemann.
- DURATION: 7 days.
- COMMON NAME: Eyebright.
- FAMILY/KINGDOM: Scrophulariaceae.
- SOURCE: Tincture of whole plant.
- SPHERES OF ACTION: mucous membrane, Particularly of the eyes, lids and respiratory tract.
- SUMMARY OF INDICATIONS: Conjunctivitis–rhinitis.

THERAPEUTIC PICTURE OF DRUG

M_{D-1} ➲ Hypochondriacal indifference; indolence.

M_{D-2} ➲ Taciturnity, and repugnance to conversation; abstraction of mind.

SO_1 ➲ Catarrhal affections of mucous membranes, especially of the eyes and nose.

SO_2 ➲ The eyes tear all the time and the lids are glued together with Pus in the morning. The margins of the lid are red, swollen and burning.

SO_3 ➲ Profuse watery coryza with violent cough and abundant expectoration.

SO_4 ➲ Inflammation and redness of the eye from being wounded.

SO_5 ➲ Inflammation and ulceration of the edges of the eyelids, with headache.

SO_6 ➲ Lancinations in the eyes (ball), excited by too bright a light.

SO_7 ➲ Photophobia, esp. in daylight and in the sunshine.

RS_1 ➲ Cough: on rising in the morning, continuing until lying down again.

RS_2 ➲ Whooping cough, only during day time, with Profuse lacrymation.

RS_3 ➲ Frequent yawning when walking in the open air.

RS_4 ➲ Interruption of breath; no cough at night; from the smoke of wood.

RS_5 ➲ Cough only during the day, with mucus in the chest; which cannot be detached; mucus frequently blood-streaked, thin; expectoration only in the morning.

FGS$_1$ ➲ Amenorrhoea, with inflammation of the eyes and ulcer on right side of the bridge of nose.

FGS$_2$ ➲ Menses painful, lasting only one hour, time regular.

FGS$_3$ ➲ Condylomata, with stitches and itching, especially when walking.

PG$_1$ ➲ Great drowsiness in the day, as from fatique of the eyes.

PG$_2$ ➲ Violent lancinations in different parts, which prevent sleep.

Modalities

Aggravation

- The evening.
- Indoors.
- Moisture.
- Light.
- In bed.
- Warmth.
- When touched.

Amelioration

- From coffee.
- In the dark.

Relations

- FOLLOWS WELL: Aco; Calc; Con; Nux-v; Phos; Puls; Rhus-t; Sil; Sulph.
- ANTIDOTES: Camph; Puls.

Eupionum

THERAPEUTIC PICTURE OF DRUG

M_{D-1} ➲ Cheerful, joyous disposition.
M_{D-2} ➲ Irritable, anger easily.
M_{D-3} ➲ Great weakness of memory.
H_{D1} ➲ Vertigo, everything turns round on sitting up in bed.
H_{D2} ➲ Sore painful spots on head.
H_{D3} ➲ Painful pulsation in forehead.
LS_1 ➲ Cramps in the calves, worse at night.
FGS_1 ➲ Burning in right ovary.
FGS_2 ➲ Gushing leucorrhoea.
FGS_3 ➲ Chronic tubal disease.
FGS_4 ➲ Uterine Flexion.
FGS_5 ➲ Menses too early and copious.
FGS_6 ➲ During menses; irritable; and disinclined to talk.
FGS_7 ➲ Burning and stitches in chest and heart.
FGS_8 ➲ After menses, yellow leucorrhoea, with severe backache.
FGS_9 ➲ When pain in back cause, the discharge gushes out.
FGS_{10} ➲ Sore between labia during urination.
FGS_{11} ➲ Pruritus pudenda, Labia swollen.
FGS_{12} ➲ Marked female symptoms and backache.
FGS_{13} ➲ Pain in back followed by a bland leucorrhoea.
LS_1 ➲ Cramps in the calves, worse at night.
PG_1 ➲ Intense sweat from slightest exertion.

Modalities

Aggravation

- In morning.
- Coughing and sneezing.
- Pain in abdomen.

Amelioration

- Rest > headache & pain in abdomen.
- Bending backwards > backache.

Relations

- COMPARE: Graph; Kreo.

Ferrum metallicum

- PROVED BY: Hahnemann.
- DURATION: 50 days.
- COMMON NAME: Iron.
- FAMILY/KINGDOM: Minerals.
- RELATION COLD/HEAT: Hot.
- MIASM: Psora.
- DIATHESIS: Haemorrhagic.
- TEMPERAMENT: Sanguine.
- SOURCE: Triturations of the Pure Metal.
- SPHERES OF ACTION: Blood, Uterus, Gastro-intestinal tract etc.
- SUMMARY OF INDICATIONS: Digestive disorders, Headache, Menstrual disorders, Bleeding disorders.

THERAPEUTIC PICTURE OF DRUG

C_{N-1} ➲ Especially adapted to women who are Pale, weak, delicate and chlorotic, yet have a fierly red face.

C_{N-2} ➲ Persons of sanguine temperament; Pettish, quarrelsome, disputative, easily excited, least contradiction angers.

M_{D-1} ➲ Irritability; Slight noises like crackling of Papper drive him to despair.

M_{D-2} ➲ Gaiety, alternating with sadness, every other day.

M_{D-3} ➲ Peevish, Passionate, and disputative.

H_{D-1} ➲ Headache on top of head, as if skull was pushed upwards.

H_{D-2} ➲ Throbbing pain in top of head when moving suddenly.

H_{D-3} ➲ Headache: occupying left side of head: with coryza; after menses.

H_{D-4} ➲ Congestion of head, pulsating hammering pains; head sensitive; worse after 12 P.M; returning periodically; feeling of an iron hand around the head; better from external pressure; face red.

H_{D-5} ➲ Vertigo on seeing flowing water.

H_{D-6} ➲ Pain in the back of head, with roaring, throbbing in the neck.

DS_1 ➲ Eructations of food after eating, without nausea.

DS_2 ➲ Nausea and vomiting after eating.

DS_3 ➲ Vomiting: at midnight, or morning after breakfast; as soon as food is taken.

DS_4 ➲ Distension and pressure in the stomach after eating.

DS_5 ➲ Heat and burning in the stomach, with momentary, cramp-like pain in splenic region.

DS_6 ➲ Soreness of the abdominal wall.

DS_7 ➲ Stools: watery, with burning at the anus; slimy, with discharge of ascarides; stools with blood and mucus.

DS_8 ➲ Costive: stools hard and different, followed by backache.

DS_9 ➲ Diarrhoea with undigested food; painless and involuntary during a meal.

DS_{10} ➲ Itching at the anus at night, from ascarides.

FGS_1 ➲ Metrorrhagia, with over-excitement of the sanguineous system.

FGS_2 ➲ Catamenia feeble and of a Pale blood.

FGS_3 ➲ During coition, smarting and pain, like that of excoriation in the vagina, with want of enjoyment.

FGS_4 ➲ Swellings and indurations of the vagina.

FGS_5 ➲ Prolapse of vagina; pain in OS tincae on lying down.

FGS_6 ➲ Milky and corrosive leucorrhoea.Tendency to abortion.

FGS_7 ➲ Menses: too early, too profuse, too long lasting, with fiery red face; ringing in the ears; intermit two or three days and then return; flow pale, watery, debilitating.

FGS_8 ➲ Face fiery red, and copious flow of blood, at one time liquid, at another black and coagulated, accompanied by Pains in the sacral region and abdomen, similar to those of child-birth.

FGS_9 ➲ Before the catamenia, shooting pains in the head, with tingling in the ears.

PG_1 ➲ Erythematous skin, worse in winter.

PG_2 ➲ Red regions become pale; lips; tongue and mucous membrane of mouth.

PG_3 ➲ Haemorrhagic diathesis; blood bright red, coagulates slowly.

PG_4 ➲ Dropsical swellings, with shooting pains.

PG_5 ➲ Violent pains, tearing and shootings, esp. at night, which compel movement of the part affected.

PG_6 ➲ Great lassitude and general weakness, produced even by speech, often alternating with anxious trembling of the whole body; she is so weak that she must lie down.

Modalities

Aggravation

- At night.
- At rest, especially while sitting still.

Amelioration

- Walking slowly.
- In summer.
- Mental exertion.

Relations

COMPLEMENTARY:	Alum; chin; Ham.
FOLLOWS WELL:	Acon; Arn; Bell; Chin; Con; Lyc; Merc; Phos; Puls; Sulph; Verat.
ANTIDOTES:	Arn; Ars; Bell; Beer; Hep; Ip; Puls; Thea; Verat.
INIMICALS:	Acet-ac.

Ferrum phosphoricum

- ➲ PROVED BY: Dr. J.C. Margan.
- ➲ COMMON NAME: Ferric Phosphate $Fe_3 (PO_4)_2$
- ➲ FAMILY/KINGDOM: Minerals.
- ➲ RELATION COLD/HEAT: Hot.
- ➲ MIASM: Psora.
- ➲ DIATHESIS: Haemorrhagic.
- ➲ SPHERES OF ACTION: The main action of this drug on relaxed muscular tissue and blood corpuscles.
- ➲ SUMMARY OF INDICATIONS: Inflammatory disorders (at the onset of illness).

THERAPEUTIC PICTURE OF DRUG

C_{N-1} ➲ Pale, anaemic with false plethora.
M_{D-1} ➲ Loss of courage & hope, better after sleep.
M_{D-2} ➲ Inability to command the right word or express himself.
M_{D-3} ➲ Indifference to ordinary matter.
H_{D-1} ➲ ill effect of sun heat.
H_{D-2} ➲ Rush of blood to head, with vertigo.
H_{D-3} ➲ Headache better by cold applications.
SO_1 ➲ Blinding headache.
SO_2 ➲ Acute otitis, when Bell. Fails, prevent suppuration.
SO_3 ➲ Nose-bleed of bright blood in children.
DS_1 ➲ Tonsil red and swollen.
DS_2 ➲ On waking, throat feels swollen and stiff.
DS_3 ➲ Vomiting of undigested food.
DS_4 ➲ Colic before stool.
DS_5 ➲ Destension in hypochondria and region of stomach.
RS_1 ➲ Congestions of lungs.

RS_2 ➲ Haemoptysis, after concussion or fall.
RS_3 ➲ Whooping cough, with retching and vomiting.
FGS_1 ➲ Menses every three weeks, with bearing down sensation.
FGS_2 ➲ Vaginismus, vagina dry & hot.
FGS_3 ➲ Pain in vagina during coition, can not bear examination.
FGS_4 ➲ Dysmenia, with accelerated pulse and red face.
FGS_5 ➲ Menses pale first half of period.
US_1 ➲ Enuresis diurenal from irritability of trigone.
US_2 ➲ Incontinence of urine.
LS_1 ➲ Rheumatism of wrist and knee.
LS_2 ➲ Nodule on dorsum of left little finger.
LS_3 ➲ Whitlow, palm hot, hand swollen and painful.
F_{R-1} ➲ Chilly daily at 1 P.M.
PG_1 ➲ Aversion to meat & milk.
PG_2 ➲ All complaints better by cold application.

Modalities

Aggravation

- ➲ At night and 4:00 to 6:00 A.M.
- ➲ Touch, Jar, Motion.
- ➲ Right side.

Amelioration

- ➲ Cold Application.

Relations

- ➲ COMPARE: Aco; China; Gels.

Gelsemium sempervirens

- PROVED BY: W.E. Payne.
- DURATION: 30 days.
- COMMON NAME: Yellow Jasamine.
- FAMILY/KINGDOM: Loganiaceae.
- RELATION COLD/HEAT: Gel is a remedy for warm climates.
- MIASM: Psora.
- TEMPERAMENT: Nervous and Hysterical.
- SOURCE: Tincture of the bark of the root.
- SPHERES OF ACTION: Brain, mucus membrane and sexual organs, spinal cord, nerves, vision & blood.
- SUMMARY OF INDICATIONS: Hysteria–Stage fright- vertigo -muscular disorder.

THERAPEUTIC PICTURE OF DRUG

C_{N-1} ➲ It has been used mostly in acute troubles.

C_{N-2} ➲ It is usually more suited to anaemic girls.

C_{N-3} ➲ Children & young people especially women of a nervous hysterical temperament.

M_{D-1} ➲ Excitable, irritable, sensitive; for the nervous affections of onanists of womens.

M_{D-2} ➲ Fear of death; utter lack of courage.

M_{D-3} ➲ Delirium in sleep; half walking, with incoherent talk; desire to be let alone.

M_{D-4} ➲ Bad effects from fright, fear, exciting news; from some unusual ordeal.

M_{D-5} ➲ Child starts, grasps the nurse and screams as if aforesaid of falling.

M_{D-6} ➲ Mental excretions cause a sense of helplessness from brain weakness; inability to attend to anything requiring thought.

H_{D-1} ➲ Vertigo, spreading from the occiput.

H_{D-2} ➲ Heaviness of head; bund like sensation around the head and occipital headache (cerebrospinal meningitis).

H_{D-3} ➲ Vertigo with pupils dilated, dim sight; general depression from heat of sun or summer.

H_{D-4} ➲ Headache preceded by blindness; better, profuse micturition.

H_{D-5} ➲ Headache with muscular soreness of the neck and shoulders (cervical spondylosis).

H_{D-6} ➲ Giddy, with loss of sight chilliness, accelerated pulse, dullness of sight or double sight.

NS_1 ➲ Paralysis of motion; muscles will not obey the will, feel bruised.

NS_2 ➲ Neuralgia, acute, sudden, darting pain; shooting, tearing along the tracks of the nerves.

NS_3 ➲ Convulsions from reflex irritation; spasm of one day.

NS_4 ➲ Complete relaxation of the entire muscular system with motor paralysis.

CVS_1 ➲ Sensation as if it is necessary to keep in motion or else the heart's action would cease.

CVS_2 ➲ Pulse frequent, soft, weak, almost imperceptible; slow and full.

CVS_3 ➲ Weak, slow pulse of old age.

CVS_4 ➲ Irregular beating of the heart; Palpitation; pain in the heart when rising from a seat.

FGS_1 ➲ Suppressed menstruation with convulsions (every morning).

FGS_2 ➲ Metrorrhagia; almost continuous flow without any pain; after ague suppressed by quinine.

FGS_3 ➲ Severe, sharp, labour-like Pains extending to back and hips.

FGS_4 ➲ Dizziness and headache with amenorrhoea.

FGS_5 ➲ Ailments from masturbation with depression and languor.

FGS_6 ➲ Spasmodic or neuralgic dysmenorrhoea.

FGS_7 ➲ Leucorrhoea; white; in gushes; with backache.

FGS_8 ➲ Spasmodic labour-Pains. Premature labour (abortion) (after fright)

FGS_9 ➲ During Pregnancy, violent pains in the uterus, headache, drowiness, double vision, obscuration of sight, giddiness, pulsation of the carotid arteries, small, slow pulse.

FGS_{10} ➲ Cramps in the abodomen and legs during Pregnancy; diplopia; drowsiness; loss of muscular power; convulsions.

MGS_1 ➲ Spermatorrhoea without erections.

MGS_2 ➲ Genital cold and relaxed.

MGS_3 ➲ Sexual power exhausted, slightest caress causes an emission.

MGS_4 ➲ Painful redness at the urethra.

PG_1 ➲ General depression from heat of sun or summer.

PG_2 ➲ Weakness and trembling: of tongue, hands, legs or of entire body.

PG_3 ➲ Lack of muscular co-ordination; confused; muscles refuse to obey the will.

PG_4 ➲ Excessive irritability of mind and body.

PG_5 ➲ Trembling and weakness; listless and languid; easily fatigued.

PG_6 ➲ Congestions, arterial or venous, with sluggish circulation.

Modalities

Aggravation

- Damp weather.
- Fog.
- Before a thunderstorm.
- Emotion or excitement.
- Bad news.
- Tobacco–smoking.
- When thinking of patient's ailments.
- At about 10 A.M.

Amelioration

- Bending forwards, by profuse urination.
- Open air.
- Continued motion.
- Stimulants.

Relations

- FOLLOWS WELL: Bapt; Ip.
- ANTIDOTES: Chin; Coff; Nat-m; Dig-Pur.
- SIMILAR: Ign; Bap; Ip.

Glonoine

- ➲ PROVED BY: Hering.
- ➲ DURATION: 1 day.
- ➲ COMMON NAME: Nitro-glycerine $C_3H_5(NO_2)O_3$.
- ➲ RELATION COLD/HEAT: Hot Patient.
- ➲ MIASM: Psora.
- ➲ TEMPERAMENT: Nervous.
- ➲ SOURCE: Nitro-glycerine dilution with alcohol.
- ➲ SPHERES OF ACTION: Brain, Pneumo-gastric and vaso-motor nerves.
- ➲ SUMMURY OF INDICATIONS: Headaches–Sinusitis–menopausal syndrome.

THERAPEUTIC PICTURE OF DRUG

C_{N-1} ➲ Nervous temperament: Plethoric, florid, sensitive women; who are very irritable and easily excited by slightest opposition.

M_{D-1} ➲ Falling down, with loss of consciousness and alternate palpitation of the heart, and congestion of the head.

M_{D-2} ➲ Usually bright and loquacious, with great flow of idias.

M_{D-3} ➲ Confusions at ideas; cannot tell where he is; well-known streets seems strange; way home too long; forgets on which side of the street he lives.

M_{D-4} ➲ Great mental agitation (with headache); fruntic, attempts to run away; to jump out of window.

H_{D-1} ➲ Sunstroke and headache. Throbbing, Pulsating frontal headache.

H_{D-2} ➲ Headache after menstruation.

H_{D-3} ➲ Head felt larger; balancing sensation, constant effort to keep head erect.

H_{D-4} ➲ Sun stroke: vertigo, violent pain; pale face, feeble pulse.

H_{D-5} ➲ Head heavy, but cannot lay in on a pillow; cannot bear any heat around the head.

H_{D-6} ➲ Shocks in the brain synchronous with the pulse.

H_{D-7} ➲ Throbbing: in temples; in vertex; occiput; in whole head.

H_{D-8} ➲ Angio-spastic neuralgia of the head and face.

H_{D-9} ➲ Headache with increased secretion of urine.

H_{D-10} ➲ Brain feels too large; bursting feeling; fullness, throbbing of arteries; all the blood seems to be pumped upwards; hold the head with the hands.

H_{D-11} ➲ Congestion to head, sudden, violent; throbbing felt with every pulse, at every step, or jarring; blood mounts from neck, throat or chest; from occiput towards eyes.

FGS_1 ➲ Menstruation suppressed by Glon.

FGS_2 ➲ Instead of menses congestion to head; face pale; worse in worm room; fainting; throbbing.

FGS_3 ➲ During menstruation congestion of blood to head and chest; headache; fainting.

FGS_4 ➲ At climaxis, flushes of heat, Pressure in head, nausea, loss of sense, vertigo, swelling of feet.

FGS_5 ➲ During Pregnancy headache, congestions of blood to the head and chest.

FGS_6 ➲ Eclampsia; unconscious; face bright-red; puffed; pulse full, hard; urine copious and albuminous.

FGS_7 ➲ Flushes of heat at the climacteric, with the catamenia.

PG_1 ➲ Convulsions: from congestions to the head; the fingers are spread apart and stretched out.

PG_2 ➲ Painless throbbing in the whole body.

PG_3 ➲ Pulsations, tingling, thrills, and a peculiar sensation of warmth through the body, extending from above downward.

Modalities

Aggravation

- ➲ In the sun, overheated room.
- ➲ Jar (Sudden movement).
- ➲ Bending head backwards.
- ➲ Stooping.
- ➲ Ascending.
- ➲ Having a haircut or wearing a hat.

Amelioration

- ➲ Brandy (cognac).
- ➲ Lying still.

Relations

- ➲ COMPARE: Amyl; Bell; Ferr; Gels; Meli; Stram.
- ➲ ANTIDOTES: Aco; Camph; Coff; Nux-v.

Graphites

- PROVED BY: Hahnemann.
- DURATION: 40-50 days.
- COMMON NAME: Black Lead (Plumbago).
- FAMILY/KINGDOM: Minerals.
- RELATION COLD/HEAT: Very Chilly.
- MIASM: Psora.
- DIATHESIS: Tubercular and cancerous.
- TEMPERAMENT: Irritable and melancholic.
- SOURCE: An allotropic modification of carbon. Trituration of prepared black lead from finest English drawing–Pencils.
- SPHERES OF ACTION: Female genital tract glands and GIT and central upon skin.
- SUMMARY OF INDICATIONS: Skin disorders–nail disorders–leucorrhoea–constipation.

THERAPEUTIC PICTURE OF DRUG

C_{N-1} ➲ Suited to women, inclined to obesity, who suffer from habitual. Constipation; with a history of delayed menstruation.

C_{N-2} ➲ Usually a lady of climacteric age, fair, anamic face, split hair, unhealthy skin.

M_{D-1} ➲ Weakness in the head, can scarcely think.

M_{D-2} ➲ Forgetfulness; dim recollection of recent events.

M_{D-3} ➲ Child impudent, teasing, laughs at reprimands.

M_{D-4} ➲ Fidgety while sitting at work.

M_{D-5} ➲ Dejection, sadness and profound melancholy with discouragement and much weeping; weeping without cause; obligate to weep at music.

DS_1 ➲ Nausea and vomiting after each meal.

DS_2 ➲ Stomach pain in temporarily relieved by eating, hot drinks especially milk and lying down.

DS_3 ➲ Fullness and hardness of the abdomen, as from incarcerated flatulence; must loosen clothing; Presses painfully at the abdominal ring.

DS_4 ➲ Constipation: large, knotty feces; chronic, with hardness in region of liver; with dryness of mucous membrane of rectum and fissure of the anus.

DS_5 ➲ Diarrhoea; stools, brownish, fluid, mixed with undigested substance (lienteric), very fetid, sour odor.

DS_6 ➲ Fissura ani; severe, sharp, cutting pain during stool, followed by constriction and aching for several hours, worse at night.

DS_7 ➲ Harmorrhoids of the rectum, with burning rhagades at the anus.

FGS_1 ➲ Menses: too scanty, pale, late with violent colic; irregular. Delayed from getting feet wet.

FGS_2 ➲ Leucorrhoea; acrid, excoriating; occurs in gushes day and night; before and after menses.

FGS_3 ➲ Vesicles and pimples on the vulva.

FGS_4 ➲ Excoriation on the vulva and between the thighs.

FGS_5 ➲ Painful swelling of the ovaries; every time she takes cold or gets her feet wet.

FGS_6 ➲ Swelling and hardness of ovaries after menses.

FGS_7 ➲ Tearing, grinding, bursting in right ovary, as if it would burst, before and during menses.

FGS_8 ➲ Suppression of catamenia, with heaviness of the limbs and congestions of blood to the head.

FGS_9 ➲ During the catamenia, flow of blood from the anus, pains in the limbs, ulcers become worse, swelling of the cheeks or of the feet, catarrh, with hoarseness and coryza, toothache, or cramps and violent cutting in the abdomen, headache, nausea, pain in the chest and weakness.

FGS_{10} ➲ Before and during the menstruation, fatiguing cough (morning and during the day).

FGS_{11} ➲ Hard cicatrices remaining after mammary abscess, retarding the flow of milk; cancer of breast, from old scars and repeated abscesses.

FGS_{12} ➲ Morning sickness during menstruation; very weak and Prostrated.

MGS_1 ➲ Uncontrollable sexual excitement; violent erections; aversion to coition.

MGS_2 ➲ Herpatic eruption on organs, with hydrocele (left side).

S_{N-1} ➲ Unhealthy skin; every injury suppurates.

S_{N-2} ➲ The nails brittle, crumbling, deformed, painful, sore, as if ulcerated; thick and crippled.

S_{N-3} ➲ Rough, hard, persistent dryness in portions of skin unaffected by eczema.

S_{N-4} ➲ Itching over various parts of body; violent itching and burning, with eruptions.

S_{N-5} ➲ Eruptions, oozing out a sticky exudation.

S_{N-6} ➲ Eczema, with profuse serous exudations, in blonds inclined to obesity; also ulternating with internal affections.

S_{N-7} ➲ Early stage of keloid and fibroma; pimples and acne.

S_{N-8} ➲ Old ulcers, with fetid pus, proud flesh, itching, stinging; old scars from ulcers.

S_{N-9} ➲ Cracks in nipples, mouth, between toes, anus.

S_{N-10} ➲ Phelgmonous erysipelas of face; burning and stinging pain; swelling of feet.

PG_1 ➲ Sensation of cobwebs on the forehead, tries hard to brush it off.

PG_2 ➲ Great tendency to take cold, and fear of the open air, and of currents of air.

PG_3 ➲ Varices, with shootings, tension and itching.

PG_4 ➲ Strong pulsation in the whole body, and esp., in the heart, augmented by the least movement.

PG_5 ➲ Cramp, like pains, cramps and contraction in different parts.

Modalities

Aggravation

- ➲ Warmth.
- ➲ At night.
- ➲ During and after menstruation.

Relations

- ➲ COMPLEMENTARY: Ars; Caust; Ferr; Hep; Lyc.
- ➲ FOLLOWS WELL: Euphr; Nat-s; Sil.
- ➲ ANTIDOTES: Aco; Ars; Nux-v.
- ➲ SIMILAR: Puls; Lyc.

Hamamelis virginiana

- ➲ PROVED BY: Hering.
- ➲ DURATION: 1-7 days.
- ➲ COMMON NAME: Witch Hazel.
- ➲ FAMILY/KINGDOM: Hamamelaceae.
- ➲ DIATHESIS: Haemorrhagic.
- ➲ SOURCE: Tincture of fresh bark of twigs and root.
- ➲ SPHERES OF ACTION: Veins, Capillaries, liver Portal system, rectum and generative organs.
- ➲ SUMMARY OF INDICATIONS: Chronic Varicose ulcers–venous disorders–bleeding heamorrhoids with burning sensation at the anus.

THERAPEUTIC PICTURE OF DRUG

M_{D-1} ➲ Forgetful, no desire to study or work.

M_{D-2} ➲ Depressed in mind; also after emissions, with regretful mind, irritable.

SO_1 ➲ Eyes inflames; vessels greatly injected; caused by a foreign substance, as melted sugar; intense soreness.

SO_2 ➲ Traumatic conjunctivitis; suggillations, or extravasations into chamber of eye.

SO_3 ➲ Epistaxis, flow passive, non-coagulable.

SO_4 ➲ Sneezing spells, watery, excoriating, burning discharge.

DS_1 ➲ Harmatemesis, blood black; sensation of trembling in the stomach, or fullness and gurgling in the abdomen; feverish by spell; weak, cold, quick pulse, profuse sweat.

DS_2 ➲ Haemorrhage; profuse, dark, grumous from ulceration of bowels.

DS_3 ➲ Piles bleeding profusely; with burning, soreness, fullness and weight; black as if it would break; urging to stool.

DS_4 ➲ Large quantities of a tar-like blood.

DS_5 ➲ Anus feels sore and raw; dysentery; pulsations in the rectum.

CVS_1 ➲ Phlebitis, varicose veins, varicose ulcers.

CVS_2 ➲ Pricking pain in region of heart and superficial veins of both arms.

CVS_3 ➲ Palpitation.

CVS_4 ➲ This is the Aconitum napellus of the venous system.

FGS_1 ➲ Menses; flow, dark and profuse; with soreness in abdomen; after a blow on ovary, or a fall; all suffering < at menstrual period.

FGS_2 ➲ Metrorrhagia, passive flow, venous blood; anaemia.

FGS_3 ➲ Amenorrhoea, vicarious bleeding from nose of stomach; costive; varices on legs.

FGS_4 ➲ Uterine, active or passive; after a fall or rough riding; vicarious Menstruation; no mental anxiety.

FGS_5 ➲ Leucorrhoea, great tenderness of vagina; flow bloody.

FGS_6 ➲ Vaginismus, intense soreness; in prurigo of ulva.

FGS_7 ➲ Uterine haemorrhage active or passive; from jolting while riding over rough roads; bearing down pain in back.

FGS_8 ➲ Dysmenorrhoea, with severe pains through the lumbar and hypogastric region and down the legs; fullness of the brain and bowels, with severe pain through the whole head, causing stupor, deep sleep; varicose veins.

FGS_9 ➲ Ovaritis after a blow; diffused agonized soreness over the whole abdomen; menses irregular; <at time of menses; retention of urine.

PG_1 ➲ It is used in venous haemorrhage from any orifice of the body; nose, lungs, bowels, uterus, bladder.

PG_2 ➲ Bruised soreness of affected parts; rheumatism, articular and muscular.

PG_3 ➲ Prickling stinging: in veins, muscles, skin.

PG_4 ➲ Takes cold easily from every exposure; but esp. to warm, moist air; subject to varicose veins.

Modalities

Aggravation

- Warmth.
- Moist Air.

Relations

- COMPARE: Arn; Calen.
- COMPLEMENTARY: Ferr.
- ANTIDOTES: Arn; Puls.

Helleborus niger

- ➲ PROVED BY: Hahnemann.
- ➲ DURATION: 20-30 days.
- ➲ COMMON NAME: Christmas Rose.
- ➲ FAMILY/KINGDOM: Ranunculaceae.
- ➲ RELATION COLD/HEAT: Chilly.
- ➲ MIASM: Psora.
- ➲ TEMPERATURE: Irritable.
- ➲ SOURCE: Tincture of dry powered root.
- ➲ SPHERES OF ACTION: Brain, Nervous system, meninges, kedney, serous membrane, digestive system and urinary organs.
- ➲ SUMMARY OF INDICATIONS: Depressed cerebral functions–hydrocephalus–disorders during dentition–diarrhoea–urinary disorders.

THERAPEUTIC PICTURE OF DRUG

C_{N-1} ➲ It is more suited to weak and delicate persons, especially children.

C_{N-2} ➲ Especially children who are Prone to brain troubles with serous effusion.

M_{D-1} ➲ Involuntary sighing; complete unconsciousness.

M_{D-2} ➲ Diminished power of mind over body; cannot fix ideas; slow in answering, stares unintelligently; muscles do not act properly if the will is not strongly fixed upon their action; as when spoken to, the attention being thereby diverted, she drops things.

M_{D-3} ➲ Constantly picking his lips and clothers.

M_{D-4} ➲ Stupidity and want of reflection, with (thoughtless) fixedness of look on one single point, much moaning and inability to think.

M_{D-5} ➲ Melancholy: silent; during Pregnancy; with anguish.

M_{D-6} ➲ Irritable; worse from consolation, does not want to be disturbed.

M_{D-7} ➲ Eclampsia: a noise or shock shortens the attack.

H_{D-1} ➲ Migraine: Headache culminate in vomiting.

H_{D-2} ➲ Meningitis: Bores head into the pillow; beats it with hands.

H_{D-3} ➲ Hydrocephalus: Dull pain in the occiput with sensation of water swashing inside.

H_{D-4} ➲ Stupefying headache, with coryza (4-8 p.m.); worse from stooping, better at rest and in the open air.

H_{D-5} ➲ Rolls head day and night; moaning, sudden screams.

H_{D-6} ➲ Painful heaviness with burning pain in the head, coldness of the fingers, sensation of general shivering, and paleness of the face.

NS_1 ➲ Convulsions with extreme coldness of body, except head or occiput, which may be hot.

NS_2 ➲ Cerebral symptoms during dentition; acute hydrocephalus, automatic motion of one arm and leg.

NS_3 ➲ Convulsive twitching of muscles; sudden relaxation of muscles.

NS_4 ➲ Epilepsy, with consciousness, followed by deep sleep.

DS_1 ➲ Mouth dry, also Palate, with cutting, scraping in Palate on moving the mouth to swallow.

DS_2 ➲ Lips dry and cracked; tongue red and dry.

DS_3 ➲ Gurgling, as if bowels were full of water; swollen painful to touch.

DS_4 ➲ Diarrhoea: during acute hydrocephalus, dentition, Pregnancy; watery, clear, tenacious, colourless mucus; white, jelly-like mucus; like frog spawn; involuntary.

DS_5 ➲ Blenorrhoea of rectum with spasm of bladder.

US_1 ➲ Frequent want to make water, with scanty emission.

US_2 ➲ Scanty urine, with sediment like coffee grounds.

US_3 ➲ Cystitis: bladder overdistended; child cannot micturate.

US_4 ➲ Feeble stream; deep-coloured urine.

US_5 ➲ Spasmodic urging, causing spasms; very little urine passes.

US_6 ➲ A large quantity of pale, watery urine is emitted.

PG_1 ➲ Convulsive twitching of the muscles during sleep.

PG_2 ➲ Relief is found in the open air, and sensations are felt as when recovering from a long illness.

PG_3 ➲ Shooting and Piercing pains in different parts, and esp. in the Periosteum, worse by fresh air, corporeal fatique, eating and drinking.

PG_4 ➲ Falling off of the hair and nails.

PG_5 ➲ All things have a freshness about them.

Modalities

Aggravation

- From evening until morning.
- From uncovering.

Amelioration

- Warmth.
- Diuresis.

Relations

- COMPARE: Apis; Apoc; Ars; Bry; Dig; Lach; Sulph; Tub; Zinc. In brain or meningeal affection.
- FOLLOWS WELL: Bell; Bry; Lyc; Nux-v; Phos; Puls; Sulph; Zinc.
- ANTIDOTES: Camph; Chin.

Helonias dioica

- PROVED BY: Tully.
- COMMON NAME: Unicorn Plant.
- FAMILY/KINGDOM: Melanthaceae.
- SOURCE: Tincture of the root. Triturations of the resinoid Helonin.
- SPHERES OF ACTION: Female sexual organs, kidney, mind, muscles, brain, nervous system, meninges, kidney, serous membrane, GIT & urinary organs.

THERAPEUTIC PICTURE OF DRUG

M_{D-1} ➲ Dull, inactive; always better when doing something, when the mind is engaged.

M_{D-2} ➲ Desire to be let alone; conversation unpleasant.

M_{D-3} ➲ Depressed mood; dull, gloomy.

M_{D-4} ➲ Irritable; cannot endure the least contradiction or receive any suggestions in relation to any subject; fault finding.

FGS_1 ➲ Loss of sexual desire and power with or without sterility.

FGS_2 ➲ Profound melancholy, deep, undefined depression, with a sensation of soreness and weight in the womb; "a consciousness of a womb."

FGS_3 ➲ Aching, dragging weakness in sacral region with Prolapsus; also at climaxis, with marked debility, profound mental gloom.

FGS_4 ➲ Prolapsus uteri and ulceration of the cervix; discharge constant, dark, badly smelling; flooding on lifting a weight and on least exertion; face sallow, having an expression of suffering; great vaginal irritation; pain in small of back.

FGS_5 ➲ Excessive uterine haemerrhage all through the Proving; Pain in back through the uterus.

FGS_6 ➲ Prolapsus uteri, leucorrhoea; the Os Protrudes externally. Uterus low down, fundus tilted forwards; the finger passes with difficultly between the Os and the rectum.

FGS_7 ➲ Menses too frequent and profuse in women who are feeble from loss of blood.

FGS_8 ➲ Flow passive: dark, coagulated, offensive.

FGS_9 ➲ Amenia, arising from or accompanied by disordered digestive apparatus and anaemic.

FGS_{10} ➲ Leucorrhoea, with atony and anaemia.

FGS_{11} ➲ Women with Prolapsus from atong, enervated by indolence and luxury; feel better when the attention in engaged, hence when doctor comes; worn out with hard work, do not care for sleep; so sleep; so tired, and the strained muscles burn and ache so.

FGS_{12} ➲ Scanty menstrual flow with heaviness, languor, drowsiness and albuminous urine.

FGS_{13} ➲ Profuse flooding, with serous leucorrhoea, much uterine and ovarian pain; climaxis.

FGS_{14} ➲ Labia and pudendum hot, red, swollen, burning and itching terribly, epidermis every morning falls off in thin, transparent exfoliations.

FGS_{15} ➲ Albuminuria during pregnancy; great weakness, drowsiness.

FGS_{16} ➲ Nipples sensitive, painful, breasts swollen; nipples tender, will not bear the pressure of ordinary dress.

US_1 ➲ Burning sensation at the kidneys; can trace their outlines by the burning. At 2.30 P.M., dull heat, and pressure in the vertex, as if skull were too full.

US_2 ➲ Burning-scalding when urinating; desire frequent and urging.

US_3 ➲ Constant aching, extreme tenderness of the kidneys, especially the right.

US_4 ➲ Involuntary discharge of urine after the bladder seemed to be emptied.

US_5 ➲ Urine: Profuse, clear, light-coloured; albuminous; diabetic.

US_6 ➲ Diabetes: first stages: Urine Profuse, clear, Saccharine; lips dry, stick together; great thirst; restlessness; emaciation; irritable and melancholic.

PG_1 ➲ Over-sensitiveness to air, worse from uncovering; better in warm air.

PG_2 ➲ Anaemia, atony from prolonged harmorrhage.

PG_3 ➲ Dropsy from albuminuria, general debility, uterine atony or after uterine haemorrhage.

Modalities

Aggravation

➲ Motion.

➲ Touch.

Amelioration

➲ When doing something (Mental diversion).

Relations

➲ COMPARE: Aletris; Lil; Phos.

➲ SIMILAR: Alet.

Hepar sulphuris

- ➲ PROVED BY: Hahnemann.
- ➲ DURATION: 40-50 days.
- ➲ COMMON NAME: Sulphurate of lime [ca.s].
- ➲ FAMILY/KINGDOM: Mineral.
- ➲ RELATION COLD/HEAT: Highly chilly.
- ➲ MIASM: Mainly anti-psoric. But all the three miasms are covered by Hepar Sulph.
- ➲ DIATHESIS: Lymphatic and scrofulous.
- ➲ TEMPERAMENT: Irritable.
- ➲ SOURCE: An impure sulphide of calcium prepared by burning in a crucible the white interior of oyster shells with pure flowers of Sulphur.
- ➲ SPHERES OF ACTION: Lymphatic, glandular system, Mucous membrane, skin, respiratory organ etc.
- ➲ SUMMARY OF INDICATIONS: Polychrest remedy–Respiratory disorders–Chronic infections–Suppurative disorders.

THERAPEUTIC PICTURE OF DRUG

C_{N-1} ➲ For torpid lymphatic constitutions.

C_{N-2} ➲ Womens with light hair and complexion, slow to act, muscles soft and flabby.

M_{D-1} ➲ Oversensitive, Physically and Mentally.

M_{D-2} ➲ The slightest cause irritates him; quick, hasty speech and hasty drinking.

M_{D-3} ➲ Anguish in the evening and night with thoughts of suicide.

M_{D-4} ➲ Excessive irritability; vexation and passion, with hasty speech and excessive weakness of memory.

M_{D-5} ➲ Anger; would have no hesitation in killing a man who offended him, only he knows better.

M_{D-6} ➲ The slightest cause irritates him and makes him extremely vehement.

DS_1 ➲ Stomach frequently and easily disordered.

DS_2 ➲ Stitching in the region of liver when walking, coughing, breathing or when touching it.

DS_3 ➲ Diarrhoeic stools: White and fetid, child has a sour smell; sour-smelling and whitish; clay-coloured; green, slimy; of sour smell; with tenesmus.

DS_4 ➲ Diarrhoea: worse during the day; after eating, and after drinking cold water.

DS_5 ➲ Dysenteric stools; difficult evacuation of soft stool or of bloody mucus with tenesmus.

RS_1 ➲ Cold beings with an irritation in the throat.

RS_2 ➲ Cough: when any part of the body is uncovered; croupy, choking, strangling; from exposure to dry west wind, the land wind.

RS_3 ➲ Hoarseness with loss of voice, choking and strangling.

RS_4 ➲ Dyspnoea with loose, rattling cough.

RS_5 ➲ Croup with loose, rattling cough; worse in the morning (Pheumonia).

RS_6 ➲ Choking cough; ratting, croaking cough; suffocative attacks; has to rise up and bend the head backwards.

RS_7 ➲ Anxious, wheezing, moist breathing, asthma worse in dry cold air; better in damp.

FGS_1 ➲ Excoriation of the vulva, and between the thighs.

FGS_2 ➲ Congestion of blood to the uterus.

FGS_3 ➲ Irritation of left ovaries; with swellings; and great sensitiveness.

FGS_4 ➲ Discharge of blood between the period, with inflation of the abdomen.

FGS_5 ➲ Catamenia too long delayed and diminished.

FGS_6 ➲ Leucorrhoea, with smarting at the vulva.

FGS_7 ➲ Cancerous ulcer on the breast, with stinging, burning of the edges, smelling like old cheese; itching nipples.

MGS_1 ➲ Itching on the penis, and at the fraenum Preputii.

MGS_2 ➲ Chancre-like ulcers on the prepuce; secondary syphilis.

MGS_3 ➲ Sexual desire increased, erections feeble.

MGS_4 ➲ Discharge of Prostatic fluid, after micturition and during hard stool, also independent of either.

US_1 ➲ Urine flow is slow and without force.

S_{N-1} ➲ Abscesses; supporting gland are very sensitive.

S_{N-2} ➲ Eruptions very sensitive, sore to touch; military rash in circles.

S_{N-3} ➲ Burning–itching on the body, with white vesicles, after scratching.

S_{N-4} ➲ Rhagades; chapped skin, with deep cracks on the hands and feet.

S_{N-5} ➲ Eczema, spreading by means of new pimples appearing just beyond the old part.

S_{N-6} ➲ Cannot bear to be uncovered, wants to be wrapped up warmly.

S_{N-7} ➲ Ulcers: discharge bloody Pus, smelling like old cheese; edges very sensitive, and have a pulsating sensation; discharge corroding.

S_{N-8} ➲ Chronic and recurring urticaria; small pox; herpes circinatus, wens and whitlows.

PG_1 ➲ The slightest injury causes suppuration.

PG_2 ➲ Extremely sensitive to cold air, drought. Feels as if the wind is blowing through some region of the body.

PG_3 ➲ Faints from even slight pain.

PG_4 ➲ Cold sores, abscesses, boils, infected ears.

PG_5 ➲ Pain, as from excoriation on bruising on various places, when they are touched.

PG_6 ➲ Swelling, inflammation, and ulceration of the glands.

PG_7 ➲ Appearance or aggravation of the pains at night, esp. during the chills.

Modalities

Aggravation

- ➲ Dry, cold winds, cool air.
- ➲ Extremely sensitive to touch.
- ➲ Lying on painful side.
- ➲ Slightest draught.
- ➲ Eating or drinking cold food or beverage.

Amelioration

- ➲ Damp wet weather.
- ➲ Warmth.
- ➲ After eating.
- ➲ Wrapping head up.

Relations

- ➲ COMPLEMENTARY: Calen.
- ➲ FOLLOWS WELL: Aco; Arn; Bell; Bryo; Iod; Lach; Merc; Nux-v., Puls; Rhus.t; Sep; Sil; Spong; Sulph; Zinc.
- ➲ ANTIDOTES: Ac-ac; Bell; Cham; Sil; Ars.
- ➲ INIMICALS: Spong .

Hydrastis canadensis

- PROVED BY: Burt.
- COMMON NAME: Golden Seal (Orange Root).
- FAMILY/KINGDOM: Ranunculaceae.
- RELATION COLD/HEAT: Not so well marked
- MIASM: Psora, Syphilis and Sycosis.
- TEMPERAMENT: Lymphatic.
- SOURCE: Tincture of the fresh root.
- SPHERES OF ACTION: Mucous membrane, especially of respiratory tract, GIT, gland and liver etc.
- SUMMARY OF INDICATIONS: Chronic bronchitis–Leucorrhoea–allays the symptoms of secondary cancer.

THERAPEUTIC PICTURE OF DRUG

M_{D-1} ➲ Forgetful; cannot remember what he is reading or talking about.

M_{D-2} ➲ Irritable: disposed to be spiteful.

M_{D-3} ➲ Gloomy, taciturn, disagreeable.

M_{D-4} ➲ Moaning with occasional outcries from the pain.

M_{D-5} ➲ Depression; sure of death and desires it.

RS_1 ➲ Hawking of yellow, tenacious mucus from posterior nares and fauces; rawness of fauces; ulcers in the throat; after mercury.

RS_2 ➲ Chest raw, sore, burning; day harsh cough.

RS_3 ➲ Feels suffocated on lying on the left side (asthma).

FGS_1 ➲ Aching pains in small of back at climaxis; uterine affections with debility and digestive disorders.

FGS_2 ➲ Hot watery discharge from uterus.

FGS_3 ➲ Leucorrhoea: tenacious, ropy, thick yellow.

FGS_4 ➲ Ulceration of the Os, Cervix and vagina; Leucorrhoea; debility; Prolapsus uteri.

FGS_5 ➲ Os uteri very tender.

FGS_6 ➲ Uterine haemorrhage; monorrhagia and metrorrhagia, with fibroid tumours; at monopouse.

FGS_7 ➲ Pruritus vulvae, with profuse leucorrhoea; sexual excitement.

FGS_8 ➲ Lancinating pain in breast extending up to shoulder and down arm.

FGS_9 ➲ Hard, irregular tumour of left breast, nipple retracted, glands in axilla enlarged and painful, calchectic appearance.

FGS_{10} ➲ Sore mouth of nursing women.

FGS_{11} ➲ Abraided, cracked and sore nipples of nursing women.

FGS_{12} ➲ For debilitated womens with viscid mucous discharges.

FGS_{13} ➲ Cachectic patient. Goiter of puberty and pregnancy.

MGS_1 ➲ Gonorrhoea, second stage, thick yellow discharge.

MGS_2 ➲ Debility, after spermatorrhoea.

MGS_3 ➲ Dragging in right groin to testicle; thence to left testicle, thence to left groin.

PG_1 ➲ Yellow string mucus from nasal passages.

PG_2 ➲ Relieves the pain of cancer.

PG_3 ➲ Weakness, physical prostration.

PG_4 ➲ Frequent sudden attacks of fainty spells, with profuse cold sweat all over.

PG_5 ➲ Mucous membranes: secretions increased tenacious, ropy; erosions.

PG_6 ➲ Clothing feels uncomfortable about the groins.

Modalities

Aggravation

- ➲ Exertion.
- ➲ Skin symptoms by warmth.

Amelioration

- ➲ By rest.
- ➲ Pressure.

Relations

- ➲ COMPARE: Xanthorrhiza apifolia; kali-bi; Ars-i, Phyt; Galium aparine, Aser; Stann; Puls.
- ➲ ANTIDOTES: Sulph.
- ➲ SIMILAR: Asterias rubens.

Hyoscyamus niger

- ➲ PROVED BY: Hahnemann.
- ➲ DURATION: 6-14 days.
- ➲ COMMON NAME: Henbane.
- ➲ FAMILY/KINGDOM: Solanaceae.
- ➲ RELATION COLD/HEAT: Chilly.
- ➲ MIASM: Psora.
- ➲ TEMPERAMENT: Sanguine, irritable, nervous and hysterical.
- ➲ SOURCE: Tincture of the fresh plant.
- ➲ SPHERES OF ACTION: Nervous system, sensorium, muscular system and mucous membrane and skin.
- ➲ SUMMURY OF INDICATIONS: Hysteria–delirium–spasms–insomnia.

THERAPEUTIC PICTURE OF DRUG

C_{N-1} ➲ Persons of sanguine temperament.

C_{N-2} ➲ Persons are usually light haired with Pale or bluish face.

M_{D-1} ➲ Womens who are irritable, nervous, hysterical.

M_{D-2} ➲ Stupor, unconsciousness; does not reply to questions; does not recognize any one. Answers properly but immediately stupor returns.

M_{D-3} ➲ Delirium continued while awake. Delirious without apparent heat; the face is pale and the limbs are cold, though the temperature is high.

M_{D-4} ➲ Delirium: talks of business; complains of imaginary wrongs. Delirium tremens, with clonic spasms; averse to light and company; visions, as if persecuted.

M_{D-5} ➲ Melancholy from unfortunate love, with rage or inclination to laugh at everything.

M_{D-6} ➲ Fears: being along; Poison; being bitten; being sold; to eat or drink; to take what is offered; suspicious of some plot.

M_{D-7} ➲ Unfortunate love, with rage and incoherent speech or inclination to laugh at everything; often followed by epilepsy.

M_{D-8} ➲ Peevish and quarrelsome humour; Jealousy.

M_{D-9} ➲ Rage, with desire to strike and to kill.

M_{D-10} ➲ Stupor, with plaintive cries, esp. on the slightest touch, and complete apathy.

M_{D-11} ➲ Lascivious mania: immodesty, will not be covered, kicks off the clothes, exposes the person; sings obscene songs; lies naked in bed and chatters.

NS_1 ➲ Spasm, without consciousness, very restless; every muscles in the body twitches, from the eyes to the toes.

NS_2 ➲ Convulsions after meals: child sickens after eating, vomits or shows distress at the stomach, sudden shriek, and then insensible.

NS_3 ➲ Paralysis after spasms, or after diphtheria.

NS_4 ➲ Epilepsy, before the attack: vertigo, sparks before eyes, ringing in ear hungry gnawing.

RS_1 ➲ Dry spasmodic cough at night, worse lying down; better sitting up, from itching in the throat.

RS_2 ➲ During cough: spasms of the larynx; painful epigastrium and hypochondria.

RS_3 ➲ Haemoptysis, bright red, with spasms, also in drunkards.

RS_4 ➲ Pneumonia: cerebral symptoms, delirium, spoor; dry, fatiquing night cough, or rattling in chest.

FGS_1 ➲ Lascivious, uncovers sexual parts.

FGS_2 ➲ Lascivious furor, without modesty.

FGS_3 ➲ Excited sexual desire without excited fancy.

FGS_4 ➲ Spasms of pregnant women, esp. during Parturition.

FGS_5 ➲ Puerperal fever.

FGS_6 ➲ Metrorrhagia, of a bright–coloured blood.

FGS_7 ➲ Metrorrhagia, the blood pale, with convulsions.

FGS_8 ➲ During the catamenia, delirium, flux of urine, sweat and convulsive trembling.

FGS_9 ➲ Before the catamenia, hysterical cramps and fits of laughter.

FGS_{10} ➲ During the menses, convulsive trembling of the hands and feet; severe headache; profuse perspiration.

MGS_1 ➲ Impotence.

MGS_2 ➲ Lascivious; exposes his person; plays with genitals during fever.

US_1 ➲ Enuresis: involuntary micturition.

US_2 ➲ Bladder paralyzed; has no will to micturate.

US_3 ➲ Urine: scanty; retained or suppressed; turbid with mucopurulent deposit; with red, sandy sediment.

PG_1 ➲ Intense sleeplessness of irritable, excitable persons from business embarrassments, often imaginary.

PG_2 ➲ Sensation of levitation; as if walking on and through air.

PG_3 ➲ Spasm and convulsions with watery diarrhoea.

PG_4 ➲ Incisive tearing, and dull pulling in the limbs and joints.

Modalities

Aggravation

- At night.
- During menses.
- Mental activity.
- Jealousy, unhappy love.
- When laying down.

Amelioration

- Stooping.

Relations

- FOLLOWS WELL: Bell; Puls; Stram; Verat.
- ANTIDOTES: Acet-ac; Bell; Chin; Cit-ac; Stram; Nit-Acid.
- SIMILAR: Bell, Stra; Ver-alb.

Ignatia amara

- PROVED BY: Hahnemann.
- DURATION: 9 days.
- COMMON NAME: St. Ignatius Bean.
- FAMILY/KINGDOM: Loganiaceae.
- RELATION COLD/HEAT: No definite.
- MIASM: Psora.
- TEMPERAMENT: Nervous temperament.
- SOURCE: Tincture and trituration of the seeds.
- SPHERES OF ACTION: Nervous system especially medulla oblongata and spinal cord.
- SUMMARY OF INDICATIONS: Emotional Problems–Chorea- headache.

THERAPEUTIC PICTURE OF DRUG

C_{N-1} ➲ Especially suited to nervous temperament.

C_{N-2} ➲ women of a sensitive, easily excited nature.

M_{D-1} ➲ Dark hair and skin but mild disposition, quick to perceive, rapid in execution.

M_{D-2} ➲ Great grief after losing persons or objects that were very dear.

M_{D-3} ➲ Changeable mood, jesting and laughing, changing to sadness, with shedding of tears.

M_{D-4} ➲ Melancholic, sad, tearful.

M_{D-5} ➲ Anger, followed by quiet grief or sorrow.

M_{D-6} ➲ Affectionate disposition, with very clear consciousness.

M_{D-7} ➲ Lachrymose and apathetic humour, with dread of exertion.

M_{D-8} ➲ Ailments from grief, mortification, bad news, or suppressed mental suffering.

M_{D-9} ➲ Children after having been reprimanded or scolded, are sent to bed and get sick.

H_{D-1} ➲ Headache as if nail is driven at the side often follows anger or grief. Worse from stooping.

NS_1 ➲ Convulsive twitching, especially after fright or grief.

NS_2 ➲ Paralysis after great mental emotion, and night watching in the sick chamber.

NS_3 ➲ Chorea after fright with grief, worse after eating; better lying on back.

NS_4 ➲ Spasms of children, preceded by hasty drinking.

NS_5 ➲ Children convulsed in sleep after having been punished.

DS_1 ➲ Inner mouth inflamed and sore; Putrid odor from mouth.

DS_2 ➲ Sensation of weakness (sinking) in the pit of the stomach, with qualmishness and flat taste, or sighing.

DS_3 ➲ Spasmodic pains in the stomach; also when better eating.

DS_4 ➲ Constipation: from carriage riding; of a paralytic origine; with excessive urging, felt more in upper abdomen; with great pain, dreads to go to closet; in women who are habitual coffee drinkers.

DS_5 ➲ Constractive sore pain in the rectum, like from blind haemorrhoids, one or two hours after stool.

DS_6 ➲ Constriction of the anus after stool, worse while standing.

DS_7 ➲ Stitching from the anus up the rectum.

DS_8 ➲ Prolapsus of the rectum, from moderate straining at stool.

FGS_1 ➲ Persons mentally and physically exhausted by long concentrated grief.

FGS_1 ➲ Catamenia premature and violent, every ten or fifteen days.

FGS_2 ➲ Blood of the catamenia black, of putrid odour, mixed with clots.

FGS_3 ➲ Cramp like and compressive pains in the region of the uterus, with fits of suffocation; Pressure and lying on the back, mitigate the pain.

FGS_4 ➲ Cramp in the uterus, during the catamenia

FGS_5 ➲ Uterine spasms, with lancinations, or like labour pains.

FGS_6 ➲ Corrosive and purulent leucorrhoea, preceded by contractive pressure in the uterus.

FGS_7 ➲ During the catamenia, heaviness, heat and pain in the head, photophobia, colic, and contractive pains, anxiety, palpitation of the heart, and great fatigue, even to fainting.

MGS_1 ➲ Lasciviousness, with weakness of genital power

MGS_2 ➲ Erections, with painful uneasiness, and aching at the pubis.

MGS_3 ➲ Much itching in the genital parts, and in the penis, in the evening after lying down, removed by scratching.

F_{R-1} ➲ Chill, with thirst; relieved by external heat.

F_{R-2} ➲ During fever, itching; nettle rash all over the body.

F_{R-3} ➲ Pulse hard, full and frequent, or very variable.

F_{R-4} ➲ Fever, with headache, and pain in the pit of the stomach, great fatique, paleness of face, or paleness and redness alternately, lips dry and cracked, nettle-rash, tongue white profound sleep with snoring.

PG_1 ➲ A remedy of great contradictions, tinnitus decreased by music, haemorrhoids decreased when walking, sore throat is better when swallowing empty feeling of the stomach not decreased by eating and aggravated by coughing.

PG_2 ➲ Involuntary sighing.

PG_3 ➲ Cannot bear tobacco: smoking, or being in tobacco smoke, produces or aggravates headache.

PG_4 ➲ Hiccough and hysterical vomiting.

PG_5 ➲ Insomnia.

PG_6 ➲ Nocturnal pains which disturb sleep.

PG_7 ➲ Complaints return at Precisely the same hour.

PG_8 ➲ Sweat slight, or only in the face; sweat when eating; and then often on a small spot on face.

PG_9 ➲ Simple and violent pain, in various parts, when they are touched.

Modalities

Aggravation

- ➲ Emotions, grief.
- ➲ Coffee.
- ➲ Morning.
- ➲ Tobacco smoke.
- ➲ Cognac.
- ➲ Light touch.

Amelioration

- ➲ Lying in the painful side.
- ➲ Walking.
- ➲ Swallowing.
- ➲ Warmth.
- ➲ Hard Pressure.

Relations

- ➲ COMPLEMENTARY: Nat-m .
- ➲ FOLLOWS WELL: Ars; Bell; Calc; Chin; Lyc; Nux-v; Puls; Rhus-t; Sep; Sil; Sulph.
- ➲ ANTIDOTES: Acet-ac, Arn; Camph; Cham; Cocc; Coff; Nux-v.
- ➲ INIMICALS: Coff.

Iodium

- PROVED BY: Hahnemann.
- DURATION: 30-40 days.
- COMMON NAME: Iodine.
- FAMILY/KINGDOM: Minerals.
- RELATION COLD/HEAT: Very hot.
- MIASM: Psora.
- DIATHESIS: Scroufulous.
- TEMPERAMENT: Irritable.
- SPHERES OF ACTION: Spleen, Breast, ovaries, Lymph gland, Dura.
- SUMMURY OF INDICATIONS: Goiter and other endocrine disorders.

THERAPEUTIC PICTURE OF DRUG

C_{N-1} ➲ Person dark or black hair and eye with low cachectic condition. Profound debility and general emaciation.

C_{N-2} ➲ Over growth body with Hypertrophy and induration of gland.

M_{D-1} ➲ Anxiety when quiet, present anxiety and depression.

M_{D-2} ➲ Sudden impulse to run and do violence. Forgetful. Must be busy. Suicidal tendency.

M_{D-3} ➲ illusions of moral feeling.

SO_1 ➲ Inflammation of the eyes, sometimes after taking cold.

SO_2 ➲ Smarting in the eyes.

SO_3 ➲ Hearing first sensitive, then dull.

SO_4 ➲ Stoppage of nose or secretion of mucus more abundant then usual

DS_1 ➲ Suffers from hunger, must eat every few hours, feels > while eating or after eating.

DS_1 ➲ Ravenous hunger, eats freely and well, yet loses flesh all the time.

DS_3 ➲ Aching in stomach after every meal.

DS_4 ➲ Gastric derangement with constipation.

DS_5 ➲ Hard, painful swelling of the spleen.

DS_6 ➲ Region of liver sore to pressure, swelling and hypertrophy of liver.
DS_7 ➲ Hard swelling of the inguinal glands.
DS_8 ➲ Constipation alternating with diarrhoea.
CVS_1 ➲ Tachycardia.
CVS_2 ➲ Palpitation from least exertion.
CVS_3 ➲ Sensation as if the heart were squeezed together.
RS_1 ➲ Pain in the larynx.
RS_2 ➲ Laryngitis, with painful roughness, worse during cough.
RS_3 ➲ Dry cough, with stitches and burning in the chest.
RS_4 ➲ Rattling of mucus in the chest, with roughness under the sternum.
RS_5 ➲ Hepatization, worse upper part of right lung.
FGS_1 ➲ Menstruation irregular, uterine Haemorrhage
FGS_2 ➲ Wedge-like pain from ovary to uterus.
FGS_3 ➲ Dwindling of mammary glands
FGS_4 ➲ Nodosities in skin of mammae.
FGS_5 ➲ Acrid Leucorrhoea, think, slimy, corroding the linen.
FGS_6 ➲ Wedge like pain in the right ovarian region.
MGS_1 ➲ Swelling and indurations of testicles, and prostrate gland.
MGS_2 ➲ Complete loss of sexual power.
MGS_3 ➲ Hydrocele, offensive sweat of genitals.
US_1 ➲ Incontinence of urine, in the aged.
US_2 ➲ Frequent and dark yellow-green urine.
LS_1 ➲ Joint inflamed and painful.
LS_2 ➲ Gonorrhoea Rheumatism.
LS_3 ➲ Oedematous swelling of feet.
LS_4 ➲ Painful corns.
PG_1 ➲ Great weakness during menses.

Modalities

Aggravation

- When quiet, in worm.
- Room, Right side.

Amelioration

- Walking about.
- In open air.

Relations

- COMPARE: Hepar; Mer-car; Phoph; Nat-Mur.
- COMPLEMENTARY: Lyco; Badiaga.
- FOLLOWS WELL: Hep; Marc; Kali-bi; Puls.
- ANTIDOTES: Hepar; Sulph; Gratiola; Thuja.

Ipecacuanha

- ➲ PROVED BY: Hahnemann.
- ➲ DURATION: 7-10 days.
- ➲ COMMON NAME: Ipecac.
- ➲ FAMILY/KINGDOM: Rubiaceae.
- ➲ RELATION COLD/HEAT: Chilly.
- ➲ MIASM: Psora.
- ➲ DIATHESIS: Haemorrhagic.
- ➲ TEMPERAMENT: Irritable.
- ➲ SOURCE: Tincture and Trituration of the dried root.
- ➲ SPHERES OF ACTION: Pneumogastric nerve, on medulla oblongata, on mucous membrane of respiratory and gastrointestinal tract.
- ➲ SUMMARY OF INDICATIONS: Gastritis–Bronchial asthma–Morning sickness–haemorrhages from orifices of the body.

THERAPEUTIC PICTURE OF DRUG

C_{N-1} ➲ It is especially suited to strong persons of lax fibre, fair people; women & children.

C_{N-2} ➲ Fair women; emphysematous (A condition of dilatation & destruction of the air passages of the lung causes breathing difficulties.) persons.

C_{N-3} ➲ Persons who have a history of epistaxis (nose bleed) and other forms of blood loss.

M_{D-1} ➲ Irritable; holds everything in contempt.

M_{D-2} ➲ Full of desire, for what they do not know.

DS_1 ➲ Persistent nausea and vomiting. Profuse saliva with a clean tongue. The nausea is not relieved by vomiting.

DS_2 ➲ Adapted to cases where the gastric symptoms.

DS_3 ➲ Vomiting: with thirst, sweat, bad breath; with diarrhoea, colic, distended abdomen; after vomit, sleepy.

DS_4 ➲ Sensation of excessive uneasiness in the stomach and epigastrium.

DS_5 ➲ Stomach feels relaxed, as if hanging down.

DS_6 ➲ Horrid, indescribable pain and sick feeling in the stomach.

DS_7 ➲ Sensation, is if the stomach were empty and flaccid.

DS_8 ➲ Dyspepsia every day, or every other day, at the same hour.

DS_9 ➲ Cutting and pinching in the abdomen; as from a hand, each finger sharply pressing into intestine, worse in the highest degree by movement, better by repose.

DS_{10} ➲ Flatulent colic, with frequent loose stools; cutting about the umbilicus.

DS_{11} ➲ Cutting pains across abdomen from left to right.

DS_{12} ➲ Asiatic cholera, first symptoms, where nausea and vomiting predominate.

DS_{13} ➲ Diarrhoea of children inclining to dysentery.

DS_{14} ➲ Desenteric evacuations, with white flocks, and followed by tenesmus.

DS_{15} ➲ Stools: yellow, painless, fermented, green as grass, with nausea and colic; green mucus; covered with red, bloody mucus; bloody; pitch-like or like frothy molasses; slimy, offensive, followed by tenesmus.

RS_1 ➲ Cough: rough, shaking; dry, from titillation in upper part of larynx; with every breath; with inclination to vomit; with spitting of blood from the least effort.

RS_2 ➲ Dyspnea; constant constriction in the chest.

RS_3 ➲ Asthma: annual attack of asthma.

RS_4 ➲ Continuous sneezing; corzya; wheezing cough.

RS_5 ➲ Chest seems full of phlegm, but does not yield to coughing.

RS_6 ➲ Suffocative cough; child becomes stiff, and blue in the face (cyanosed).

RS_7 ➲ Whooping-cough, with nosebleed, bleeding from mouth, vomiting; losses breath, turn pale or blue, and becomes rigid.

RS_8 ➲ Phthisis: haemoptysis from the slightest exertion.

FGS_1 ➲ Leucorrhoea: acrid, corrosive, staining and corroding the linen; most abundant to times of menses.

FGS_2 ➲ Cancerous degeneration of the cervix; cutting pains in abdomen and haemorrhage at every stool.

FGS_3 ➲ Trouble some sensation, as of bearing down towards the genital parts, and towards the anus.

FGS_4 ➲ Metrorrhagia, with discharge of bright red and coagulated blood, with oppressed breathing.

FGS_5 ➲ Metrorrhagia, much depression and pain in right half of head; soreness about womb and pain in left hip and back; weight across forehead, and phlegm in back of throat, causing sickness; skin yellowish and very irritable, dark round eyes.

FGS_6 ➲ In labour and threatened miscarriage pains fly from left to right with nausea.

PG_1 ➲ In all diseases with constant and continual nausea.

PG_2 ➲ Gushing of bright, red blood from any orifice of the body.

PG_3 ➲ Pale patient; cold sweat. Intermittent fever.

PG_4 ➲ Too great sensibility to cold and to heat.

PG_5 ➲ Fits of uneasiness, with dislike to all food, and excessive and sudden debility.

PG_6 ➲ Chlorosis, menses scanty; skin and mucous surfaces pale, anaemic.

PG_7 ➲ Pain, as from a bruise, in all the bones; tingling in the joints, as when numbed.

Modalities

Aggravation

- Lying down.
- Slightest motion.
- Moist warm wind periodically.

Amelioration

- By rest.
- Pressure.
- Closing eyes.

Relations

➲ COMPLEMENTARY:	Cupr.
➲ FOLLOWS WELL:	Ant-t; Arn; Ars; Bell; bry; Codm; Calc. Cham; Chin; Cupr; Ign; Nux-v; Phos. Puls; Rheum; Sep; Sulph; Tab; Verat.
➲ ANTIDOTES:	Arn; Ars; Chin; Nux-v; Tab.
➲ SIMILAR:	Puls.

Kalium bichromicum

- ➲ PROVED BY: Drysdale.
- ➲ DURATION: 30 days.
- ➲ COMMON NAME: Potassium Bichromate ($K_2Cr_2O_7$).
- ➲ FAMILY/KINGDOM: Minerals.
- ➲ RELATION COLD/HEAT: Chilly.
- ➲ MIASM: Psora, sycosis & Syphilis.
- ➲ SPHERES OF ACTION: On mucous membrane, skin fibrous tissue, gland, kidney.
- ➲ SUMMURY OF INDICATIONS: Conjunctivitis–rhinitis–bronchitis–gastroenteritis–polymyossitis.

THERAPEUTIC PICTURE OF DRUG

C_{N-1} ➲ Fatty person having light hair, fine complexion and suffering from catarrhal affection.

M_{D-1} ➲ ill–humoured, low spirited and indifferent.

M_{D-2} ➲ Easily excited.

M_{D-3} ➲ Anxiety arises from chest, with distress in stomach.

H_{D-1} ➲ Stitches in bones of head, as from a sharp needle.

H_{D-2} ➲ Morning headache.

H_{D-3} ➲ Headache from suppression of discharge from the nose.

SO_1 ➲ Headache–Blurred vision or blindness precedes the attack.

SO_2 ➲ Nose pressive pain in root of nose, discharge of plugs, clinkers.

SO_3 ➲ Oedematous, bladder-like appearance of uvula.

DS_1 ➲ Feeling of coldness in stomach and bowels.

DS_2 ➲ Gastritis, rough ulcer of stomach.

DS_3 ➲ Dislikes water, cannot digest meat.

DS_4 ➲ Chronic intestinal ulceration.

DS_5 ➲ Jelly-like, gelatinous, worse morning.
DS_6 ➲ Sensation of a plug in anus.
RS_1 ➲ Profuse, yellow expectoration, very glutinous and sticky.
RS_2 ➲ Viocehoarse, worse, evening.
RS_3 ➲ Catarrhal Laryngitis cough has a brassy sound.
FGS_1 ➲ Yellow, tenacious leucorrhoea.
FGS_2 ➲ Pruritus of vulva, with great burning and excitement.
FGS_3 ➲ Prolapsus uteri, worse in hot weather.
MGS_1 ➲ Constriction at root of penis, at night on awakening.
MGS_2 ➲ Sexual desire absent in fleshy people.
MGS_3 ➲ Itching in hairy part of genitals.
US_1 ➲ After urinating a drop seems to remain which cannot be expelled.
US_2 ➲ During micturition heat in urethra.
US_3 ➲ Painful drawing from perineum into urethra.
LS_1 ➲ Great weakness of the hand.
LS_2 ➲ Rheumatic pain in the finger-joints.
LS_3 ➲ Pain in the right hip, extending to the knee.
S_{N-1} ➲ Acne, papular eruptions.
S_{N-2} ➲ Skin hot, dry and red.
S_{N-3} ➲ Dry eruption like measles.

Modalities

Aggravation

➲ Beer, morning.
➲ Hot weather.
➲ Undressing.

Amelioration

➲ From heat.

Relations

➲ COMPARE: Tart, Brom, Hepar, Calc, Ant-Crud.
➲ COMPLEMENTARY: Ars.
➲ FOLLOWS WELL: Ant-t, Ber-b, Puls.
➲ ANTIDOTES: Ars. Lach.
➲ INIMICALS: Calc-carb.

Kalium bromatum

- ➲ COMMON NAME: Potassium Bromide (K.Br.).
- ➲ FAMILY/KINGDOM: Minerals.
- ➲ RELATION COLD/HEAT: Patients is neither hot nor chilly.
- ➲ MIASM: Psora & Syphilis.
- ➲ TEMPERAMENT: Patient is depressed melancholic and weepy.
- ➲ SOURCE: K Br solution Trituration.
- ➲ SPHERES OF ACTION: Mind, Cerebro spinal nervous system and female sexual organs & skin.
- ➲ SUMMURY OF INDICATIONS: Nervous disorders–Spasms–Epilepsy–Colic–Acne–Nephritis, loss of memory (Alzheimer's Syndrome)

THERAPEUTIC PICTURE OF DRUG

C_{N-1} ➲ More particularly adapted to persons inclined to obesity.

M_{D-1} ➲ Fits of uncontrollable weeping and profound melancholic delusions.

M_{D-2} ➲ Loss of memory; forgets how to talk; absentiminded; has to be told the word before she could speak it.

M_{D-3} ➲ Depressed, low spirited, anxious, "feel as if they would lose their mind."

M_{D-4} ➲ Restlessness and sleeplessness due to worry and grief. Loss of property or reputation, from business embarrassments.

SO_1 ➲ Smell lessened

SO_2 ➲ Sounds echo in ears, headache.

SO_3 ➲ Ringing in ears.

SO_4 ➲ Vision dim, pupils dilated, with heavy lids and drowsiness.

NS_1 ➲ Spasms: From fright, anger or other emotions in nervous, plethoric persons; during parturition, teething, whooping–cough.

NS_2 ➲ Epilepsy: Congenital, syphilitic, tubercular; usually a day or two before menses; at new moon; headache follows attack.

DS_1 ➲ Sensation as if bowels were falling out.

DS_2 ➲ Internal coldness of abdomen.

DS_3 ➲ Abdominal spasms, walls retracted, convulsive motion of eyes and limbs.

- DS_4 ➲ Constipation, stools dry, hard, infrequent.
- RS_1 ➲ Spasmodic, dry croup, occurring suddenly from reflex.
- RS_2 ➲ Whooping-cough, with spasmodic, dry cough.
- RS_3 ➲ Cough worse at night and when lying down.
- FGS_1 ➲ Ovarian neuralgia from ungratified sexual desire; nervous unrest.
- FGS_2 ➲ Neuralgia of ovaries; pain, swelling, tenderness of left ovary, diminution of sexual desire.
- FGS_3 ➲ Epilepsy from ovarian irritation.
- FGS_4 ➲ Metrorrhagia from reflex irritation, or of nervous origin.
- FGS_5 ➲ Menorrhagia from ovarian irritation caused by strong sexual desire.
- FGS_6 ➲ Flooding, especially in young women.
- FGS_7 ➲ Epileptic attacks at or near menstrual periods.
- FGS_8 ➲ Nymphomania.
- FGS_9 ➲ Sterility from excessive sexual indulgence.
- FGS_{10} ➲ Aversion to coition; menses scanty.
- FGS_{11} ➲ During menses: epileptic spasms, nymphomania, itching, burning, and excitement in-vulva, pudenda, and clitoris.
- MGS_1 ➲ Desire lessened even to impotence.
- MGS_2 ➲ Sensual and lascivious fancies and dreams.
- MGS_3 ➲ Spermatorrhoea, before paralytic symptoms have set in.
- US_1 ➲ Diabetes, the urine is loaded with sugar.
- US_2 ➲ Dribbling of urine at beginning of stool.
- US_3 ➲ Incontinence of urine.
- LS_1 ➲ Fidgety hands, busy twitching of fingers.
- LS_2 ➲ Cannot stand erect, leg weak.
- S_{N-1} ➲ Acne of face, pustules.
- S_{N-2} ➲ Psoriasis.
- PG_1 ➲ Diminished sensation in fauces, larynx, urethra, entire body; staggering, uncertain gait; feels as if the legs are uncontrollable when walking.

Modalities

Aggravation

- ➲ Mental exertions.
- ➲ Emotions.
- ➲ Sexual excess.

Amelioration

- ➲ When occupied mentally or physically.

Relations

- ➲ FOLLOWS WELL: Cact.
- ➲ ANTIDOTES: Camph; Helon; Nux-v; Zinc.

Kali carbonicum

- PROVED BY: Hahnemann.
- DURATION: 40-50 days.
- COMMON NAME: Potassium Carbonate ($K_2O_2 Co_2$).
- FAMILY/KINGDOM: Minerals.
- RELATION COLD/HEAT: Chilly.
- MIASM: Psora.
- DIATHESIS: Tubercular.
- TEMPERAMENT: Irritable.
- SOURCE: Tincture of $K_2O_2 Co_2$.
- SPHERES OF ACTION: Respiratory, mucus membrane, ovaro–uterine system.
- SUMMARY OF INDICATIONS: Pain syndromes–low backache–menstrual disorders–bronchitis.

THERAPEUTIC PICTURE OF DRUG

C_{N-1} ➲ For disease of old people, dropsy and paralysis With dark hair. Lax fibre, inclined to obesity.

M_{D-1} ➲ Great aversion to being alone.

M_{D-2} ➲ Despondent, Alternating moods.

M_{D-3} ➲ Very Irritable, Full of fear & imaginations.

H_{D-1} ➲ One-sided headache, with nausea.

H_{D-2} ➲ Pressing pain in back of head.

H_{D-3} ➲ Dreat dryness of hair, falls out.

H_{D-4} ➲ Headache from riding in cold wind.

SO_1 ➲ Bag-like swelling between the upper eyelids and eyebrows.

SO_2 ➲ Weak eye after coition, pollution, abortion, measles.

SO_3 ➲ Stitching in ears.

SO_4 ➲ Noises in the ear after a cold drink.

DS_1 ➲ Stitching in the pit of stomach, anxiety.

DS_2 ➲ Pit of stomach swollen, tense, sensitive to touch.
DS_3 ➲ Cutting, shooting, darking all over the abdomen.
RS_1 ➲ Cough on moving arm.
RS_2 ➲ Dry cough esp. at night and evening.
RS_3 ➲ Cough with sputum of masses of blood and pus.
RS_4 ➲ Hydrothorax.
RS_5 ➲ Cough: Spasmodic with gagging or vomiting of Ingesta.
FGS_1 ➲ Feels, badly, weak before menstruation, backache before and during menses.
FGS_2 ➲ Labour pain insufficient, violent backache, wants the back press (Caust.).
FGS_3 ➲ Pruritus.
FGS_4 ➲ Exaggerated sexual desire.
FGS_5 ➲ Cystic tumors of ovaries.
MGS_1 ➲ Sexual desire excessive with burning sensation.
MGS_2 ➲ After coition, weak esp. the eyes.
MGS_3 ➲ Scrotum feels as if bruised.
US_1 ➲ Pressure on bladder long before urine comes.
US_2 ➲ After micturition, burning in urethra.
LS_1 ➲ Backs and legs give out.
LS_2 ➲ Soles very sensitive.
LS_3 ➲ Pain from hip to knee, pain in knee.
B_{K-1} ➲ Small of back feels weak.
B_{K-2} ➲ Severe backache during pregnancy.
B_{K-3} ➲ Hip disease.
PG_1 ➲ Pain-stitiching, darting, worse lying on affected side.

Modalities

Aggravation

- ➲ Afer coition, At rest in cold weather.
- ➲ From soup & coffee.

Amelioration

- ➲ When occupied mentally or physically.
- ➲ Warm weather.
- ➲ By rocking.

Relations

- ➲ COMPARE: Bry; Lyc; Nat-m; Nit-acid.
- ➲ COMPLEMENTARY: Carb-veg; Nux.
- ➲ FOLLOWS WELL: Ac- Nit; Ac-flour; Ars; Lyco.
- ➲ ANTIDOTES: Camph; Helon; Coff; Dulc.

Kalium hydriodicum

- ➲ DURATION: 20-30 days.
- ➲ COMMON NAME: Iodide of Potassium.
- ➲ FAMILY/KINGDOM: Minerals.
- ➲ DIATHESIS: Haemorrhagic.
- ➲ SOURCE: K.I. Solution. Trituration of K.I.
- ➲ SPHERES OF ACTION: Fibrous & Connective tissues.

THERAPEUTIC PICTURE OF DRUG

M_{D-1} ➲ Sad, anxious, harsh temper.
M_{D-2} ➲ Irritable.
H_{D-1} ➲ Congestion of the head, heat and throbbing.
H_{D-2} ➲ Falling out of hair.
H_{D-3} ➲ Headache, at 5: 00 A.M., inability to find a resting-place.
H_{D-4} ➲ Hard lumps on skull with headache.
SO_1 ➲ Burning in the eyes, they secrete a purulent mucus.
SO_2 ➲ Oedema of eyelids, with lachrymation.
SO_3 ➲ Violent epistaxis, after mercury.
DS_1 ➲ Food tasteless.
DS_2 ➲ Hiccough, gulping up of large quantities of air.
DS_3 ➲ Cutting and burning around umbilicus.
DS_4 ➲ Faintness at epigastrium.
RS_1 ➲ Expectoration like soap-suds, greenish.
RS_2 ➲ Inclination to cough.
RS_3 ➲ Spasmodic croup in morning.
RS_4 ➲ Provocation in larynx to dry cough.
RS_5 ➲ Dry, hacking cough, afterwards copious, greenish-exectoration.
FGS_1 ➲ Menses late, profuse.

FGS_2 ➲ During menses Uterus feels as if squeezed.

FGS_3 ➲ Corrosive leucorrhoea with subacute inflammatory conditions of the womb in young married women.

FGS_4 ➲ Fibroid tumors, metritis, subinvolution, hypertrophy, [1x or 1gr. Crude, 3 times a day]

FGS_5 ➲ Menstruation that had been suppressed six months flowed profusely, with pain in abdomen and diarrhoea.

FGS_6 ➲ Pressure in uterus when walking> sitting, with dragging pain.

LS_1 ➲ Rheumatism of knees with effusion.

LS_2 ➲ Left shoulder feels bruised.

LS_3 ➲ Pain as if bruised in the left instep.

LS_4 ➲ Sciatica, cannot stay in bed.

S_{N-1} ➲ Acne, hydroa.

S_{N-2} ➲ Purple spots, worse on legs.

S_{N-3} ➲ Rough nodules all over, worse any covering, heat of body intense.

Modalities

Aggravation

- ➲ Warm clothing.
- ➲ Warm room.
- ➲ At night.
- ➲ Damp weather.

Amelioration

- ➲ Motion.
- ➲ Open air

Relations

- ➲ COMPARE: Mez; Sulph; Merc; Iod.
- ➲ ANTIDOTES: Am-m; Ars; Chin; Merc; Rhus.t; Sulph; Valer.

Kalium muriaticum

➲ PROVED BY: Central Council for research in Homoeopathy, Govt. of India.
➲ COMMON NAME: Potassium Chloride Kel.
➲ SPHERES OF ACTION: On blood carpuscles, muscles Nerve–Brain cells.

THERAPEUTIC PICTURE OF DRUG

M_{D-1} ➲ Patient imagines, he must starve.
H_{D-1} ➲ Crusta Lactea, Dandruff.
H_{D-2} ➲ In meningitis.
SO_1 ➲ Parenchymatous keratitis, cataract.
SO_2 ➲ Deafness from swelling of external ear.
SO_3 ➲ Closed Eustachian tubes.
DS_1 ➲ Mapped tongue.
DS_2 ➲ Sensation as if a tumour growing on tongue.
DS_3 ➲ Want of appetite.
DS_4 ➲ Constipation, light coloured stools denoting want to bile, sluggish action of liver.
DS_5 ➲ Diarrhoea after fatty food.
FGS_1 ➲ Menses too late or suppressed, checked or too early, excessive discharge, dark clotted, or tough black blood like tar.
FGS_2 ➲ Leucorrhoea–discharge of milky- white mucus, thick, non–irritating bland.
FGS_3 ➲ Morning sickness, with vomiting of white phlegm.
FGS_4 ➲ Bunches in breast feel quite soft and are tender.
MGS_1 ➲ In bubo for the soft swelling, and in soft chancres.
MGS_2 ➲ Gonorrhoea and orchitis resulting from a suppression of same.
S_{N-1} ➲ Acne, erythema, eczema and other eruption on skin.
S_{N-2} ➲ Burns of all degrees.

S_{N-3} ➲ Warts on hands.

S_{N-4} ➲ Dry flour-like scales in skin.

Modalities

Aggravation

➲ Rich food.

➲ Fat.

➲ Motion.

Relations

➲ COMPARE: Bell; Bry; Mercur; Puls.

Kreosotum

- ➲ PROVED BY: Wahle.
- ➲ DURATION: 15-20 days.
- ➲ COMMON NAME: Kreosote.
- ➲ RELATION COLD/HEAT: Chilly.
- ➲ MIASM: Psora and syphilis.
- ➲ DIATHESIS: Haemorrhagic & Scorbutic.
- ➲ TEMPERAMENT: Irritable.
- ➲ SOURCE: A product of distillation of wood Tar. ($C_3H_{10}O_2$).
- ➲ SPHERES OF ACTION: Lymphatic system and mucous membrane of female generative organs and digestive tract, skin and teeth.
- ➲ SUMMARY OF INDICATIONS: Skin and gum disease–menstrual disorders–incontinence of urine.

THERAPEUTIC PICTURE OF DRUG

C_{N-1} ➲ Ladies having dark complexion.

C_{N-2} ➲ Tall, slender, ill developed, overgrown, very tall for her age.

C_{N-3} ➲ Children are old looking, wrinkled, scrofulous with rapid emaciation and difficult dentition.

M_{D-1} ➲ Music causes weeping and Palpitations.

M_{D-2} ➲ Vanishing of thought; stupid, forgetful, Peevish, irritable.

DS_1 ➲ Toothache: extending to the temples and to the left side of face; drawing, extending to inner ear and temples.

DS_2 ➲ Very painful dentition; teeth being to decay as soon as they appear; dark specks on teeth, commencing decay.

DS_3 ➲ Nausea; vomiting of food several hours after eating; of sweetish water in the morning.

DS_4 ➲ Sensation of coldness, as if ice water is in the stomach.

DS_5 ➲ Nausea, during pregnancy; constant inclination to vomit with doing so.

DS_6 ➲ Cholera infantum in connection with painful dentition, green stools, nausea, dry skin, exhaustion etc.

DS_7 ➲ Diarrhoea; very offensive; dark brown; bloody, fetid stool.

FGS_1 ➲ Post climacteric diseases of women.

FGS_2 ➲ Menses: too early, profuse, protracted; Pain during, but < after it; flow on lying down, cease on sitting or walking about; cold drinks relieve menstrual Pains; flow intermits, at times almost ceasing, then commencing again.

FGS_3 ➲ Leucorrhoea acrid, corrosive, offensive, worse between periods; has the odour of green corn; stiffens like starch, stains the linen yellow.

FGS_4 ➲ Lochia: dark, brown, lumpy, offensive, acrid; almost ceases, then freshens up again.

FGS_5 ➲ Violent corrosive itching of Pudenda and Vagina.

FGS_6 ➲ Desire for coition, in females, especially in morning.

FGS_7 ➲ After coition, pain, as of excoriatiation, and hard knottiness in neck of uterus, or swelling of the genital parts with burning pains.

FGS_8 ➲ After coition discharge of dark blood the next day.

FGS_9 ➲ Before and during menses: Roaring in the head; also humming and difficulty of hearing.

US_1 ➲ Diminished secretion; though drinking much; frequent urging, especially at night, must rise, though but small quantity passes.

US_2 ➲ Frequent urging with copious pale discharge; at night cannot get out of bed quick enough.

US_3 ➲ Wets bed at night; dreams he is urinating properly.

US_4 ➲ Urine: chestnut brown; clouded; reddish, with red sediment; depositing white sediment; colourless; fetid.

US_5 ➲ During micturition, burning between the labia.

PG_1 ➲ Burning pains; worse taking or exertion, better lying on the unaffected side; nervous excitable.

PG_2 ➲ Haemorrhages; small wounds bleed much.

PG_3 ➲ Pains, as from excoriation and ulceration; painful paralytic sensation; pulling and shooting pains.

PG_4 ➲ Corrosive, foetid, ichorous discharges from mucus membranes; vitality greatly depressed.

Modalities

Aggravation

- ➲ In the open air.
- ➲ Cold weather.
- ➲ When exposed to cold.

- From washing or bathing with cold water.
- Especially when lying down.

Amelioration

- Generally better from warmth, warm food.
- Motion.

Relations

FOLLOWS WELL:	Ars; Bell; Calc; Kali-C; Lyc; Nit-ac; Nux-v; Rhus-t; Sep; Sulph.
ANTIDOTES:	Aco; Nux-v.
INIMICALS:	After carb-v.

Lac canium

- ➲ PROVED BY: Swan.
- ➲ TEMPERAMENT: Irritable.
- ➲ COMMON NAME: Dog's milk.
- ➲ SPHERES OF ACTION: Mucous membrane, female urogenital system, uterus, cervix, throat and mind.
- ➲ SUMMARY OF INDICATIONS: Anxiety–amnesia–tonsillitis–pharyngitis–Priapism–for termination of lactation–mastitis.

THERAPEUTIC PICTURE OF DRUG

M_{D-1} ➲ Vary forgetful, In writing, makes mistakes.
M_{D-2} ➲ Despondent, thinks her disease incurable.
M_{D-3} ➲ Attack of Rage, vision of snakes. Thinks himself of little consequence.
M_{D-4} ➲ Very forgetful, absent minded.
H_{D-1} ➲ Blurred vision, nausea and vomiting at height of attack of headache.
H_{D-2} ➲ Sharp pain like a stab in right temple, at 7.00 P.M.
H_{D-3} ➲ Pain in forehead, afternoon, first left side.
SO_1 ➲ Noises in ears.
SO_2 ➲ Nose, bloody pus discharged.
SO_3 ➲ Drooling in diphtheria.
SO_4 ➲ Watery discharge, followed by dry sensation in nose.
DS_1 ➲ Cracking of jaw while eating.
DS_2 ➲ Pain in abdomen intermittent.
DS_3 ➲ Sensation while walking as if abdomen would burst.
DS_4 ➲ Profuse diarrhoea with colic pain.
DS_5 ➲ Frequent desire for stool all through provings.
DS_6 ➲ Sinking at epigastrium, faintness in stomach.
FGS_1 ➲ Menses too early, profuse, flow in gushes.
FGS_2 ➲ Breasts swollen, painful before and better on appearance of menses.

- FGS_3 ➲ Mastitis, worse, least jar.
- FGS_4 ➲ Helps to dry up milk.
- FGS_5 ➲ Sexual organ easily excited.
- MGS_1 ➲ Sexual desire quite marked.
- US_1 ➲ Urination causes intense pain in the urethra soon passing off.
- US_2 ➲ Nocturnal enuresis, a specific.
- LS_1 ➲ Sciatica right side.
- LS_2 ➲ Pain in arms of fingers.
- LS_3 ➲ Burning in palm and soles.
- LS_4 ➲ Backache, spine very sensitive to touch or pressure.
- PG_1 ➲ Chronic "Blue" condition, everything seems so dark that it can grow to darker.

Modalities

Aggravation

- ➲ Morning of one day & the evening of next.

Amelioration

- ➲ Cold & cold drinks.
- ➲ Rest & lying down.

Relations

- ➲ COMPARE: Lach; Con; Lac-felinum.
- ➲ SIMILAR: Apis; Lachesis; Murex.

Lac vaccinum defloratum

- ➲ PROVED BY: Dr. Swan.
- ➲ COMMON NAME: Skimmed Milk (Cow's).
- ➲ RELATION COLD/HEAT: Chilly.
- ➲ MIASM: Psora and Syphilis.
- ➲ SUMMARY OF INDICATIONS: Headache–vomiting–constipation–globus hystericus–menstrual disorders.

THERAPEUTIC PICTURE OF DRUG

C_{N-1} ➲ Pale, sickly, anaemic look, wornout, wasted womens with sallow complexion.

M_{D-1} ➲ Despondent, she does not care to live and has no fear of death, but is sure he is going to die.

H_{D-1} ➲ Migraine: Intense throbbing, with nausea, vomiting, blindness and obstinate constipation; worse, noise, light, motion, during menses with great prostation and better by pressure and bandaging the head tightly.

H_{D-2} ➲ Despondent; Pain begins in the forehead and radiates to the occiput, in the morning, on rising.

DS_1 ➲ Nausea and vomiting and a sensation of deathly sickness, worse from movement or rising up in bed.

DS_2 ➲ Vomiting first of undigested food, intensely acid, then of bitter water; of pregnancy.

DS_3 ➲ Violent pain in pit of stomach, seldom lower, brought on by fatique.

DS_4 ➲ Constipation: with chronic headache; most powerful purgatives were of no avail; faeces dry and hard, passed with great straining, lacerating anus, extorting cries and passing considerable blood.

FGS_1 ➲ Menses delayed a week with congestion of blood to head, coldness of hands, nausea, and vertigo.

FGS_2 ➲ After putting hands in cold water sudden suppression on menses; pains all over, especially in head.

FGS_3 ➲ Irregular menstruation, sometime very dark and scanty, sometimes colourless water.

FGS_4 ➲ Slight yellowish leucorrhoea.

FGS_5 ➲ Morning sickness during pregnancy; deathly sickness at stomach on waking; vertigo and waterbrash on rising; constipation.

FGS_6 ➲ Decrease in size of breast.

FGS_7 ➲ Diminished secretion of milk.

PG_1 ➲ Great lassitude and disinclination to exertion.

PG_2 ➲ Disease with faulty and defective nutrition with reflex affections of nervous centers.

PG_3 ➲ Great restlessness and extreme and protracted suffering from loss of sleep at night.

PG_4 ➲ Sensation: as if cold air was blowing on her, even while covered up; as if sheets were damp.

PG_5 ➲ Feels completely tired out and exhausted, whether she does anything or not; great fatique from walking.

Modalities

Aggravation

- ➲ In morning on rising.
- ➲ Noise, light, motion.
- ➲ During menses.
- ➲ Conversation.

Amelioration

- ➲ Pressure, tight bandaging.
- ➲ Profuse urination.
- ➲ Cold application.

Relations

- ➲ COMPARE: Nat–Mur.

Lachesis mutus

- ➲ PROVED BY: Hering.
- ➲ DURATION: 20-30 days.
- ➲ COMMON NAME: Surukuku Snake Poison.
- ➲ FAMILY/KINGDOM: Ophidia.
- ➲ RELATION COLD/HEAT: Hot.
- ➲ MIASM: Psora.
- ➲ DIATHESIS: Haemorrhagic.
- ➲ TEMPERAMENT: Melancholic & sad.
- ➲ SPHERES OF ACTION: Mind, cardio–vascular, skin, mucus membrane, heart, respiratory organ, female genital organ.
- ➲ SUMMURY OF INDICATIONS: Headache–Constipation–epilepsy–narcolepsy–snake bite.

THERAPEUTIC PICTURE OF DRUG

C_{N-1} ➲ Thin emaciated subject during & after climacteric age, who have changed both mentally & physically by these, illness, to women having disposition to low spirit, blue and purple look.

M_{D-1} ➲ Mental excitability, ecstasy with almost prophetic, perceptions, with a vivid imagination, great loquacity, want to walk all the time, jumps from one idea to another, one word often leads into another story.

M_{D-2} ➲ Mania after over studying.

M_{D-3} ➲ Proud, jealous, suspicious.

M_{D-4} ➲ Suicidal mood, tired to life

H_{D-1} ➲ Pain at root of nose.

H_{D-2} ➲ Vertigo chiefly on waking in morning.

H_{D-3} ➲ Intoxication, stupor and loss of consciousness.

H_{D-4} ➲ Momentary vertigo on closing the eye.
H_{D-5} ➲ Softening of brain and its membranes.
SO_1 ➲ Haemorrhages into interior chamber.
SO_2 ➲ Photophobia, over-sensitive to light.
SO_3 ➲ Ear sensitive to wind.
SO_4 ➲ Dryness of ear, cerumen, scanty, too hard and too pale.
SO_5 ➲ Nose-bleed in amenorrhoea, typhus.
SO_6 ➲ Redness of the point of nose.
DS_1 ➲ Sore, worse left side, swallowing liquids.
DS_2 ➲ Pain into the ear.
DS_3 ➲ Collar and neck band must be vary loose.
DS_4 ➲ Burning like fire in hypogastric and lumber region.
DS_5 ➲ Thin offensive stools.
DS_6 ➲ Rectum prolapsed and tumefied.
RS_1 ➲ Has to cough hard and long before he can raise.
RS_2 ➲ Spiting large quantities of rope mucus.
RS_3 ➲ Breathing almost stops on falling asleep.
RS_4 ➲ Chest feels contricted.
FGS_1 ➲ Menses at regular time, too short, scanty, feebly pains all relieved by the flow, always better during menses.
FGS_2 ➲ Climacteric troubles, palpitation, flashes of heat, haemorrhages, vertex headache, fainting spells, worse, pressure of clothes.
FGS_3 ➲ Left ovary very painful & swollen, indurated.
FGS_4 ➲ Mammae inflamed, bluish.
MGS_1 ➲ Sexual excitement.
MGS_2 ➲ Onanism with epilepsy.
LS_1 ➲ Coccyx and sacrum pain, especially on rising from sitting posture.
B_{K-1} ➲ Neuralgia of coccyx, worse rising from sitting posture.
B_{K-2} ➲ Pain in small of back, with constipation.
F_{R-1} ➲ Chill, runs up the back to head.
F_{R-2} ➲ Chill at night, flushes of heat by day.
F_{R-3} ➲ Sweat cold, stain, yellow, bloody, staining red.
PG_1 ➲ All symptoms worse after sleep, or the aggravation wakes him from sleep, sleep into the aggravation, in morning on waking.
PG_2 ➲ Left side principally affected, disease begin on the left and go to the right side.

Modalities

Aggravation

- After sleep.
- Heat in general, extremes of Tap.
- Alcohol, acid, quinine, mercury.
- Summer & heat of sun.

Amelioration

- With appearance of discharge & cold application.

Relations

- COMPLEMENTARY: Hepar; Lyco; Nitric acid.
- FOLLOWS WELL: Acon; Ars; Carb-v; Lyco; Nux.
- ANTIDOTES: Alum; Bell; Hepar; Marc; Nit Acid.
- INIMICALS: Ac-acid; Ac-carbol; Ac-Nitric; Dulc; Psor.

Ledum palustre

- PROVED BY: Hahnemann.
- DURATION: 30 days.
- COMMON NAME: Marsh Tea.
- FAMILY/KINGDOM: Ericaceae.
- RELATION COLD/HEAT: Chilly.
- MIASM: Boric and Syphilitic.
- DIATHESIS: Rheumatic and gouty.
- SOURCE: Tincture of dried small twings and leaves collected after flowering begins.
- SPHERES OF ACTION: Skin, serous and mucous membranes, fibrous tissues, circulatory system and joints.
- SUMMARY OF INDICATIONS: Puncture wounds–confusions–rheumatic disorders. Prevents tetanus.

THERAPEUTIC PICTURE OF DRUG

C_{N-1} ➲ Constitutions abused by alcohol.

M_{D-1} ➲ Imperturbable gravity; morose and peevish humor.

M_{D-2} ➲ Tendency to anger and rage; vehement angry mood.

SO_1 ➲ Aching in eyes.

SO_2 ➲ Extravasations of blood in the lids, conjunctiva, aqueous or vitreous.

SO_3 ➲ Confused wounds; cataract with gout.

LS_1 ➲ Rheumatic pain in the joints of the arms.

LS_2 ➲ Gouty nodosities on the hand and finger-joints; drawing pain from hands upward.

LS_3 ➲ Rheumatic pains going from below upward, joints pale, swollen, tense, hot; with stinging, drawing pains; worse from warmth of bed and bed covering, from motion, and in the evening before 12 P.M.

LS_4 ➲ Swelling of the feet and up to the knees.

LS_5 ➲ Pain of the soles of the feet, as if bruised, when walking.

LS_6 ➲ Ball of great toe painful, swollen, soles very sensitive; tendons stiff.

S_{N-1} ➲ Itching and gnawing in skin, with burning after having scratched; itching worse by scratching.

S_{N-2} ➲ Eruption, like rot in sheep, with desquamation; bluish spots over body, like Petechiae.

S_{N-3} ➲ Oedematous swellings, also of skin of whole body.

PG_1 ➲ Emaciation of affected parts.

PG_2 ➲ Coldness and want of vital heat.

PG_3 ➲ Complaints of people who are cold all the time, in bed, in the house; they always feel cold and chilly.

PG_4 ➲ Long-remaining discolouration after injuries; "black and blue" places become green.

Modalities

Aggravation

- ➲ Warm applications.
- ➲ Heat of the bed.
- ➲ Night.

Amelioration

- ➲ Cold applications.

Relations

- ➲ COMPARE: Arn; Crot-t; Ham; Bellis, Ruta.
- ➲ FOLLOW WELL: Aco; Bell; Bry; Chel; Nux-v; Puls; Rhus-t; Sulph.
- ➲ ANTIDOTES: Camph.
- ➲ INIMICAL: Chin.

Lilium tigrinum

- ➲ PROVED BY: W. Payne.
- ➲ DURATION: 14-20 days.
- ➲ COMMON NAME: Tiger Lily.
- ➲ FAMILY/KINGDOM: Liliaceae.
- ➲ RELATION COLD/HEAT: Hot.
- ➲ MIASM: Psora.
- ➲ TEMPERAMENT: Irritable.
- ➲ SOURCE: Tincture of fresh stalk, leaves and flowers.
- ➲ SPHERES OF ACTION: On Pelvic organ such as uterus, Fellopian tubes ovaries, brain.
- ➲ SUMMARY OF INDICATIONS: Hysteria-mental depression-tachycardia-Palpitation- menstrual disorders.

THERAPEUTIC PICTURE OF DRUG

C_{N-1} ➲ Especially suited to unmarried women who suffer from uterine trouble.

M_{D-1} ➲ Weeping disposition, can hardly avoid weeping.

M_{D-2} ➲ Vary much timid and fearful.

M_{D-3} ➲ Profound depression of spirit, consolation aggravates the complaints.

M_{D-4} ➲ Anxious, fear some organic and incurable diseases.

H_{D-1} ➲ Wild, crazy feeling on vertax.

H_{D2} ➲ Heavy feeling in the head, with morning diarrhoea.

H_{D3} ➲ Fullness of head, heavy, dull.

SO_1 ➲ Hypermetropia, presbyopia.

SO_2 ➲ Eyes painful, sensitive to light.

SO_3 ➲ Frequent sneezing, at 10 A.M.

DS_1 ➲ Test of blood, congestion to chest.

DS_2 ➲ Loss of appetite, Aversion to bread and coffee.

DS_3 ➲ Bloated abdomen after a meal.

DS_4 ➲ Abdomen sensitive to pressure or jarring.
DS_5 ➲ Empty feeling of Abdomen and stomach.
DS_6 ➲ Tenesmus and great desire for stool but every effort resulted only in voiding a little urine.
CVS_1 ➲ Sensation as if heart was grasped in a vise.
CVS_2 ➲ Pulsations over whole body.
CVS_3 ➲ Cold feeling about heart.
CVS_4 ➲ Angina pectoris with pain in right arm.
FGS_1 ➲ Menses early, scanty, dark, clotted, offensive.
FGS_2 ➲ Flow only when moving about.
FGS_3 ➲ Bearing down sensation with urgent desire for stool, as though all organs would scape.
FGS_4 ➲ Congestion of uterus, prolapse and anteversion.
FGS_5 ➲ Constant desire to support parts externally.
FGS_6 ➲ Pain in ovaries and down thighs.
FGS_7 ➲ Acrid down leucorrdoea.
FGS_8 ➲ Smarting in labia.
FGS_9 ➲ Pruritus pudendi.
FGS_{10} ➲ Must kept busy to repress sexual desire.
LS_1 ➲ Dull pain in left shoulder.
LS_2 ➲ Arms and hands stiff and hot, as if parched.
LS_3 ➲ Pain in right hip, extending down the thigh.
LS_4 ➲ Cannot walk on uneven ground.
LS_5 ➲ Pain in ankle joint.
PG_1 ➲ Aimless, harried motion.

Modalities

Aggravation

➲ Consolation.

➲ Warm Room.

Amelioration

➲ Fresh air.

Relations

➲ COMPARE: Cact; Helon; Murex; Sep.

➲ ANTIDOTES: Helon; Nux; Puls; Plat.

Lycopodium clavatum

- PROVED BY: Hahnemann.
- DURATION: 40-50 days.
- COMMON NAME: Wolf's Claw (Club Moss).
- FAMILY/KINGDOM: Lycopodiaceae.
- RELATION COLD/HEAT: Sensitive to cold.
- MIASM: Anti-psoric, anti-syphilitic and anti-sycotic.
- DIATHESIS: Lithic and uric acid diathesis.
- SOURCE: Trituration of spores.
- SPHERES OF ACTION: Mucous membrane of genito-urinary tract, respiratory tract, digestive system, kidney etc.
- SUMMARY OF INDICATIONS: Chronic gastritis–constipation–sexual disorders.

THERAPEUTIC PICTURE OF DRUG

C_{N-1} ➲ It has Grauvogl's carbonitrogenoid constitution.

C_{N-2} ➲ Suited to especially for extremes of life, both for children and old people.

C_{N-3} ➲ For womens intellectually keen, but physically weak.

C_{N-4} ➲ Upper part of body emaciated, lower part semi-dropsical.

C_{N-5} ➲ Predisposed to lung and hepatic affections.

M_{D-1} ➲ Weak memory, confused thoughts; spells or writes wrong words and syllables.

M_{D-2} ➲ Failing brain power; cannot bear to see anything new; cannot read what he writes.

M_{D-3} ➲ Sadness in the morning on awaking.

M_{D-4} ➲ Silent, melancholy, and Peevish humour; despair of eternal salvation.

M_{D-5} ➲ Dread of men; desires to be alone, or else aversion to solitude.

M_{D-6} ➲ Irritability and susceptibility, with tears.

M_{D-7} ➲ Avaricious, greedy, miserly, malicious, pusillanimous.

M_{D-8} ➲ Weeps all day, cannot calm herself; very sensitive even cries when thanked.

DS_1 ➲ Tongue is darted out and oscillates to and fro (Angiana; Tonsillitis).

DS_2 ➲ Tongue distended, giving patient a silly expression (Angina; Diphtheria).

DS_3 ➲ Swelling and suppuration of tonsils, going from right to left.

DS_4 ➲ Vomits: food and bile; coagulated blood; sour substances; dark greenish masses after eating or drinking.

DS_5 ➲ Gastric affections: excessive accumulation of flatulence; constant sensation of satiety; good appetite, but a few mouthfuls fill up to the throat, and he feels bloated.

DS_6 ➲ Great fermentation in the abdomen; rumbling, croaking, rattling; also with colic and discharge of much flatus; brown spots on the abdomen.

DS_7 ➲ Hernia (right side); crural hernia, females.

DS_8 ➲ Constipation: since Puberty; since last confinement; when away from home; of infants; with stool hard; ineffectual urging from a contraction of the sphincter ani; after stool feeling as if much remained unpassed, or great distress in the rectum; much flatulence.

DS_9 ➲ Discharge of blood from genitals during every stool.

DS_{10} ➲ Excessive accumulation of flatus.

DS_{11} ➲ Good appetite, but a few mouthfuls fill up to the throat and then patient feels bloated and uncomfortable.

RS_1 ➲ Cough excited by a tickling, or as if produced by the vapour of sulphar or, by taking a deep inspiration, generally with a yellowish grey and saltiest expectoration, sometime with great weakness of stomach, fever nocturnal sweat, and emaciation.

RS_2 ➲ Cough with expectoration through the day and without expectoration during the night; cough worse: from 4 to 8 P.M., on alternate days.

RS_3 ➲ Catarrh of the chest in infants seems full of mucus, rattling.

RS_4 ➲ Neglected Pneumonia; especially with continuing hepatization and Purulent sputum. (Typhoid Pheumonia).

RS_5 ➲ Fauces brownish-red; diphtheritic Patches spreading from right tonsil to left, or descending from the nose; worse from cold drinks and after sleep.

RS_6 ➲ Continuous pressure on the chest; raw feeling in ternallyl tearing under clavicles, tension.

FGS_1 ➲ Dryness of vagina; burning in; during and after coition; Physometra.

FGS_2 ➲ Foetus appears to be turning somersaults.

FGS_3 ➲ Menses too late; last too long; too profuse.

FGS_4 ➲ Pain in the right ovarian region.

FGS_5 ➲ Varicose veins of Pudenda.

FGS_6 ➲ Leucorrhoea, acrid, with burning in the vagina.

FGS_7 ➲ Discharge of blood from genitals during stool.

FGS_8 ➲ Swelling of the breasts with nodosites.

FGS_9 ➲ Excoriation and moist scabs on nipples.

FGS_{10} ➲ Stinging in nipples.

FGS_{11} ➲ Milk in breasts without being pregnant.

MGS_1 ➲ Impotence: Penis small, cold and relaxed; also from Poisoning with chlorine; after onanism.

MGS_2 ➲ Erections feeble; during and embrace falls asleep.

MGS_3 ➲ Soreness between the scrotum and thigh.

MGS_4 ➲ Excessive and exhausting pollutions.

MGS_5 ➲ Itching of inner surface of the Prepuce; yellowish tumor behind the corona glandis.

US_1 ➲ Pain in the back before micturating; ceases after flow; slow in coming, must strain.

US_2 ➲ Turbid, milky urine, with an offensive, purulent sediment.

US_3 ➲ Urine: scanty, dark red, albuminous with strangury; deposits a red, sandy sediment; frequent and copious at night, scanty by day; pale.

US_4 ➲ Haematuria, from gravel or chronic catarrh.

US_5 ➲ Child cries before micturating.

PG_1 ➲ Deep-seated, progressive, chronic disease.

PG_2 ➲ Pains: aching–pressure, drawing: Chiefly right sided, 4 to 8 P.M.

PG_3 ➲ Affected on the right side and pain radiates from right to left.

PG_4 ➲ Hunger at night when waking.

PG_5 ➲ Child sleeps all day and cries all night.

PG_6 ➲ Great desire for, or marked repugnance to fresh air, with excessive sensitiveness to cool air.

PG_7 ➲ Total Prostration of strength, with feeling of the lower jaw, eyes cloudy and half closed, and slow respiration through the mouth.

PG_8 ➲ Excoriated places on the skin of children; the sore places are humid.

Modalities

Aggravation

- ➲ Nearly all diseases from 4 P.M. to 8 P.M.
- ➲ Right side.
- ➲ Heat, warmth.

Amelioration

- ➲ Warm food and drinks.
- ➲ From uncovering the head.
- ➲ Loosening the garments.

- Passing flatus.
- Motion.
- After midnight.

Relations

- COMPLEMENTARY: Iod; Lach.
- FOLLOWS WELL: Anac; Bell; Bry. Calc, Colch; Dros; Graph; hyos; Kali-c; Lach; Led; Nux-v; Phos; Puls; Sep; Sil; Stram; Ther; Verat.
- ANTIDOTES: Aco; Camph; Caus; Chamo; Coff; Graph; Puls.
- INIMICALS: After sulph; Except in cycle of sulph; Calc; Lyc; Sulph.

Lyssinum

- ➲ PROVED BY: Dr. Hering.
- ➲ COMMON NAME: The Saliva of a Rabid Dog.
- ➲ FAMILY/KINGDOM: Nosode.
- ➲ SPHERES OF ACTION: Nervous system then Oesophagus, female gnitalia.
- ➲ SUMMARY OF INDICATIONS: Hysteria–Convulsions–Sore throat–Prolapsed uterus.

THERAPEUTIC PICTURE OF DRUG

M_{D-1} ➲ Memory for single words much improved.
M_{D-2} ➲ During convulsions, mental illusions and hallucinations.
M_{D-3} ➲ Hyper sensitiveness of all the senses.
M_{D-4} ➲ Mental emotion or mortifying news, always makes her worse.
M_{D-5} ➲ Craving for salt Aversion to fat food.
H_{D-1} ➲ Headache, < by noise of running water or bright light.
H_{D-2} ➲ Headache from bites of dogs, rabid or not.
H_{D-3} ➲ Violent headache and backache.
H_{D-4} ➲ Scalp feels contracted and pinched.
SO_1 ➲ Swelling of eyelids after bits of dog.
SO_2 ➲ Fals vision, dullness of sight.
SO_3 ➲ Hearing water poured out in next room makes him very irritable and nervous.
SO_4 ➲ The great sensibility to smell of tobacco.
DS_1 ➲ Nausea and vomiting after diarrhoea.
DS_2 ➲ Vomiting throughout three days with prostration.
DS_3 ➲ Rigidity of muscles of abdomen.
DS_4 ➲ Tenesmus during and after stool.
DS_5 ➲ Stool of bloody mucus-involuntary stools.

- FGS_1 ➲ Prolapsus uteri, many cases of years' standing cure. (Sensitiveness of vagina, rendering coition, painful).
- FGS_2 ➲ Constant desire of urinate on seeing running water.
- FGS_3 ➲ Pain in left ovarian region.
- FGS_4 ➲ Severe leucorrhoea with pain in back and lower part of bowels.
- FGS_5 ➲ Catamenia, during pregnancy.
- MGS_1 ➲ Strong erections, without sexual excitement.
- MGS_2 ➲ Increased sexual desire with frequent seminal emission.
- MGS_3 ➲ Hydrocele, a trophy of testicles.
- LS_1 ➲ A pressive pain in Rt. Hip bone.
- LS_2 ➲ Cramp in arm.
- LS_3 ➲ Hand tremble so much, he can scarcely write.
- PG_1 ➲ Cannot bear heat of sun.

Modalities

Aggravation

- Sight or sound of water.
- Bright, Dazzling light.
- Carriage riding.

Relations

- COMPARE: Bell; Canth; Stram.
- ANTIDOTES: Nux-v; Bell; Camph.

Magnesia carbonica

- PROVED BY: Hahnemann.
- DURATION: 40-50 days.
- COMMON NAME: Carbonate of Magnesium $(Mg\,Co_3)_4\,Mg\,(OH)_2 + 5H_2O$.
- FAMILY/KINGDOM: Minerals.
- RELATION COLD/HEAT: Very much sensitive to cold air.
- MIASM: Psora.
- TEMPERAMENT: Nervous.
- SPHERES OF ACTION: Female genital organs and gastro-intestinal system and liver.
- SUMMARY OF INDICATIONS: Digestive disorders–diarrhoae–Menstrual disorders.

THERAPEUTIC PICTURE OF DRUG

C_{N-1} ➲ Especially suited to women having broken–down or worn–out constitution with uterine.

C_{N-2} ➲ Climacteric disorders and with lax fibres.

C_{N-3} ➲ Sour smell of the whole body.

C_{N-4} ➲ Children of irritable disposition, nervous temperament.

M_{D-1} ➲ Inquietude and fear, with trembling and heat.

M_{D-2} ➲ Anxious with perspiration all day.

M_{D-3} ➲ Uneasiness, with trembling of hands and absence of mind.

M_{D-4} ➲ Sad mood with indisposition to talk.

M_{D-5} ➲ Anxious and warm through whole body especially in head, while eating warm food.

M_{D-6} ➲ Trembling anguish, and fear, as if some accident would happen all day, going off after going to bed.

M_{D-7} ➲ Ill humour in evening.

DS_1 ➲ Spasmodic affections of the stomach and intestines, increase secretion from mucous membranes.

DS_2 ➲ Constrictive pain in the stomach.

DS_3 ➲ Pressing, spasmodic, contractive, colicky pains; relieved by green stools.

DS_4 ➲ Colic, followed by leucorrhoea. Cutting about nabel, better from emitting flatus.

DS_5 ➲ Greenish, frothy and mucous diarrhoea esp. in children, which looks like the green on a frog pond, with cutting pains.

DS_6 ➲ Stools with white floating limps, like fallow; always preceded by griping, worse on right side.

DS_7 ➲ Diarrhoea of a sour smell of children.

FGS_1 ➲ Sore throat before menses appear.

FGS_2 ➲ Before menses, coryza and nasal obstruction.

FGS_3 ➲ Menses too late and scanty, thick, dark, like Pitch; mucoid Leucorrhoea.

FGS_4 ➲ Menstrual flow only during sleep; more profuse at night, or when lying down; ceases when walking.

FGS_5 ➲ Toothache, during Pregnancy $<$ at night.

FGS_6 ➲ Heartburn: sour, belching, eructations, taste and vomiting; of pregnancy.

FGS_7 ➲ Constant headache, at each excessive menstrual period.

PG_1 ➲ Unrefreshing sleep, more tired on rising than when retiring.

PG_2 ➲ Pains: neuralgic, lightning–like, increased left side. During pregnancy increased at night.

PG_3 ➲ Pain on the vertex as if the hairs were pulled.

PG_4 ➲ Dazed feeling, packs and unpacks her clothes on a journey, without consciousness of having done so.

PG_5 ➲ Painful sensitiveness of whole body.

Modalities

Aggravation

- ➲ Milk.
- ➲ Every three weeks.
- ➲ Change of temperature.
- ➲ Rest.

Amelioration

- ➲ Warm air, but worse in warmth of bed

Relations

- ➲ COMPLEMENTARY: Cham.
- ➲ FOLLOWS WELL: Caust; Phos; Puls; Sep; Sulph.
- ➲ ANTIDOTES: Cham; Rheum; Nux-v; Puls; Merc-Viv; Ars.

Magnesia muriatica

- ➲ PROVED BY: Hahnemann.
- ➲ DURATION: 40-50 days.
- ➲ COMMON NAME: Magnesium Chloride ($MgCl_2$).
- ➲ FAMILY/KINGDOM: Mineral.
- ➲ RELATION COLD/HEAT: Chilly Patient.
- ➲ MIASM: Psora.
- ➲ SOURCE: Trituration of $MgCl_2$.
- ➲ SUMMARY OF INDICATIONS: Women's disorders–Constipation–Liver disorders.

THERAPEUTIC PICTURE OF DRUG

C_{N-1} ➲ Especially adopted to disease of women, spasmodic and Hysterical complaints, complicated with uterine disease, who suffered for year for attack of indigestion.

M_{D-1} ➲ Anxious in the room, relived in the open air.

M_{D-2} ➲ Disinclined to talk, prefers solitude.

M_{D-3} ➲ Tearful, inclined to weep.

H_{D1} ➲ Heaviness in head, with a dizziness, which causes falling down.

H_{D-2} ➲ Congestion, with heat, painful humming and ebullition in head.

H_{D-3} ➲ Much sweating in the head.

SO_1 ➲ Nocturnal agglutination of eyelids.

SO_2 ➲ Loss of smell and taste, following catarrh.

SO_3 ➲ Shooting, acute pullings, and boring in ears.

DS_1 ➲ Throbbing in the pit of stomach.

DS_2 ➲ Regurgitation while waling.

DS_3 ➲ Diarrhoea of mucus and blood.

DS_4 ➲ Flatulent colic, forcing patient to bend double, relived by rubbing, warmth, pressure.

DS_5 ➲ Constipation–Stool hard scanty, crumbling at verge of anus, of Infants during dentition.

FGS_1 ➲ Wore from sexual exertion.

FGS_2 ➲ Menses black clotted

FGS_3 ➲ Pain in back and thighs

FGS_4 ➲ Metrorrhagia, worse at night

FGS_5 ➲ Great excitement at every period.

FGS_6 ➲ Leucorrhoea with every stool and after exercise.

LS_1 ➲ Heaviness in the leg.

LS_2 ➲ Twitching, tearing in the hip.

LS_3 ➲ Foot sweat

LS_4 ➲ Cramp in calves, at night.

LS_5 ➲ Uneasiness and tension in thighs.

LS_6 ➲ Writers' and player's cramp.

PG_1 ➲ Indurations after inflammations.

PG_2 ➲ Liability to take cold.

PG_3 ➲ Uneasiness in evening in bed on closing the eyes.

Modalities

Aggravation

- ➲ From sea bathing.
- ➲ Immediately after eating.
- ➲ Lying on right side.

Amelioration

- ➲ From pressure.
- ➲ Motion, open air (except headache).

Relations

- ➲ COMPARE: Chamomilla.
- ➲ ANTIDOTES: Cham; Camph; Nux; Ars.

Magnesia phosphorica

- ➲ PROVED BY: Hahnemann.
- ➲ COMMON NAME: Phosphate of Magnesium [$MgHPO_4 7H_2O$].
- ➲ FAMILY/KINGDOM: Minerals.
- ➲ RELATION COLD/HEAT: Chilly Patient.
- ➲ MIASM: Psora.
- ➲ TEMPERAMENT: Nervous.
- ➲ SPHERES OF ACTION: Brain, Nerves, muscles, uterus and intestine.
- ➲ SUMMARY OF INDICATIONS: Analgesic–Teething disorders–Colic–Occupational cramps–Neuralgias–Fever–Muscular weakness–Student's examination anxieties.

THERAPEUTIC PICTURE OF DRUG

C_{N-1} ➲ Especially adapted to the affection of thin, emaciated Women of a highly nervous organization.

C_{N-2} ➲ Dark complexion.

M_{D-1} ➲ Laments all the time about pain.

M_{D-2} ➲ Inability to think clearly.

M_{D-3} ➲ Sleepless on account of indigestion.

H_{D1} ➲ Headache due to excessive studying.

H_{D-2} ➲ Sensation as if the contents of the skull were liquid, as if the parts of brain were changing places or as of a cap was on the head.

H_{D-3} ➲ Vertigo on moving, falls forward on closing the eyes, better walking in open air.

H_{D-4} ➲ Aches after mental labour, with chilliness; always better by warmth and worse from 10 to 11 A.M. or 4 to 5 P.M.

DS_1 ➲ Colic with distention, better with gentle pressure and warmth.

DS_2 ➲ Colic with belching, which gives no relief.

DS_3 ➲ Toothache relieved by heat.

DS$_4$ ➲ Toothache: while riding in a carriage, worse in the cold; at night, compelling one to rise and walk about, the pain is unsupportable while at rest; during pregnancy; mostly burning, tearing, drawing, twitching, or great ulcerative pain, with twitching in the fingers and feet.

DS$_5$ ➲ Spasms or cramp of stomach, with clean tongue, as if a band was drawn tightly around the body.

FGS$_1$ ➲ Menstrual colic; Pain precedes flow.

FGS$_2$ ➲ Menses six to nine days too soon.

FGS$_3$ ➲ With menses: great weakness; intensely sore, bruised feeling all through abdomen, could hardly be up at all but was much <lying down.

FGS$_4$ ➲ Labiae swollen and at times intensely painful

FGS$_5$ ➲ Flow dark, fibrinous stringy.

FGS$_6$ ➲ Dysmenia; Pain (cutting, drawing, pressing, cramping) severe, intermittent <right side, > from heat; >by flow.

PG$_1$ ➲ This is popularly called the "homoeopathic aspirin". Magnesia phosphorica relieves any spasmodic pain, such as calf muscle cramps, menstrual cramps, biliary or intestinal colic. The pain is better with warmth.

PG$_2$ ➲ Intermittent, spasmodic pains and neuralgia.

PG$_3$ ➲ Frequent hiccoughs with heartburn.

PG$_4$ ➲ Symptoms usually worse on the right side.

PG$_5$ ➲ General muscular weakness. Writer's cramp and other occupational cramps.

PG$_6$ ➲ Sensation of a constricting band around the body, which is worse with dry or cold air.

PG$_7$ ➲ Anxieties of students and public performers.

Modalities

Aggravation

- Cold touch, cold bath.
- Motion.
- Night.
- Light touch.

Amelioration

- Warmth.
- Bending double.
- Friction, Pressure;

Relations

- COMPARE: Bell; Caul; Colo; Lyc; Puls.
- ANTIDOTES: Bell; Gels; Lach.
- SIMILAR: Kalium-Phos; Colo; Silic; Zinc-met; Dio-vill.

Medorrhinum

- PROVED BY: Swan.
- DURATION: 40 days.
- COMMON NAME: The Gonorrhoal Cocci.
- FAMILY/KINGDOM: A-Nosode.
- RELATION COLD/HEAT: Hot.
- MIASM: Sycosis.
- DIATHESIS: Rheumatic & Gouty Diathesis.
- TEMPERAMENT: Weeping, Peevish.
- SUMMARY OF INDICATIONS: Chronic arthritis–Chronic diarrhoea–infective disorders of the genito–Urinary system–nervous system disorders–impotence.

THERAPEUTIC PICTURE OF DRUG

C_{N-1} ➲ Constitutioal effects of maltreated or suppressed gonorrhoea with trembling all over, weak, fatigued and emaciated.

M_{D-1} ➲ Weakness of memory, cannot remember names, words or initial letters, has to ask name of most intimate fried, even forgets his own name.

M_{D-2} ➲ Constantly loses the thread of conversation.

M_{D-3} ➲ Anticipates death, always anticipating, feels matters most sensitively before they occur and generally correctly.

M_{D-4} ➲ Time passes too slowly.

H_{D-1} ➲ Pain circling through head and around crown.

H_{D-2} ➲ Intense headache for three days, with inflammation of eye.

H_{D-3} ➲ Pain in back of head and in right eye.

H_{D-4} ➲ Weight and pressure in vertex.

SO_1 ➲ Total deafness of both ears, with very little noise, had to used a trumpet.

SO_2 ➲ Entire loss of smell for several days.

SO_3 ➲ Nose inflamed swollen.

SO_4 ➲ Coldness of end of nose.

NS_1 ➲ Trembling allover (subjective).

DS_1 ➲ Ravenous hunger soon after eating.

DS_2 ➲ Violent pain in liver and spleen.

DS_3 ➲ Hiccough, nausea, with frontal headache, after drinking water.

DS_4 ➲ Beating as a pulse in abdomen vertically.

DS_5 ➲ Intense itching of stomach.

RS_1 ➲ Soreness in larynx, as if ulcerated.

RS_2 ➲ Sensate of lump in larynx.

FGS_1 ➲ Menses–profuse, very dark, clotted, stains difficult to washout.

FGS_2 ➲ For women, with chronic ovaritis, salpingitis, Pelvic immflamtary diseases.

FGS_3 ➲ Cellulites, fibroids, cysts, and other morbid growth of the uterus and ovaries, especially if symptoms points to malignancy, with or without sycotic origin.

FGS_4 ➲ Intense pruritus of labia & vagina < by thiniking, of it.

FGS_5 ➲ Breast & nipple sore and sensitive to touch.

FGS_6 ➲ Intense menstrual colic, with drawing up of knees and terrible bearing down labour like pain, must press feet against support, as in labour.

FGS_7 ➲ Metrorrhagia at climacteric, profuse for week &, flow, dark, clotted, offensive.

MGS_1 ➲ Emissions during sleep.

MGS_2 ➲ Intense and frequent erection day and night.

US_1 ➲ Noctural enuresis.

LS_1 ➲ Leg heavy ache all night, cannot keep them still.

LS_2 ➲ Soreness of sole.

LS_3 ➲ Rheumatic pain in right shoulder and arm.

LS_4 ➲ Small yellow spot on hand.

PG_1 ➲ Intensely restless and fidgety leg and feets. (Zinc)

PG_2 ➲ Burning of hand & feet (Lach, Sulph, want them covered and fanned).

PG_3 ➲ In satiate craving–for liquor, for sweets. (Sulph), ice, oranges, green fruits.

Modalities

Aggravation

- When thinking of it (Helon ox – avc) heat covering, thunderstorm, least movement, sweet.

Amelioration

- At the sea shore (Rev-to-Nat-mur).
- Lying on stomach.
- Damp weather.

Relations

- COMPARE: Ipecac.
- ANTIDOTES: Ipec.
- INIMICALS: Sulpher.

Mercurius solubilis

- ➲ COMMON NAME: Hahnemannis soluble mercury (Black oxide of mercury)
- ➲ FAMILY/KINGDOM: Minerals.
- ➲ SOURCE: Dimercuros ammonium nitrate Z (NH_2Hg_2) NO_3H_2O.
- ➲ SUMMURY OF INDICATIONS: Chronic infections–diarrhoea–Oral disorders–Genito–urinary disorders.

THERAPEUTIC PICTURE OF DRUG

M_{D-1} ➲ Slow in answering questions.
M_{D-2} ➲ Memory weakness and loss of will power.
M_{D-3} ➲ Weary of life.
M_{D-4} ➲ Mistrustful.
M_{D-5} ➲ Thinks she is losing her reasons.
H_{D-1} ➲ Congestion to the head.
H_{D-2} ➲ Tension about scalp, as if bandaged.
H_{D-3} ➲ Hydrocephalus, body bathed in sweat.
H_{D-4} ➲ Constant rotary motion of head, even when lying.
H_{D-5} ➲ Nocturnal aphalalgia.
SO_1 ➲ Otorrhoea: bloody, offensive discharge, with stabbing tearing pain; increased right side, at night and lying on affected side.
SO_2 ➲ Profuse, burning, acrid discharge.
SO_3 ➲ Iritis, with hypopyon.
SO_4 ➲ Pain and swelling of nasal bone and caries, with greenish fetid ulceration.
SO_5 ➲ Nose bleed at night.
DS_1 ➲ Teeth feel loose, fall out.
DS_2 ➲ Taste, bitter, sweetish, saltish.
DS_3 ➲ Inflamed, with burning, aphthous ulcers, copious, fetid, ropy salivation.
DS_4 ➲ Swelling and hardness of liver
DS_5 ➲ Complete icterus.

DS_6 ➲ Pain in abdomen, as if a caused by chill.
DS_7 ➲ Greenish, bloody stoal worse at night.
RS_1 ➲ Short-breathed on ascending or walking.
RS_2 ➲ Convulsive cough, with retching.
RS_3 ➲ Burning and tickling in the larynx with hoarseness.
DS_8 ➲ Morning sickness, with profuse salivation.
DS_9 ➲ Gums are swollen, spongy and bleeding. Tongue swollen and profuse salivation occurs, dysentery with colic and tenesmus. Epistaxis.
FGS_1 ➲ Menses profuse, with abdominal pain (dysmenorrhoea).
FGS_2 ➲ Leucorrhoea excoriating, greenish and bloody.
FGS_3 ➲ Sensation of rawness in parts.
FGS_4 ➲ Stinging pain in the ovaries.
MGS_1 ➲ Lascivious excitement, with painful nightly erections.
MGS_2 ➲ Testicles swollen, hard, shining.
MGS_3 ➲ Ulceration in the gland, with cheesy base, chancroids.
US_1 ➲ Frequent urging, greenish discharge from urethra.
US_2 ➲ Itching and burning; worse, after micturating; better, washing with cold water.
LS_1 ➲ Red and hot swelling from the elbow to the wrist.
LS_2 ➲ Nails drop off.
LS_3 ➲ Cold sweat on the feet, twitching of arm and leg.
S_{N-1} ➲ General tendency to free perspiration, but patient is not relieved thereby.
S_{N-2} ➲ Itching all over, worse at night, when arm in bed.
S_{N-3} ➲ Scabies, if some of the vesicles become pustular.

Modalities

Aggravation

- Night.
- Sleeping.
- Warmth of bed (itching aggravated).

Relations

- COMPARE: Zez; Phos; Syph; Kali-m.
- COMPLEMENTARY: Badiaga.
- ANTIDOTES: Camphora officinarum; Hep; Aur.

Murex purpurea

- ➲ PROVED BY: Petroz.
- ➲ COMMON NAME: Purple fish.
- ➲ FAMILY/KINGDOM: Muricidae.
- ➲ TEMPERAMENT: Melancholic.
- ➲ SPHERES OF ACTION: Acts esp. upon female genital organ-uterus, ovaries, gential organs.
- ➲ SUMMARY OF INDICATIONS: Female genital disorders- climacteric disorders.

THERAPEUTIC PICTURE OF DRUG

C_{N-1} ➲ Best adapted to lively affectionate women.

M_{D-1} ➲ Person of a melancholy temperament.

H_{D-1} ➲ Pain in occiput, some times very acute.

H_{D-2} ➲ Pain in left temple.

DS_1 ➲ Awful hunger and emptiness, even after a meal.

DS_2 ➲ Tensive pain in right hypochondrium.

DS_3 ➲ During stoal, bloody leucorrhoea.

FGS_1 ➲ For the suffering during climacteric (Lach., Sep., Sulph.)

FGS_2 ➲ Least contact of parts, causes violent sexual Exitement (Zin, orig).

FGS_3 ➲ Sorepain in uterus, a distinct sensation of a womb (Helon, Lyss).

FGS_4 ➲ Violent excitement in sexual organs and excessive desire for an embrace (rev. of sep).

FGS_5 ➲ Bearing down sensation, as if internal organs would be pushed out, must sit down and crossed limbs > pressure (But no sexual desire-Sepia.

FGS_6 ➲ Menses–Irregular, early, profuse, protracted large clots.

FGS_7 ➲ Leucohhoea, < Mental depression, happier when Leucorrhoea is worse.

US_1 ➲ Frequent want to urinate during day, at night with emission of colourless urine.

US_2 ➲ Slight discharge of blood when making water.

LS_1 ➲ Pain in forearm, below elbow.

LS_2 ➲ Intolerable creeping pain in right hip.

S_{N-1} ➲ Skin dry, as if about to cracked.

Modalities

Aggravation

➲ From least touch.

Amelioration

➲ When leucohhoea.

Relations

➲ COMPARE: Platina; Lilium; Sepia.

Natrum carbonicum

- PROVED BY: Hahnemann.
- DURATION: 30 days.
- COMMON NAME: Carbonate of Sodium [$Na_2 CO_3 10H_2O$].
- FAMILY/KINGDOM: Minerals.
- RELATION COLD/HEAT: Chilly Patient.
- MIASM: Psora.
- SOURCE: Sodium carbonate trituration.
- SPHERES OF ACTION: Mucous membrane and skin of the body.
- SUMMARY OF INDICATIONS: Exhaustion (physical and mental debility)–sunstroke–headaches.

THERAPEUTIC PICTURE OF DRUG

C_{N-1} ➲ Suited to women of leucophlegmatic constitution.

C_{N-2} ➲ The patient has aversion to open air and dislike of exercise, either mental or physical.

C_{N-3} ➲ Imbecility.

C_{N-4} ➲ Face pale with blue ring around the eyes.

M_{D-1} ➲ Inability to think or to perform any mental labour; causes headache; feels stupefied if she tries to exert himself; comprehension slow, difficult, imbecility.

M_{D-2} ➲ Aversion to man and society.

M_{D-3} ➲ Sadness; depression of spirits; hypochondrical mood.

M_{D-4} ➲ Irritable, excitable mood; avarice; maliciousness.

M_{D-5} ➲ Restlessness, with attacks of anxiety, especially during a thunder-storm worse from music.

M_{D-6} ➲ Sensitive to the presence of certain individuals.

H_{D-1} ➲ Headache: from slightest mental exertion; from sun or working under artificial light; with tension, in nape or occiput before menses; head feels too large, sensation as if it would burst.

H_{D-2} ➲ Headaches with the return of hot weather; vertigo from exposure to sun.

H_{D-3} ➲ Pain on the head at certain hours of the day.

RS_1 ➲ Accumulation of mucus in throat, and in Posterior nares.

RS_2 ➲ Dry cough, when coming into a warm room from out doors.

RS_3 ➲ Throat painful when swallowing and gaping.

RS_4 ➲ Cough with coldness of the left breast or chest.

RS_5 ➲ Thick, yellow, green offensive, musty, hard discharge from nose; often ceasing after a meal.

FGS_1 ➲ Induration of the cervix.

FGS_2 ➲ Pudenda sore.

FGS_3 ➲ Bearing down as if everything would come out (Prolapse) heaviness, <sitting,> by moving.

FGS_4 ➲ Menses late, scanty, like meat washings.

FGS_5 ➲ Leucorrheal discharge, offensive, irritating, preceded by colic.

FGS_6 ➲ Discharge of mucus from vagina after an embrance, causing sterility.

PG_1 ➲ Chronic effects of sunstroke; headaches with return of hot weather.

PG_2 ➲ Inclination to perspire, which may be caused by any exertion.

PG_3 ➲ Great debility: caused by heat of summer; exhaustion from least effort, mental or physical.

PG_4 ➲ Emaciation, with pale complexion, dilated Pupils, and deep coloured urine.

PG_5 ➲ Falling out of the hair.

Modalities

Aggravation

➲ Sitting.

➲ From music.

➲ In the sun.

➲ Excessive summer heat.

➲ Mental exertion.

➲ A thunderstorm, draught, change of weather.

Amelioration

➲ By moving.

➲ By boring in ears or nose.

Relations

➲ FOLLOWS WELL: Calc; Nit.ac; Nux-v; Puls; Sep; Sulph.

➲ ANTIDOTES: Ars; Camph; Nitri-spir-dul.

Natrium hypochlorosum

- ➲ COMMON NAME: Natrum Chloratum Liquor Sodae Chloratae.
- ➲ FAMILY/KINGDOM: Minerals.
- ➲ SOURCE: Liquor sodae chloratae.

THERAPEUTIC PICTURE OF DRUG

C_{N-1} ➲ Flabby, debilitated constitution.

M_{D-1} ➲ Much distressed, laugh & cries, talk in sleep.

M_{D-2} ➲ Keep her hasband awake.

M_{D-3} ➲ Very low spirited and depressed, could cry all days.

H_{D-1} ➲ Pain across forehead, extending down nose.

H_{D-2} ➲ Pain darting from temple to temple coming and going, suddenly.

SO_1 ➲ Epistaxis, dark-coloured blood comes away inclots by day and night.

SO_2 ➲ Pain in right side of face.

DS_1 ➲ Drowsy after meals.

DS_2 ➲ Swelling low in abdomen going up to chest and causing dyspnoea.

DS_3 ➲ Bloating, tight feeling across upper abdomen.

DS_4 ➲ Constipation for three days.

DS_5 ➲ Cutting pain like knives in anus, coming between 6 and 7 a.m.

FGS_1 ➲ Feeling as if uterus were pushed up on sitting down (Ferr-iod).

FGS_2 ➲ Feels as if it opened and shut.

FGS_3 ➲ Violent metrorrhagia.

FGS_4 ➲ Leucorrhoea & backache.

FGS_5 ➲ Passive, bearing down from heavy condition of uterus.

FGS_6 ➲ Womb is heavy, sodden, with tendency to prolapse.

LS_1 ➲ Pain in both hip joints and calves of legs with tingling extending to toes.

LS_2 ➲ Hand swollen every morning.

LS_3 ➲ Extreme weakness in ankles and knees.

Modalities

Aggravation

- In night.
- After meals.
- Before menstrual period.

Amelioration

- Loosening clothes.

Relations

- COMPARE: Aur; Calc; Sepia.
- ANTIDOTES: Pulsat; Guaiacum.

Natrium muriaticum

- PROVED BY: Hahnemann.
- DURATION: 40-50 days.
- COMMON NAME: Common Salt (Nacl).
- FAMILY/KINGDOM: Minerals.
- RELATION COLD/HEAT: Hot Patient.
- MIASM: Psora, Syphilis & Sycosis.
- DIATHESIS: Scrofulous.
- TEMPERAMENT: Nervous.
- SOURCE: Nacl-Trituration.
- SPHERES OF ACTION: Skin, mind, genital organs, alimentary tract, blood & lymphatic system.
- SUMMARY OF INDICATIONS: Anxiety–Migraine–Constipation–Skin disorders.

THERAPEUTIC PICTURE OF DRUG

C_{N-1} ➲ Emaciated people having shiny, oily and waxy look of the face, as if greased.

C_{N-2} ➲ Emaciation is well marked in neck with losing of flesh while living well.

C_{N-3} ➲ Cachectic appearance having blue ring around the eye.

M_{D-1} ➲ Awkward, hasty, drops things from nervous weakness.

M_{D-2} ➲ Marked disposition to weep; sad weeping mood; without cause, but consolation from other < her troubles.

M_{D-3} ➲ Phychic causes of disease; ill effects of grief, fright, anger etc.

M_{D-4} ➲ Depressed, particularly in chronic diseases.

M_{D-5} ➲ Irritable; gets into a passion about trifies.

H_{D-1} ➲ Headache: beginning with blindness with zig-zag dazzling, like lightning in eyes, ushering in a throbbing headache, which is worse from eye strain.

H_{D-2} ➲ Bursting headache; beating or stitches through to neck or chest; face red; nausea, vomiting.

H_{D-3} ➲ Throbbing as from little hammers; awakens with the headache every morning; worse from reading or talking.

H_{D-4} ➲ Headache in school-girls.

H_{D-5} ➲ Headache from sunrise till sunset, worse at midday; right eye congested; worse from light.

DS_1 ➲ Tongue: mapped with red insular patches; like ring worm on sides.

DS_2 ➲ Tongue: heavy, difficult speech; children slow in learning to talk.

DS_3 ➲ Sensation of a hair on the tongue.

DS_4 ➲ Vesicles and ulcers in mouth and on tongue, smarting and burning when touched by food.

DS_5 ➲ Constipation from inactivity of the rectum. Stool hard, difficult or crumbling; anus contracted; anus torn, bleeding, smarting, burning afterward; stitches in rectum.

DS_6 ➲ Dryness and smarting of rectum and anus; passes blood with stool.

DS_7 ➲ Haemorrhoids, with stinging pains; moisture oozes from the anus; herpetic eruption about the anus.

FGS_1 ➲ Menses irregular; usually profuse. Vagina dry.

FGS_2 ➲ Leucorrhoea acrid, watery.

FGS_3 ➲ Bearing down pains; worse in the morning.

FGS_4 ➲ Prolapsus uteri, with cutting in the urethra.

FGS_5 ➲ Vulvitis with falling off of hair.

FGS_6 ➲ Itching of external parts with falling of hair.

FGS_7 ➲ Pimples on mons veneris.

FGS_8 ➲ Nausea and vomiting during pregnancy; morning sickness with vomiting of frothy, watery phlegm.

FGS_9 ➲ During pregnancy: dysuria; albuminuria; craves salt; congestion to chest; palpitation; haemorrhoids; cough; escape of urine.

FGS_{10} ➲ Child refuses of breast; nursing sore mouth.

FGS_{11} ➲ Dull stitch beneath right nipple, also in abdomen.

FGS_{12} ➲ Breast sensitive to slightest touch.

MGS_1 ➲ Impotence with retarded emission.

MGS_2 ➲ Emission, even after coitus.

MGS_3 ➲ Excessive irritability of the sexual instinct, but with physically weakness.

MGS_4 ➲ Erections in the morning, without sexual excitement.

MGS_5 ➲ Itching, soreness and moisture between scrotum and thighs; Pus-like smegma on the glans.

US_1 ➲ Increased, involuntary when walking, coughing etc.

US_2 ➲ Pain just after maturating.

US_3 ➲ Polyuria, thirst for large quantities of water.

US_4 ➲ Has to wait long for urine to pass, especially if others are near him.

US_5 ➲ Urinal sediment like brick-dust; dark; like coffee.

US_6 ➲ After urination, burning, and cutting in urethra; Haematuria.

S_{N-1} ➲ Eczema; raw, red, inflamed, especially in edges of hair; increased from eating too much salt, at sea-shore or from an ocean voyage.

S_{N-2} ➲ Skin of hands, esp. about nails, dry, cracked; hang-nails.

S_{N-3} ➲ Whitish hives on arms and hands.

S_{N-4} ➲ Military eruption, with shooting pain.

S_{N-5} ➲ Rash over whole body, with stinging sensation in skin.

S_{N-6} ➲ Exanthema on mouth; lips; in intermittent fever where there are large exanthematous spots looking like large Peas, on lips (cold sores); lips look puffy.

S_{N-7} ➲ Warts; on Palms of hands.

S_{N-8} ➲ Urticaria, acute or chronic; over whole body, especially after violent exercise.

F_{R-1} ➲ Chill Predominates, mostly internal; hands and feet icy-cold.

F_{R-2} ➲ Intermittent Paroxysms at about 10 A.M. or 11 A.M.

F_{R-3} ➲ Heat; violent thirst, increases with fever.

F_{R-4} ➲ Coldness of the body and continuous chilliness very marked.

F_{R-5} ➲ Hydremia in chronic malarial states with weakness, constipation, loss of appetite etc.

F_{R-6} ➲ Sweats on every exertion; sweat relieving headache and other pains; though it weakness.

F_{R-7} ➲ Apyrexia: stitches about liver; great languor; emaciation; sallow complexion.

PG_1 ➲ Symptoms worse from sunrise to sunset.

PG_2 ➲ The hair falls out when touched, in nursing women.

PG_3 ➲ Great emaciation; losing flesh while living well.

PG_4 ➲ Craving for salt; great aversion to bread.

PG_5 ➲ Great liability to take cold.

PG_6 ➲ Dreams of thieves in the house, making so strong an impression that patient wakes up and can not go to sleep again until the house has been searched; fantastic dreams.

PG_7 ➲ Great relaxation of all physical and moral powers, after fatique.

Modalities

Aggravation

- At about 10 A.M. or 11 A.M.
- At thc sea-shore or from sea air.
- Heat of sun or stove.

- Mental exertion talking, writing, reading, noise, music.
- Lying down, consolation.

Amelioration

- In the open air; cold bathing.
- Missing regular meals.
- Lying on right side.
- Tight clothing, pressure on back.

Relations

- COMPLEMENTARY: Apis; Sep.
- FOLLOWS WELL: Bry; Calc; Kali-C; Puls; Rhus-t; Sep; Sulph.
- ANTIDOTES: Ars-alb; Camph; Nit-s-d; Phos.

Natrium phosphoricum

- PROVED BY: E.A. Farrington.
- COMMON NAME: Sodium Phosphate $Na_2 HPo_4 12H_2O$.
- FAMILY/KINGDOM: Minerals.
- SOURCE: Trituration & Solution of $Na_2HPO_4.12H_2O$.
- SPHERES OF ACTION: on G.I. tract, bones, glands, lungs, abdominal organ.

THERAPEUTIC PICTURE OF DRUG

M_{D-1} ➲ Imagines on walking at night, that pieces of furniture and person that he hear a foot step in the next room.

M_{D-2} ➲ Fear bad news.

M_{D-3} ➲ Easily startled, irritable, memory lost.

SO_1 ➲ Shooting pain in right cheek.

SO_2 ➲ Intense itching of face especially nose.

SO_3 ➲ Discharge of golden-yellow, creamy matter from the eyes.

SO_4 ➲ Fullness in ears, aching in right meatus.

DS_1 ➲ Thin moist coating on the tongue.

DS_2 ➲ Dyspnoea from the fat food.

DS_3 ➲ Heaviness and pressure in epigastrium.

DS_4 ➲ Sharp cutting in hypochondria and left iliac region.

DS_5 ➲ Sticking as from splinter in anus on walking.

DS_6 ➲ After coition (man) urging to stool and urination.

FGS_1 ➲ Sterility, with acrid secretion from vagina.

FGS_2 ➲ Leucorrhoea, discharge creamy or Honey-coloured or acid and watery.

FGS_3 ➲ Sour smelling, discharge from uterus.

FGS_4 ➲ Morning sickness with sour vomiting.

FGS_5 ➲ Menses too early, pale, thin watery.

MGS_1 ➲ Drawing in testes and cords.

MGS_2 ➲ Emission at night with vivid dream.

MGS_3 ➲ Great itching of scrotum, pressure anus.

LS_1 ➲ Rheumatism of knee joint.

LS_2 ➲ Synovial crepitation.

LS_3 ➲ Shooting pain from neck over right shoulder.

LS_4 ➲ Numbness of right finger, occasional darting.

Modalities

Aggravation

- ➲ Thunder & Storm, during menses.
- ➲ Afternoon and evening.

Relations

- ➲ COMPARE: Carb-Veg; Kali-c; Nux.
- ➲ ANTIDOTES: Sep.

Natrium sulphuricum

- ➲ PROVED BY: Schreter.
- ➲ DURATION: 30-40 days.
- ➲ COMMON NAME: Sodium Sulphate Glauber's Salt = ($Na_2SO_4 + 10H_2O$).
- ➲ FAMILY/KINGDOM: Minerals.
- ➲ RELATION COLD/HEAT: Very chilly patients.
- ➲ MIASM: Sycosis.
- ➲ TEMPERAMENT: Bilious.
- ➲ SOURCE: Na_2SO_4 Trituration.
- ➲ SPHERES OF ACTION: Gastro-intestinal tract, mind and genital organs, meninges, respiratory system and slain.
- ➲ SUMMARY OF INDICATIONS: Suicidal depression–Skin affections–Toothache–Post-traumatic Syndrome (PTS).

THERAPEUTIC PICTURE OF DRUG

C_{N-1} ➲ Hydrogenoid constitution, where the complaints are due to living in damp houses, basement, cellers etc.

M_{D-1} ➲ Inability to think.

M_{D-2} ➲ Satiety of life; must use all self control to prevent shooting himself.

M_{D-3} ➲ Depressed; tearful; music makes her sad.

M_{D-4} ➲ Cheerfulness, happy mood; after stool.

M_{D-5} ➲ Irritable, worse mornings.

SO_1 ➲ Eyes: granular lids; very small blisters; green pus and photophobia.

SO_2 ➲ Nosebleed during menses.

NS_1 ➲ Violent crushing gnawing pains at base of brain. (Spinal meningitis).

NS_2 ➲ Violent congestion of blood to head; delirium; opisthotonos.

NS_3 ➲ Spasms with mental irritability and delirium; head drawn back.

DS_1 ➲ Toothache better with cold water, cool air.

DS_2 ➲ Dirty, greenish-gray or brown coating on tongue.

DS_3 ➲ Diarrhoea: sudden urging, gushing, much flatus; on first rising and standing on the feet; after a spell of wet weather; living or working in basements or a damp environment.

RS_1 ➲ Sycotic Pneumonia: lower lobe of left lung; great soreness of chest, during cough, has to sit up in bed and hold the chest with both hands.

RS_2 ➲ Asthma in children, as a constitutional remedy.

RS_3 ➲ Humid asthma; rattling in the chest between 4 and 5 A.M.

RS_4 ➲ Dyspnoea during damp weather; must hold the chest when coughing.

RS_5 ➲ Cough with thick ropy, greenish expectoration; all gone sensation in the chest; constant desire to take deep, long breaths.

FGS_1 ➲ Catamenia scanty; retarded, with colic, and suppressed stools, or hard faeces.

FGS_2 ➲ Headache, and epistaxis, during catamenia.

FGS_3 ➲ The blood of the catamenia is acrid and corrosive, or coagulated, and flows only in morning.

FGS_4 ➲ Leucorrhoea: acrid, corrosive; parts inflamed, swollen, covered with vesicles, size of lentiles, filled with Pus (after Parturition).

PG_1 ➲ Sensitivity for every change of climate from dry to wet; cannot tolerate sea air or eat plants that thrive near water; suited for recovers slowly from every illness.

PG_2 ➲ Every spring skin affections reappear.

Modalities

Aggravation

- Damp basements or dwellings.
- Damp weather.
- Rest, lying down, music.

Amelioration

- Dry weather.
- Pressure.
- Changing position.
- Open air.
- Must change position frequently, but it is painful and gives some relief.

Relations

➲ COMPLEMENTARY:	Ars; Thuj.
➲ ANTIDOTES:	Nux-v.
➲ SIMILAR:	Nat-mur; Sulph-Const.

Nitricum acidum

- DURATION: 40-60 days.
- COMMON NAME: Nitric acid Aqua fortis (HNO_3).
- FAMILY/KINGDOM: Minerals.
- RELATION COLD/HEAT: Chilly Patient.
- MIASM: Psora, Syphilis, Sycosis.
- DIATHESIS: Haemorrhagic.
- TEMPERAMENT: Nervous & Irritable.
- SOURCE: Solution HNO_3.
- SPHERES OF ACTION: Blood; Mucous membrane, skin, glands, bones and gastro-intestinal tract.
- SUMMARY OF INDICATIONS: Chronic diarrhoea–Chronic Cystitis.

THERAPEUTIC PICTURE OF DRUG

C_{N-1} ➲ Ugly looking appearance; with broken down cachectic constitution.

C_{N-2} ➲ Especially suited to thin persons of rigid fibre, dark complexions, black hair and eyes, the brunette rather than the blonde-nervous temperament.

C_{N-3} ➲ Persons suffering with chronic diseases who take cold easily; are easily disposed to diarrhoea; to those who suffer with constipation.

M_{D-1} ➲ Irritable, hateful, vindictive, head strong.

M_{D-2} ➲ Hopeless despair.

M_{D-3} ➲ Sensitive to noise, pain, touch, jar.

M_{D-4} ➲ Fear of death.

M_{D-5} ➲ Great anxiety about his disease; constantly thinking about her past troubles; morbid fear of cholera (Ars.); depressed and anxious in the evening.

SO_1 ➲ Nosebleed, mornings; black, clotted; also when weeping; blood acrid.

SO_2 ➲ Ozaena, with ulcers; dirty, blood mucous from Posterior nares.

SO_3 ➲ Green casts from the nose every morning.

SO_4 ➲ Cracking in the ears when masticating.

SO_5 ➲ Hardness of hearing, from induration and swelling of tonsils; after abuse of mercury.

SO_6 ➲ Very sensitive to noise, like the rattle of wagons over pavements.

DS_1 ➲ Ulceration of tongue, with tough, ropymucus; painful pimples on the sides of the tongue.

DS_2 ➲ Cadaverous smell from the mouth; saliva fetid, acrid, makes lips sore.

DS_3 ➲ Mucous membrane of mouth, swollen ulcerated; with pricking pains, especially after abuse of mercury.

DS_4 ➲ Before stool: colic; cutting; constant pressure in rectum; constant but fruitless desire.

DS_5 ➲ During stool: nausea; tenesmus; spasm of anus; cutting in anus and rectum; acute pain in abdomen; sensation as if faeces remained and cold not be expelled; splinter-like pains in rectum with ineffectual urging; burning; tearing; palpitation of heart.

DS_6 ➲ After stool: continued urging; exhaustion; irritation, anxiety, general uneasiness; anus sore, raw; cutting, straining, shooting in rectum, continuing for hours.

DS_7 ➲ Diarrhoea: great straining but little passes, as if faces remained and cannot be expelled.

DS_8 ➲ Hemorrhage bright red, not clotted; faint from least motion; ulcer in ileo-coecal region.

DS_9 ➲ Piles: old, pendulous, ceased bleeding, but pain when touched, worse in warm weather; slimy, fissured, bleed after every stool.

DS_{10} ➲ Fissures in rectum; tearing spasmodic symptoms during stool; lancination after, even after soft stools.

FGS_1 ➲ External parts sore, with ulcers (Hep; Merc; Thuj).

FGS_2 ➲ Leucorrhoea brown, flesh coloured, watery, or stringy, offensive.

FGS_3 ➲ Hair on genitals fall out (Nat-m; Zinc).

FGS_4 ➲ Uterine haemorrhages.

FGS_5 ➲ Menses early, profuse, like muddy water, with pain in the back, hips and thighs.

FGS_6 ➲ Stitches through vagina.

FGS_7 ➲ Metrorrhagia after parturition.

FGS_8 ➲ Hard nodosities on breast. Atrophy of breasts.

US_1 ➲ Urine: scanty, dark-brown, strong-smelling, "like horse's urine;" cold, when voided; turbid, looks like the sediment of a cider barrel.

US_2 ➲ Alternation of cloudy, phosphatic urine with profuse urinary secretion in old prostatic cases.

PG_1 ➲ Great physical irritability.

PG_2 ➲ Sensation as if a band were around affected parts.

PG_3 ➲ Pains: sticking, pricking as from splinters; suddenly appearing and disappearing.

Modalities

Aggravation

- ➲ Evening and at night.
- ➲ After midnight.
- ➲ Contact.
- ➲ Change of temperature or weather (cold or hot weather).
- ➲ During sweating.
- ➲ On waking.
- ➲ While walking.

Amelioration

- ➲ While riding in a vehicle.

Relations

- ➲ COMPLEMENTARY: Ars; Calad;
- ➲ FOLLOWS WELL: Arn; Bell; Calc; Carb-v; Kali-c; Kreos; Merc; Phos; Puls; Sec; Sep; Sil; Sulph; Thuj.
- ➲ ANTIDOTES: Calc, Con; Hep; Merc; Mez; Sulph; Aco;
- ➲ INIMICALS: Lach; After Calc–Hahnemann.

Nux moschata

- PROVED BY: Helbig.
- DURATION: 40 days.
- COMMON NAME: Nutmeg.
- FAMILY/KINGDOM: Myristicaceae.
- RELATION COLD/HEAT: Chilly.
- MIASM: Psora & Sycosis.
- DIATHESIS: Rheumtic.
- TEMPERAMENT: Nervous & hysterical.
- SPHERES OF ACTION: Nervous system, mucous membrane uterus and ovaries.
- SUMMARY OF INDICATIONS: Disorders of old age- Amnesia–Insomnia–Dyspepsia–Peptic ulcers.

THERAPEUTIC PICTURE OF DRUG

C_{N-1} ➲ It is suited especially to women & children with dry skin who rarely perspire, weak old women who are delicate, sensitive and dyspeptic having hydrogenoid constitution.

M_{D-1} ➲ Weakness or loss of memory (Anac, Lac-c, Lyc).

M_{D-2} ➲ Changeable humour–one movement laughing, the next crying (Croc.; Ign) sudden change from grave to gay, from lively to serene.

M_{D-3} ➲ Thinks she has two head.

H_{D-1} ➲ Painless pulsating in head, fears to go to sleep.

H_{D-2} ➲ Apoplexy, softening of the brain.

H_{D-3} ➲ Feeling of expansion, with sleepiness.

H_{D-4} ➲ Bursting headache, better hard pressure.

SO_1 ➲ Blindness, then fainting.

SO_2 ➲ Lids heavy, stiff, feels sick, faint.

SO_3 ➲ Over sensitiveness of smell.

- SO_4 ➲ Hearing over sensitiveness, buzzing in ears.
- DS_1 ➲ Sliva like cotton.
- DS_2 ➲ Heat and burning in stomach.
- DS_3 ➲ Cramps in stomach.
- DS_4 ➲ Flatulent dyspepsia.
- DS_5 ➲ Sensation of weight in hypochondria and upper abdomen.
- DS_6 ➲ Abdomen enormously distended, after meals.
- DS_7 ➲ Diarrhoea of fried egg.
- DS_8 ➲ Great dryness of mouth, tongue so dry it adheres to roof of mouth.
- FGS_1 ➲ Pain, nausea and vomiting during pregnancy, from weaning pessaries.
- FGS_2 ➲ Menses too long, dark, thick.
- FGS_3 ➲ Leucorrhoea in place of menses (cocc), patient awakened with dry tongue (Lech) Physometra (Lac-c, Lyc).
- FGS_4 ➲ Variableness of menstruation, irregularity of time and quantity.
- FGS_5 ➲ At every menstrual nisus, mouth, throat and tongue become intolerably dry, especially when sleeping.
- US_1 ➲ Renal colic.
- US_2 ➲ Pain from stone in the bladder or gravel.
- US_3 ➲ Urine with a violent-like smell.
- LS_1 ➲ Pain in right hip to knee.
- LS_2 ➲ Rheumatism from getting feet wet.
- LS_3 ➲ Feet cold with appearance of menses.
- PG_1 ➲ All the ailments are accompanied by drowsiness and sleepiness (op) or an inclination to faint (Hep) complaints cause sleepiness.

Modalities

Aggravation

- ➲ Cold, wet windy weather (Rhod).
- ➲ Lying on painful side.
- ➲ Weather change, cold food & water.

Amelioration

- ➲ Warm weather, warm room.
- ➲ Wrapping up warmly.

Relations

- ➲ COMPARE: Nux-v; Puls; Rhus; Asaf.
- ➲ ANTIDOTES: Murcurial inhalation camph; Op.

Nux vomica

- ➲ PROVED BY: Hahnemann.
- ➲ DURATION: 15-21 days.
- ➲ COMMON NAME: Poison Nut.
- ➲ FAMILY/KINGDOM: Loganiaceae.
- ➲ RELATION COLD/HEAT: Very chilly remedy.
- ➲ MIASM: Psora.
- ➲ TEMPERAMENT: Bilous, Sanguine, irritable and impatient temperament.
- ➲ SOURCE: Tincture and Trituration of imported seeds.
- ➲ SPHERES OF ACTION: Every organ is susceptible to the action of Nux-vomica.
- ➲ SUMMARY OF INDICATIONS: Diseases due to spicy foods, drinks and lack of exercise. A good remedy to commence treatment of patients who have had an excess of allopathic medication. This remedy is best administered before bed time. One of the most commonly used Polychrests.

THERAPEUTIC PICTURE OF DRUG

C_{N-1} ➲ Nux Vomica is ideally suited to thin spare subjects with dark hair and dark complexion.

C_{N-2} ➲ Who lead a sedentary life, nervous, extremely susceptible to external impressions, habituated to over study, debauches, jealous and hypochondriac.

C_{N-3} ➲ Persons of all walks of life, from the highest to the lowest standard, richest or poorest, civilized or uncivilized.

M_{D-1} ➲ "Nux is chiefly successful with persons of an ardent character; of an irritable, impatient temperament, disposed to anger, spite or deception."– Hahnemann.

M_{D-2} ➲ Very irritable; sensitive to all impression and inclination to commit suicide, but is afraid to die.

M_{D-3} ➲ Does not want to be touched.

M_{D-4} ➲ Ugly, malicious; can not bear noises, odors, light, etc.

M_{D-5} ➲ Even the least ailment affects him greatly.

M_{D-6} ➲ Hypochondriac: literary, studious persons, who are too much at home, suffer from want to exercise, with gastric, abdominal complaints and costiveness; especially in drunkards.

H_{D-1} ➲ Headache in the occiput area or over the eyes, as if nail is driven in.

SO_1 ➲ Nose stuffed up, especially at night and in the open air. Nose drips during the day and in a warm room.

DS_1 ➲ Eructations: sour or bitter; putrid in the morning.

DS_2 ➲ Hiccough from overeating, or from cold drinks.

DS_3 ➲ Nausea: early in the morning; with fainting; after eating; from tobacco.

DS_4 ➲ Weight and pain in the stomach; worse, eating, some time after.

DS_5 ➲ Ravenous hunger, especially, about a day before an attack of dyspepsia.

DS_6 ➲ Epigastrium bloated, with pressure, as of a stone, several hours after, eating.

DS_7 ➲ Dyspepsia from drinking strong coffee.

DS_8 ➲ Strangulated hernia, especially umbilical.

DS_9 ➲ Alternate constipation and diarrhoea, in persons who have taken purgatives all their lives.

DS_{10} ➲ Constipation, with rush of blood to the head; obstructed portal circulation; frequent, ineffectual urging; stools may be in hard masses.

DS_{11} ➲ Stools: small slimy, bloody, with urging, ceasing after stool; mucous or watery, from indigestion or cold; like pitch with blood.

DS_{12} ➲ Haemorrhoids, blind or flowing; abdominal plethora; congestion to the head; worse from high living or sedentary habits.

DS_{13} ➲ Burning and sticking in rectum; anus burning, smarting and feels as if cut, some hours after stool.

FGS_1 ➲ Menses too early, last too long; always irregular, blood black (cycl.; Lach.; Puls.) with fainting spells.

FGS_2 ➲ Dysmenorrhoea with pain in the sacrum, and constant urging to stool.

FGS_3 ➲ Metrorrhagia with sensation as if the bowels wanted to move.

FGS_4 ➲ Labour Pains: violent, spasmodic; cause urging to stool or to urinate; <in back; prefers a warm room.

FGS_5 ➲ During the catamenia, spasmodic colic, Nausea and vomiting. Vomitus is sour and bitter. Belching, especially after improper eating or over-indulgence in spicy foods or alcoholic drinks. Worse in the mornings and about one hour after eating.

FGS_6 ➲ Pains as from excoriation in mammae.

MGS_1 ➲ Spermatorrhoea with dreams, backache, burning in the spine, weakness and irritability.

MGS_2 ➲ Constrictive pain in the testicles; orchitis.

MGS_3 ➲ Emissions during sleep; especially after onanism or from too high living.

MGS_4 ➲ Bad effects of sexual excesses.

MGS_5 ➲ Easily excited desire, painful erections, especially in the morning; often excitable but power is weak.

F_{R-1} ➲ Paroxysms anticipated in the morning; cold stage predominates.

F_{R-2} ➲ Chilly; must be covered in every stage of fever.

F_{R-3} ➲ Chilliness on being uncovered, yet he does not allow being covered.

F_{R-4} ➲ Perspiration sour; only one side of the body and dry heat of the body.

F_{R-5} ➲ Aching in limbs and back, and gastric symptoms.

PG_1 ➲ Nux is popularly called the "hangover remedy", because it often relieves the person who has over-indulged in food or alcohol. It is also helps the regular users of laxatives to break the habit.

PG_2 ➲ Dizziness. Colds from dry, cold weather.

PG_3 ➲ Insomnia after mental strain, abuse of coffee, alcohol, tobacco.

PG_4 ➲ Wakes up between 3 and 4 A.M. falls asleep at day break, unrefreshed on walking. Needs a siesta.

PG_5 ➲ Excitability of whole nervous system, with too great sensitiveness of all the organs, principally those of sight and hearing.

Modalities

Aggravation

- Early morning.
- Anger.
- Dry weather.
- Spices.
- Cold.
- Narcotics.
- Aphrodisiacs.
- Mental exertion.
- Eating (one hour after).
- Touch.
- Stimulants.
- Open air.
- Alcohol.

Amelioration

- Rest
- Strong pressure
- Warmth
- Massage
- Evening
- Uninterrupted sleep
- Masturbation

Relations

- COMPLEMENTARY: Kali-c; Sep; Sulph.
- FOLLOWS WELL: Act-sp; Ars.; Bell; Cact; Carb-v; Cocc; Colch; Hyos; Lyc; Phos; Puls; Rhus-t; Sep; Sulph.
- ANTIDOTES: Acon; Ars; Cham; Cocc; Coff; Ign; Op; Puls; Thuj.
- INIMICALS: Aceton; Zinc.

Onosmodium virginianum

- ➲ PROVED BY: W.E. Green.
- ➲ COMMON NAME: Onosmodium or Virginianum or False Gromwell.
- ➲ FAMILY/KINGDOM: Boraginaceae.
- ➲ SOURCE: Tincture of entire fresh plant including root.

THERAPEUTIC PICTURE OF DRUG

M_{D-1} ➲ Talkative, but in a disconnect way.
M_{D-2} ➲ Irritable, Irresolute.
M_{D-3} ➲ Minutes seems like hours.
M_{D-4} ➲ Fear to look down let she might fall down stair.
M_{D-5} ➲ Listless and Apathetic.
H_{D-1} ➲ Eyes heavy and dull, ocular muscles tense.
H_{D-2} ➲ Pain in eye ball & between orbit and ball.
H_{D-3} ➲ Occipito-frontal pain in morning on waking.
H_{D-4} ➲ Pain in mastoid.
SO_1 ➲ Pain in and over left eye.
SO_2 ➲ Optic disc hyperaemic.
SO_3 ➲ Fullness in ears, hearing impaired.
DS_1 ➲ Constriction of pharynx when swallowing.
DS_2 ➲ Throat perfectly dry and stiff.
DS_3 ➲ Appetite increased.
DS_4 ➲ Craving for Ice-water and cold drinks.
DS_5 ➲ Abdomen feels bloated.
FGS_1 ➲ Sexual desire completely destroyed.
FGS_2 ➲ Feels as if menses would appear.
FGS_3 ➲ Aching in breast.
FGS_4 ➲ Nipple itch.

FGS_5 ➲ Menses too early and too prolonged.

FGS_6 ➲ Severe uterine pains, bearing-down pains, do pain return.

FGS_7 ➲ Soreness in uterine region.

FGS_8 ➲ Leucorrhoea, yellow, acrid, profuse.

LS_1 ➲ Tired and numb feeling in legs.

LS_2 ➲ Trembling of arm and hands.

LS_3 ➲ Shooting in joints of left fingers.

LS_4 ➲ Pain in left scapular region.

Modalities

Aggravation

- Lying down.
- In dark, motion, jar.
- Tight clothing.

Amelioration

- From sleep.
- From cold drinks & eating.

Relations

- COMPARE: Nazt-mar.; Gels; Ruta.

Opium

- ➲ PROVED BY: Hahnemann.
- ➲ DURATION: 7 days.
- ➲ COMMON NAME: Poppy.
- ➲ FAMILY/KINGDOM: Papaveraceae.
- ➲ RELATION COLD/HEAT: Hot.
- ➲ SOURCE: Opium is the gummy exudation of the unripe capsule of the Poppy.
- ➲ SPHERES OF ACTION: Mind, senses, nerves, skin mucous membranes, respiratory, digestive and urinary system.
- ➲ SUMMARY OF INDICATIONS: Polyneuropathy–Stroke–Constipation–The unconscious state.

THERAPEUTIC PICTURE OF DRUG

C_{N-1} ➲ Persons with light hair, lax muscles, and want of bodily irritability.

C_{N-2} ➲ It is especially adopted to diseases of first and second childhood eg. to children and old people.

M_{D-1} ➲ Think she is not at home (Bry.); this is continually in her mind.

M_{D-2} ➲ Picking of bed clothes during sleep (while awake, Bell; Hyos).

M_{D-3} ➲ Delirium with frightful vision, of mice, scorpions, etc and with desire to run away.

M_{D-4} ➲ Loquacious delirium, with open eyes and red face; furious delirium.

M_{D-5} ➲ Grief over insults is followed by convulsions.

M_{D-6} ➲ Carelessness, or great anxiety and uneasiness.

NS_1 ➲ Disorders with insensibility and partial or complete Paralysis.

NS_2 ➲ Spasms: from emotion, fright, anger etc; from approach of strangers (children); from crying.

NS_3 ➲ Twitching, trembling of head, arms, hands.

NS_4 ➲ Numbness and insensibility.

DS_1 ➲ Obstinate constipation; no desire to go to stool.

DS_2 ➲ Spasmodic retention of faeces in small intestines.

DS_3 ➲ Violent pain in the rectum, as if pressed as under.

DS_4 ➲ Stool: involuntary, especially after fright (Gels.); black and offensive; from Paralysis of sphincter.

DS_5 ➲ Opium renders the intestines so sluggish that the most active purgatives lose their power–Hering.

DS_6 ➲ Persistent diarrhoea in those treated with large doses of the drug-Lippe

FGS_1 ➲ Severe labour-like pains in uterus; with urging to stool; >bending double (and by warmth).

FGS_2 ➲ Bearing down with right grain pain, bloated abdomen, apathetic and drowsy, confined bowels, menses too soon, aching all over.

FGS_3 ➲ Menses: irregular; Profuse; violent colic forcing her to bend over; urging to stool; suppressed.

FGS_4 ➲ Suppressed, false or spasmodic labour-pains.

FGS_5 ➲ Puerperal spams, during and after parturition with loss of consciousness and drowsiness or coma between the Paroxysms.

FGS_6 ➲ Violent movements of the foetus.

MGS_1 ➲ Violent erections; or impotence.

MGS_2 ➲ Excitement of the sexual organs.

US_1 ➲ Retention of urine: from paralysis of fundus of bladder; from spasm of sphincter; from nursing after passion of nurse.

US_2 ➲ Emission of blood in urinating.

US_3 ➲ Acute, spasmodic constriction of urethra, with passage of blood urine.

PG_1 ➲ Great excitement of sexual organs, with sexual desire and orgasm.

PG_2 ➲ Perfect loss of sexual desire from lack of nutrition.

PG_3 ➲ All complaints: with great sopor; painless, complains of nothing; wants nothing.

PG_4 ➲ Want of susceptibility to remedies; lack of vital reaction the well chosen remedy makes no impression (Carb-v; Laur. Valer.).

PG_5 ➲ Bed feels so hot she cannot lie on it. (bed feels hard, Arn., Bry.; Pyrog.); more often in search of a cool place; must be uncovered.

PG_6 ➲ Sleeplessness, with acuteness of hearing; clocks striking and cocks crowing at a great distance, keep her awake.

Modalities

Aggravation

➲ During and after sleep (Apis; Lach).

➲ While Perspiring.

- Warmth.
- Stimulants.

Amelioration

- Cold.
- Constant walking.

Relations

- FOLLOWS WELL: Aco; Ant-t; Bell; Bry; Hyos; Nux-m; Nut-v.
- ANTIDOTES: Dell; Ipec; Nux-v; Chaml Verat; wine.

Palladium metallicum

- ➲ COMMON NAME: Trituration Palladium.
- ➲ FAMILY/KINGDOM: Minerals.

THERAPEUTIC PICTURE OF DRUG

M_{D-1} ➲ Weeping mood, Love of approbation. Pride, easily offended. Inclined to use violent language.

M_{D-2} ➲ Keeps up brightly when in company.

M_{D-3} ➲ Easily wounded pride.

M_{D-4} ➲ Exited and impatient

H_{D-1} ➲ Pain across top of head from ear to ear.

H_{D-2} ➲ Sallow complexion

H_{D-3} ➲ Headache causing irritability and impatience.

DS_1 ➲ Pain and soreness in liver.

DS_2 ➲ Sensation in flanks as if viscera gone.

DS_3 ➲ Shooting pains from navel to pelvis.

DS_4 ➲ Constipation, stools hard, frequently whitish.

DS_5 ➲ Frequent soft stool.

Ds_6 ➲ Intestines feel strangulated.

FGS_1 ➲ Pain & swelling in region of right ovary.

FGS_2 ➲ Uterine prolapses and retroversion.

FGS_3 ➲ Cutting pain in uterus, relieved after stool.

FGS_4 ➲ Shooting or burning pain in pelvis and bearing down, relived by rubbing.

FGS_5 ➲ Soreness and shooting pain from navel to breast.

FGS_6 ➲ Menstrual discharge while nursing.

FGS_7 ➲ Glairy Leucorrhoea.

US_1 ➲ Frequent micturition, bladder feels full but little urine is passed.

US_2 ➲ Muddy urine, urine like water mixed with blood.

LS_1 ➲ Sudden stitches in right shoulder joint.

LS_2 ➲ Pain in right arm and temple.

LS_3 ➲ Itching in left ankle.

Modalities

Aggravation

- ➲ From exertion and while standing.
- ➲ Before & after menstruation.

Amelioration

- ➲ By rubbing.
- ➲ Lying on left side.

Relations

- ➲ COMPARE: Arg; Lil; Apis; Helon
- ➲ COMPLEMENTARY: Plat.
- ➲ ANTIDOTES: Chin; Bell; Glon.

Petroleum

- PROVED BY: Hahnemann.
- DURATION: 40-50 days.
- COMMON NAME: Coal oil (Rock Oil).
- FAMILY/KINGDOM: Anthracite.
- RELATION COLD/HEAT: Very Chilly.
- MIASM: Psora.
- DIATHESIS: Scrofulous
- TEMPERAMENT: Irritable, quarrelsome.
- SPHERES OF ACTION: Mucous membrane, skin, GIT, heart meninges and cerebrum.
- SUMMARY OF INDICATIONS: Travel sickness–Peptic Ulcer–Skin disorders.

THERAPEUTIC PICTURE OF DRUG

C_{N-1} ➲ Adapted to persons of light hair and light skin who suffer from cutaneous eruptions and gastro-intestinal disorders.

M_{D-1} ➲ Anxious and timorous disposition; sadness and mental dejection.

M_{D-2} ➲ Great irresolution; uneasiness respecting the future.

M_{D-3} ➲ Loss of memory; does not know where she is in the street.

M_{D-4} ➲ During sleep or delirium; imagines that one leg is double; that another person lies alongside of him in same bed; that there are two babies in the bed (Valer).

M_{D-5} ➲ Imagines he has a third leg which will not keep quite.

H_{D-1} ➲ Vertigo on stooping, or on rising from bed, or from a seat with bilious vomiting.

H_{D-2} ➲ Occipital headache, with general spasms and screaming; loss of appetite, constipation.

H_{D-3} ➲ Sensation as if everything in the head were alive.

H_{D-4} ➲ Head feels numb, as if made of wood or as if bruised.

DS_1 ➲ Drawing pains whenever stomach is empty; relived by constant eating (Anac.-ori.; cheli-m., sep.).

DS_2 ➲ Sensation of emptiness and weakness in stomach; weakness of digestion.

DS_3 ➲ Diarrhoea: often preceded by cultings colic only during the day.

DS_4 ➲ Diarrhoea: from cabbage, sour-krout; after riding in a carriage.

DS_5 ➲ Diarrhoea: yellow, watery, gushing; during Pregnancy, stormy weather; always in the day time.

FGS_1 ➲ Before menses, throbbing, in the head (Kreos.). Leucorrhoea. Profuse, albuminous (Alum.; oox.; Bor.; Cal-p).

FGS_2 ➲ Genitals sore and moist.

FGS_3 ➲ Sensation of moisture(Eup-pur.)

FGS_4 ➲ Itching and mealy, coating of nipple.

MGS_1 ➲ Prostate inflamed and swollen (Prostatitis).

MGS_2 ➲ Itching in a urethra.

MGS_3 ➲ Herpetic eruptions on the Perineum.

LS_1 ➲ Tearing in hands; burning sensation in palms of hands.

LS_2 ➲ Sweating of hands.

LS_3 ➲ Pain in wrist joint as if sprained.

S_{N-1} ➲ Skin of hands rough, cracked; tips of fingers rough, cracked, fissured, especially in the cold; tenderness of the feet, which are bathed in foul smelling sweat (Graph., sani aqua, sil.,)

S_{N2} ➲ Great sensibility of the surface of skin.

S_{N3} ➲ Miliary urticaria; itching tetters; itching, excoriated and running spots on skin.

S_{N4} ➲ Painful, itching chilblains and chapped hands < in cold weather; decubitus.

S_{N5} ➲ Herpes: of genital organs extending to Perineum and thighs.

S_{N6} ➲ Thick, greenish crusts, burning and itching; redness, raw; cracks bleed easily.

S_{N7} ➲ Exanthema corroding and spreading; very difficult to heal.

PG_1 ➲ Swelling and induration of glands, also after a contusion.

PG_2 ➲ Many of the symptoms appear, or are worse, during stormy weather.

PG_3 ➲ Great lassitude morning and evening; tendency to take cold.

PG_4 ➲ Several symptoms manifest them selves in mornings.

PG_5 ➲ Disorders when riding in an auto, railroad car or in a ship (cocc; sani).

Modalities

Aggravation

- Carriage riding (Cocc, Sani).
- During a thunderstorm.
- In winter (Alumina).

Relations

- FOLLOWS WELL: Bry; Calc; Lyc; Nit-ac; Nux-v.; Puls; Sep; Sil; Sulph.
- ANTIDOTES: Acon; Nux-vom; Cocc.

Phosphoricum acidum

- PROVED BY: Hahemann.
- DURATION: 40 days.
- COMMON NAME: Glacial Phosphoric acid (H_3PO_4).
- FAMILY/KINGDOM: Minerals.
- RELATION COLD/HEAT: Chilly.
- MIASM: Psora, Syphilis, Sycosis.
- TEMPERAMENT: Mild disposition and xiedling temperament.
- SOURCE: In U.S. the first solution is made of glacial phosphoric acid.
- SPHERES OF ACTION: Brain, nerve, blood, kidneys, sex organs, mucous membrane.
- SUMMARY OF INDICATIONS: Emotion disorders–Debilitation due to sexual excesses.

THERAPEUTIC PICTURE OF DRUG

C_{N-1} ➲ Best suited to person of originally strong constitutions, who have become debilitated by loss of vitual fluid.

C_{N-2} ➲ Pale sickly complexion.

M_{D-1} ➲ Is listless, indifferent to the affairs of life, Apathetic, Prostrated and stupefied with grief.

M_{D-2} ➲ Low muttering delirium, lies in a stupor, unconscious of all that's going on around him.

H_{D-1} ➲ Great heaviness of the head.

H_{D-2} ➲ School girl's headache, from overuse of eyes.

H_{D-3} ➲ Periosteal pains compel motion.

H_{D-4} ➲ Itching of scalp.

SO_1 ➲ Nervous deafness, after typhoid disease.

SO_2 ➲ Discharge of bloody pus for the nose.

SO_3 ➲ Burning in skin of cheeks.

SO_4 ➲ Hairs of the beard fall out, especially after grief and sorrow.
SO_5 ➲ Eye sunken and surrounded by blue margins.
DS_1 ➲ Pressure as from a weight, with sleepiness after eating.
DS_2 ➲ Craves juicy things.
DS_3 ➲ Shooting and cutting in abdomen.
DS_4 ➲ Swelling of inguinal glands.
DS_5 ➲ Intolerable pain in haemorrhoids when sitting.
DS_6 ➲ Diarrhoea–Painless, nat debilitating, white or yellow
FGS_1 ➲ Menses too early & profuse, with pain in liver.
FGS_2 ➲ Itching, yellow leucorrhoea after menses.
FGS_3 ➲ Milk scanty health deteriorated from nursing.
MGS_1 ➲ Eruption on penis and scrotum.
MGS_2 ➲ Gnawing pain in testes.
MGS_3 ➲ Emission at night and at stoal.
MGS_4 ➲ Prostatorrhoea even when passing stool.
MGS_5 ➲ Emission, frequent and debilitation, several in one night.
MGS_6 ➲ Onanism, when patient is distressed by the culpability of his indulgence.
MGS_7 ➲ Hair of sexual parts fall off.
MGS_8 ➲ Fig warts, complication with chancre.
US_1 ➲ Urine–profuse urination at night of clear, watery urine which form a white, cloud at once.
US_2 ➲ Constant urging to urinate.
US_3 ➲ Fetid urine, flow of urine with spasmodic pain in loins.
US_4 ➲ Involuntary urination
LS_1 ➲ Stiffness and cramp in joints.
LS_2 ➲ Hand trembling when writing.
LS_3 ➲ Ulcer on lower leg.
LS_4 ➲ Pain in tibia at night.
LS_5 ➲ Pain at night in bones of limb.

Modalities

Aggravation

- From mental affections.
- Loss of vital fluid.
- Self abuse, sexual excess.

Amelioration

- By sitting.
- Standing and warmth of bed.

Relations

- COMPARE: Phos; Puls; Pic- acid; Sil; Mur-ac.
- FOLLOWS WELL: Ars; Bell; Chin; Nux; Lyco; Sele; Phos; Sulph.
- ANTIDOTES: Camph; Staph; Coff.

Phosphorus

- ➲ PROVED BY: Hahnemann.
- ➲ DURATION: 40 days.
- ➲ COMMON NAME: Phosphorus.
- ➲ FAMILY/KINGDOM: Minerals.
- ➲ RELATION COLD/HEAT: Chilly.
- ➲ MIASM: Psora.
- ➲ DIATHESIS: Tubercular.
- ➲ TEMPERAMENT: Sanguine, Bilious, Irritable.
- ➲ SOURCE: Trituration of red amorphous phosphorus.
- ➲ SPHERES OF ACTION: Every tissue of the body eg. Skin, mucous membrane, bones, blood, spinal cord, nerves, heart, liver, kidney and lungs.
- ➲ SUMMARY OF INDICATIONS: Haemorrhage–Gastritis–Respiratory disorders–Alopecia areata–dandruff–Hypertension.

THERAPEUTIC PICTURE OF DRUG

C_{N-1} ➲ Good and beautiful look.

C_{N-2} ➲ Having fair, thin, transparent skin, delicate eyelashes, fine blond or brownish red hair.

C_{N-3} ➲ Young persons who grow too rapidly and are inclined to stoop.

C_{N-4} ➲ Chlorotic anaemia at the time of Puberty.

C_{N-5} ➲ Phosphorus is best suited for tall, selender person.

M_{D-1} ➲ Fearfulness, as if something were creeping out of every corner.

M_{D-2} ➲ Great depression of spirits; easily vexed

M_{D-3} ➲ Anxious, restless: at twilight; when alone; about the future; during a thunder storm; with Palpitation.

M_{D-4} ➲ Oversensitive to external impression, light odours, touch, noise etc.

M_{D-5} ➲ Great apathy, very sluggish; dislike to talk; answers slowly or not at all.

M_{D-6} ➲ Irritability of mind and body; prostrated from the least unpleasant impression.

M_{D-7} ➲ Melancholy sadness and melancholy, sometimes with violent weeping, or interrupted by fits of involuntary laughter.

DS_1 ➲ Necrosis of the (left) lower jaw.

DS_2 ➲ Thirst for ice-cold drinks, which are vomited as soon as they become warm in the stomach.

DS_3 ➲ Burning pains in stomach, intestines and between shoulder blades.

DS_4 ➲ During Pregnancy; unable to drink water; sight of it causes vomiting; must close her eyes while bathing.

DS_5 ➲ Constipation, feces slender, long, dry, tough and hard, like a dog's; voided with difficulty.

DS_5 ➲ Chronic painless diarrhoea of undigested food with much thirst for water during the night.

DS_7 ➲ Frequent diarrhoea, during cholera time.

DS_8 ➲ Painless, debilitating diarrhoea, worse mornings.

DS_9 ➲ Severe, watery diarrhoea with a sensation as if the anus remains open permanently.

RS_1 ➲ Hoarseness, loss of voice.

RS_2 ➲ Painful laryngitis; tight, heavy chest (as if a weight is lying on it.)

RS_3 ➲ Croupy, dry, vasping, tickling, pain cough, which is very exhausting.

RS_4 ➲ Worse when laughing, talking or breathing cold air.

FGS_1 ➲ Leucorrhoea profuse, smarting, corrosive, instead of menses.

FGS_2 ➲ Amenorrhoea, with vicarious menstruation (Bry.).

FGS_3 ➲ Tearing in genital organs and stiches upwards from vagina in uterus.

FGS_4 ➲ Metritis, chlorosis, phlebitis.

FGS_5 ➲ Discharge of blood from uterus during Pregnancy.

FGS_6 ➲ Catamenia of too long duration, with toothache and colic.

FGS_7 ➲ On appearance of menses; incisive, griping pains in the back and vomiting.

FGS_8 ➲ After menses: Weakness, blue circles round eyes, and anxiety.

FGS_9 ➲ During menses: shooting headaches; fermentation in abdomen; expectoration of blood; Pains in back; soreness of limb; great lassitude and fever; or Palpitation of heart; shiverings; swelling of gums and cheeks, and many other sufferings.

FGS_{10} ➲ Hard and painful nodosities in breast. (Stiching pain).

FGS_{11} ➲ Inflammation (erysipe latous) of breast, even after formation of Pus.

FGS_{12} ➲ At 3.30 P.M. Pain from left nipple to right nipple, hence to right shoulder and right little finger.

FGS_{13} ➲ Fistulous tracks after mammary abscess.

MGS_1 ➲ Irresistible desire; involuntary emissions, with lascivious dreams.

MGS_2 ➲ Impotence after excessive excitement and onanism.

MGS_3 ➲ Hydrocele after gonorrhoeal orchits, with sexual weakness, also, after seminal losses.

PG_1 ➲ Symptoms are usually worse on the left-side.

PG_2 ➲ Appears to be well despite a high temperature.

PG_3 ➲ Sweats at night. Perspiration has the odour of sulphur.

PG_4 ➲ Dandruff. Alopecia areata.

Modalities

Aggravation

- Evening.
- Lying on the left (or painful side).
- Physical or mental exertion.
- Thunder storms.
- Changes of weather.
- Warm food or warm drinks.
- Touch.

Amelioration

- Open air.
- Lying on the right-side.
- Sleep, in dark.
- Being rubbed.
- Cold food or cold drink (until it gets warm).
- Washing with very cold water.

Relations

- COMPLEMENTARY: All-c; Ars; Carb-v.
- FOLLOWS WELL: Ars; Bell; Bry; Calc; Carb-v; Chin.; Kali-c; Lyc.; Nux-v; Puls; Rhus-t; Sep; Sil; Sulp.
- ANTIDOTES: Camph; Coff; Nux-v; Ter.
- INIMICALS: Apis; Caust.

Phytolacca decandra

- PROVED BY: Allentown College.
- COMMON NAME: spoke Root (Red Ink Plant).
- FAMILY/KINGDOM: Phytolaccaceae.
- RELATION COLD/HEAT: Chilly.
- MIASM: Syphilitic and Sycotic.
- DIATHESIS: Rheumatic & Gouty.
- SOURCE: Tincture of fresh root during in winter.
- SPHERES OF ACTION: Chiefly upon glandular system particularly on the throat and mammary gland.
- SUMMARY OF INDICATIONS: Anorexia- mammary disorders.

THERAPEUTIC PICTURE OF DRUG

C_{N-1} ➲ Emaciated patient, chlorotic with loss of fat.

C_{N-2} ➲ Face sunken, pale, Hippocratic, blue rings around the eye with yellow complexion.

M_{D-1} ➲ Entire Indifference to life, sure she will dye.

M_{D-2} ➲ Indisposition to mental exertion.

M_{D-3} ➲ Loss of personal delicacy, disregard of surround objects.

H_{D-1} ➲ Pain in back of head and neck.

H_{D-2} ➲ Sensation of soreness deep in brain.

SO_1 ➲ Shooting pain from left eye to top of head.

SO_2 ➲ Irritation in one eustachian tube.

SO_3 ➲ Total obstruction of nose when riding must breath through mouth.

SO_4 ➲ Nasal discharge acrid, excoriating.

SO_5 ➲ Great pain in root of tongue when swallowing burning, as from a coal of fire or red hot iron, dryness.

DS_1 ➲ Metallic taste.

DS_2 ➲ Throat feels rough, narrow hot.

- DS_3 ➲ Quinsy, tonsils and fauces swollen, with burning pain, cannot swallow even water.
- DS_4 ➲ Throat feel very hot, pain at root of tongue extending to ear.
- DS_5 ➲ Sore spot in right hypochondrium.
- DS_6 ➲ Intense thirst, canine hunger soon after eating.
- DS_7 ➲ Vomits undigested food.
- DS_8 ➲ Burning, gripping pain in umbilical region.
- DS_9 ➲ Rheumatism extending to abdomen.
- RS_1 ➲ Respiration difficulty, oppressed.
- RS_2 ➲ Aching pain in chest and side, with cough.
- FGS_1 ➲ Mammae full of hard, painful nodosites.
- FGS_2 ➲ Breast, shows on early tendency to cake, is feel, Stony hard and painful.
- FGS_3 ➲ When child nurses pain goes from nipple all over body.
- FGS_4 ➲ These is mastitis with enlaged nuxillary gland.
- FGS_5 ➲ Mammary abscess, fistula, gaping, angey ulcers, Ichorous, foetid, unhealthy.
- FGS_6 ➲ Nipple, sensitive, sore fissured (Graph), < Intensely by nursing, pain radiates over whole body.
- FGS_7 ➲ Tumefied breast neither heals nor suppurates, is of a purple hue and " hard as old cheese" (Bryo) (Lac-c, Phel).
- LS_1 ➲ Finger-joints swollen, hard, shining.
- LS_2 ➲ Lame feeling in the arms.
- LS_3 ➲ Chronic rheumatism of left hip.
- LS_4 ➲ Ulcers and nodes on legs.
- PG_1 ➲ Can not drink hot fluid.

Modalities

Aggravation

- ➲ When it rains.
- ➲ Exposure to damp clod weather.
- ➲ Motion, at night and rt. Side.

Amelioration

- ➲ Warm, dry weather and rest.

Relations

- ➲ COMPARE: Bry; Rhus; Kali-hyd; Merc; Phytolacco; Berry.
- ➲ ANTIDOTES: Milk and salt; Bell.
- ➲ INIMICALS: Mercurius.

Platina metallicum

- ➲ PROVED BY: Stapf.
- ➲ DURATION: 35-40 days.
- ➲ COMMON NAME: Platinum.
- ➲ FAMILY/KINGDOM: Minerals.
- ➲ RELATION COLD/HEAT: Hot.
- ➲ MIASM: Psora.
- ➲ TEMPERAMENT: Hysterical and Sanguine.
- ➲ SOURCE: Trituration of Pt.
- ➲ SPHERES OF ACTION: Nerve centers, genital tendency to anesthesia, Paralysis in womens.
- ➲ SUMMARY OF INDICATIONS: Headache–Dysmenorrhoea–Sexual disorders of womens–Constipation.

THERAPEUTIC PICTURE OF DRUG

C_{N-1} ➲ Especially suited to women of dark hair, dark complexion.

C_{N-2} ➲ Womens having rigid muscular fibres.

C_{N-3} ➲ Womens suffers from too early & too profuse menses.

M_{D-1} ➲ Arrogant, proud, contemptuous; "looking down" on people usually venerated; a kind of "casting them off" unwillingly.

M_{D-2} ➲ Low-spirited, inclined to shed tears, worse in the morning; weeps with the pains.

M_{D-3} ➲ Mental delusions, as if everything about (her) was small.

M_{D-4} ➲ All persons physically and mentally inferior, but she feels physically large and superior.

M_{D-5} ➲ A sensation of growing larger in every direction.

M_{D-6} ➲ Much anguish; she feels as if she would lose her senses and die soon.

M_{D-7} ➲ Trifling things produce profound vexation (Ign.am; Staph.) for a long period.

M_{D-8} ➲ Distisfied with life, but fear of death (Aco, Ars).

M_{D-9} ➲ Mental disturbances after fright, grief, vexation, onanism, pride.

M_{D-10} ➲ Mania, with great pride; fault-finding; unchaste talk; trembling and clonic spasms; caused by fright or anger.

M_{D-11} ➲ Mental symptoms appear as physical symptoms disappears and vice versa.

H_{D-1} ➲ Neuralgic headache in sensitive or hysterical persons; cramp-like pressing inwards with hot and red face, and roaring in head.

H_{D-2} ➲ Sensation of numbness in head and externally on vertex, preceded by a sensation of contraction of brain and scalp.

H_{D-3} ➲ Constriction around the forehead and nigh temples.

DS_1 ➲ Sensation of constriction in pit of the stomach and in abdomen.

DS_2 ➲ Pressing and bearing down in abdomen, extending into Pelvis.

DS_3 ➲ Constipation; especially while traveling (at sea: Bry.); similar to lead poisoning; from inertia of bowels; frequently unsuccessful urging; stools adhere to the rectum and anus like soft clay (alumina); during pregnancy.

FGS_1 ➲ Before catamenia, cuttings and pain like those of labour in hypogastrium.

FGS_2 ➲ Menses too early, too profuse and too short-lasting; flow dark, clotted; Preceded by spasms, much bearing down, desire for stool, or backache.

FGS_3 ➲ Metrorrhagia the body feels as if growing large; genitals very sensitive.

FGS_4 ➲ Haemorrhages like clots, with uterine cancer, fibroids, etc; even the fibroid may be cured.

FGS_5 ➲ Leucorrhoea like white of egg, only by day, after urination and after rising from a seat.

FGS_6 ➲ Severe stitches in right ovarian region.

FGS_7 ➲ The external sexual organs are exceedingly sensitive; cannot bear the napkin to touch her; will go into spasms from an examination; vulva painfully sensitive during coitus; will faint during, or cannot endure, coitus (compare, Murx; Orig).

FGS_8 ➲ Nymphomania, worse in the lying-in; tingling or titillation from genitals up into abdomen.

FGS_9 ➲ Abnormal sexual appetite and melancholia.

PG_1 ➲ Pains slight at commencement, increase gradually, often at regular intervals, and diminish in same manner.

PG_2 ➲ Moral and physical affections, appearing alternately.

PG_3 ➲ Face changing colour frequently; dark haired females.

Modalities

Aggravation

- Sitting and standing.
- Evening.

Amelioration

- Walking.

Relations

- COMPARE: Aur; Croc; Ign; Kali-p; Puls; Sep; Stann; Valer.
- FOLLOWS WELL: Anac; Arg-Met; Bell; Ign; Lyc; Puls; Rhus-t; Sep; Verat.
- ANTIDOTES: Puls; Nit-s-d; Bell.

Plumbum metallicum

- ➲ PROVED BY: Hartlaub.
- ➲ DURATION: 20-30 days.
- ➲ COMMON NAME: Lead (Pb).
- ➲ FAMILY/KINGDOM: Minerals.
- ➲ RELATION COLD/HEAT: Chilly.
- ➲ MIASM: Syphilis.
- ➲ SOURCE: Trituration of Pb.
- ➲ SPHERES OF ACTION: Esp Nervous System, blood, alimentary tract, uterus etc.
- ➲ SUMMARY OF INDICATIONS: Amnesia-muscular dystrophies-abdominal colic constipation- anaemias.

THERAPEUTIC PICTURE OF DRUG

C_{N-1} ➲ Excersive and Rappid emaciation, with extreme weakness and analmia.

C_{N-2} ➲ Look of Face/greasy, shiny, pale, yellow and Hippo-Cratic.

C_{N-3} ➲ Complexion: Pale, ash-coloured, corpse-like, cheek sunken.

M_{D-1} ➲ Mental Depression.

M_{D-2} ➲ Fear of being assassinated.

M_{D-3} ➲ Slow of perception, Intellectual torpor, gradually increas Apathy.

M_{D-4} ➲ Weakness & loss of memory, unable to fire proper word.

NS_1 ➲ Sclerosis of the brain or progressive muscular atrophy; alternating with colic.

NS_2 ➲ Paralysis: Proceeded by mental derangement.

NS_3 ➲ Adopted to diseases from spinal origin.

NS_4 ➲ Epelipsy, chronic forms; before the spell, legs heavy and numb, tongue swollen.

DS_1 ➲ Distinct blue line along margin of gums.

DS_2 ➲ Gums: swollen; show a lead colored line; painful, with head tubercles.

DS_3 ➲ Abdomen herd as a stone; knots in recti muscles; anxious, with cold sweat and deathly faintness.

DS_4 ➲ Cutting, contractive pains, with restlessness tossing; better from rubbing, or hard pressure.

DS_5 ➲ Large, hard swelling in ileo-coecal region, painful to touch and motion (Typhilitis).

DS_6 ➲ Colic alternates with delirium and pain in atrophied limb.

DS_7 ➲ Violant colic, sansation as if Abdominal wall was drawn as if by a string to the spire.

DS_8 ➲ Stools hard, lampy, black like Sheep dung.

DS_9 ➲ Most obstinate constipation; stools blackish; continued and ineffectual want to evacuate.

DS_{10} ➲ Intolerable pain from spasms of rectum, with every evacuation lasting on hour or two; horrible constriction much worse if stool solid.

DS_{11} ➲ Prolapsus ani, with Paralysis; fissures of anus.

FGS_1 ➲ Feels a lack of room for foetus in uterus, inability of uterus to expand, threatening abortion.

FGS_2 ➲ Vulva & vagina Hypersensitive.

FGS_3 ➲ Stitches and burning pain in breasts.

FGS_4 ➲ Vaginismus, with emaciation and constipation.

FGS_5 ➲ Induration of mammary glands.

FGS_6 ➲ Menorrhagia with sansation of string pilling from Abdomen to back.

MGS_1 ➲ Testicles drawn up, feel constricted.

MGS_2 ➲ Loss of sexual power.

MGS_3 ➲ Genitals swollen and inflamed.

US_1 ➲ Chronic interstitial nephritis, with severe pain in the abdomen.

US_2 ➲ Urine scanty; tenesmus of the bladder; emission drop by drop; dribble, is high-coloured and fetid.

US_3 ➲ Morbus brightii, contracted kidney.

PG_1 ➲ Affections in lower teeth; tongue; sweetish taste, as in expectoration of cough with sweetish taste.

PG_2 ➲ Burning sensation in various parts of body.

PG_3 ➲ General emaciation, esp. in Paralysed parts, followed by swelling of those parts.

Modalities

Aggravation

➲ At Night.

➲ From Motion.

Amelioration

- By Rubbing.
- Hard Pressure.
- Physical exertion.

Relations

COMPARE:	Alumina; Platina; Opium.
FOLLOWS WELL:	Ars; Bell; Lyc; Phas; Puls.
ANTIDOTES:	Alum; Coce; Krcos; Op; Plat; Stram; Zinc.

Podophyllum peltatum

- PROVED BY: JEANES.
- DURATION: 30 days.
- COMMON NAME: May Apple (Wild lemon).
- FAMILY/KINGDOM: Berberidaceae.
- RELATION COLD/HEAT: Affected by extremes of Heat and Cold.
- MIASM: Psora and syphilis.
- TEMPERAMENT: Bilious temperament.
- SOURCE: Tincture of root gathered after fruit has ripened; of whole fresh plant; of ripe fruit.
- SPHERES OF ACTION: Digestive tract mucous membrane e.g. duodenum, rectum, glandular structure and liver.
- SUMMARY OF INDICATIONS: Acute & chronic diarrhoea-teething problems- Prolapsea uterus.

THERAPEUTIC PICTURE OF DRUG

C_{N-1} ➲ Children who suffer from diarrhoea during the time of dentition in hot weather.

C_{N-2} ➲ Adapted to womens of bilious temperament.

C_{N-3} ➲ Womens, who suffer from gastro-intestinal derangement.

C_{N-4} ➲ Especially after abuse of mercury, "bilious attacks".

M_{D-1} ➲ Loquacity and delirium from eating and fruits.

M_{D-2} ➲ Depression of spirits, also, in gastric affections.

M_{D-3} ➲ Most dipression; Imagines, he is going to die or be very ill (Ars.).

M_{D-4} ➲ Disgust for life; headache.

DS_1 ➲ Difficult dentition: moaming, grinding the teath at ninght; intense desire to press the gums together (Phyto-deca.).

DS_2 ➲ Cramp-like pain in bowels, with retraction of abdominal muscles, 10 p.m., and again at 5 A.m. until 9 A.m.; lead colic.

DS_3 ➲ Patient is constantly rubbing and shaking the region of liver with is hand.

DS_4 ➲ Cholera infantum and morbus.

DS_5 ➲ Diarrhoea; of long standing, early in the morning, during dentition, with hot, glowing cheeks while being bathed or washed; in hot weather after acid fruits.

DS_6 ➲ Morning, painless diarrhoea which is not due to venous stasis or intestinal ulceration.

DS_7 ➲ Diarrhoea, with great sinking at epigastrium, sensation as if everything would drop through the pelvis.

DS_8 ➲ Stools: frequent, painless, watery, fetid discharges, gushing out; yellow-colored, with meal-like sediment; green sour, with flatulence; morning, during dentition; greenish-yellow, slimy, bloody, gelatinuous, mixed with feces; tenemus and prolapsus ani.

DS_9 ➲ Constipation alternating with diarrhoea; internal and external piles.

FGS_1 ➲ Suppressed menses in young girls.

FGS_2 ➲ Symptoms of prolapsus uteri, with pain in sacrum, muco-gelatinous stools.

FGS_3 ➲ Prolapsus uteri: with diarrhoea; from washing; after over-lifting or straining; after parturition.

FGS_4 ➲ Bearing down in abdomen and back during menses; ovarian pains running into thighs.

FGS_5 ➲ During Pregnancy: swelling of labia; can lie comfortably only on stomach, early months; excessive vomiting.

FGS_6 ➲ Haemorrhoids and Protapsus ani after confinement; Pendulous abdomen.

F_{R-1} ➲ Fever Paroxysmal at 7 a.m., with great loquacity during chill and heat.

F_{R-2} ➲ Chill with pain in hypochondria, knees, ankles and wrists.

F_{R-3} ➲ Sweat: Profuse, dropped off prover's fingers; of feet in evening; bathed in cold; warm on head and legs.

PG_1 ➲ Sudden shock of jerking pains.

PG_2 ➲ Stiffness on beginning to move.

PG_3 ➲ Prostration with the pain; faintness and emptiness after stool.

PG_4 ➲ Thrist for large quantities of cold water.

Modalities

Aggravation

- ➲ In early morning (Aloe-soc; Nuc-v; Sulph).
- ➲ In Hot weather.
- ➲ During dentition

Relations

- ➲ COMPARE: Aloe; Chel; Coll; Lit-t; Merc; Nux-v; Sulph.
- ➲ COMPLEMENTARY: Sulph.
- ➲ ANTIDOTES: Colocy; Nux-v; Lept-vir; Lac-ac.

Psorinum

- PROVED BY: Hering.
- DURATION: 30-40 days.
- COMMON NAME: A product of Psora.
- FAMILY/KINGDOM: A Nosode.
- RELATION COLD/HEAT: Extremely Chilly.
- MIASM: Psora.
- SPHERES OF ACTION: All the Psoric manifesation mind, gland, skin etc.
- SUMMARY OF INDICATIONS: Skin disorders- chronic diarrhoea-chronic leucorrhoea allergic disorders.

THERAPEUTIC PICTURE OF DRUG

C_{N-1} ➲ Lean, thin person with skin eruption & having filthy smell of body which-persists even after washing.

C_{N-2} ➲ Children are pale, delicate, sickly.

M_{D-1} ➲ Anxious, full of fear, evil forebodings.

M_{D-2} ➲ Extremely Psoric patients, nervous, restless, easily Sad suicidal thoughts.

M_{D-3} ➲ Religious melancholy, very depressed, despairs of salvation of Recovery (Meli).

H_{D-1} ➲ Chronic headaches; hungry during attacks; with vertigo.

H_{D-2} ➲ Morning headache, with pressing in forehead, stupefaction, staggering, eyes feels sore.

H_{D-3} ➲ Hammering Pain; brain feels too large; worse change of weather.

H_{D-4} ➲ Humid eruptions on the scalp (crusta lacteal); hair matted (plica plonica); hair dry.

SO_1 ➲ Photophobia when walking in open air.

SO_2 ➲ Inflamed lids; cannot open the eyes; lies with face buried in Pillow.

SO_3 ➲ External ears, raw, red, oozing; scabs form; sore pain behind ears.

SO_4 ➲ Otorrhoea very offensive, Purulent (watery, stinking diarrhoea).

DS_1 ➲ Diarrhoea preceded by colic; green, bilious, mixed with mucus; four times; of green mucus, mixed with blood; frequent liquid.

DS_1 ➲ Eructions like a bad eggs.

DS_2 ➲ Very hungry all the time, must have something to eat in the middle of the night.

DS3 ➲ Obstinate constipation, with severe pains.

DS_4 ➲ Diarrhoea preceded by colic; green, bilious, mixed with mucus; four times a day without pain.

DS_5 ➲ Stool: fluid, fetid smell like a rotten eggs or carrion; worse at night, of green mucus, mixed with blood, frequent, liquid.

RS_1 ➲ Asthma with dyspnoea; worse, sitting up; better, lying down and keeping arms spread wide apart.

RS_2 ➲ Dry, hacking, from titillation in trachea; dry, with weakness, heaviness, or soreness in chest; evenings, pains in threat and chest.

RS_3 ➲ Chronic blenorrhoea of the lungs, threatening phthisis.

RS_4 ➲ Hay fever returning irregularly every year.

FGS_1 ➲ Leuorrhaea foetid, large, lumby.

FGS_2 ➲ With much backache & debility, during clamaxis.

FGS_3 ➲ Mammae swollen & painful.

FGS_4 ➲ Pimples oozing and acrid fluid that burn and excoriates the glands.

FGS_5 ➲ During pregnancy most obstinate vomiting foetus move too violently, when the best selected remedy fails to Relieve, to correct the Psoric diathesis of the unborn.

MGS_1 ➲ Prostatic fluid discharged before urinating.

MGS_2 ➲ Sycotic excrescences on edges of prepuce, with itching and burning.

MGS_3 ➲ Impotence, want of emissions during coitus.

S_{N-1} ➲ Skin dirty, greasy-looking, with yellow blotches here and there.

S_{N-2} ➲ Herpetic eruptions, especially on the scalp and in the bends of joints with itching; worse from warmth of bed.

S_{N-3} ➲ After suppressed itch; Urticaria, in attacks, after every exertion; tuberculosis; single Pustules often appear.

S_{N-4} ➲ Indolent ulcers, slow to heal; eczema behind the ears.

PG_1 ➲ Hungry in the middle of the night.

PG_2 ➲ Feels unusually well day before attack.

PG_3 ➲ Great sensitiveness to cold air or change of weather.

PG_4 ➲ Body has filthy smell, even after bathing.

Modalities

Aggravation

- Coffee.
- Changes of Weather.
- In hot, Sunshine.
- Dread of least cold air or draft.

Amelioration

- Heat, Warm.
- Clothing, even in summer.

Relations

- COMPLEMENTARY: Sulph; Tubercul.
- FOLLOWS WELL: Allum; Borax; Carb-V; Chin; Sulph.
- ANTIDOTES: Coff.
- INIMICALS: Sep.

Pulsatilla pratensis (Anemone pratensis = Pulsatilla nigricans)

- ➲ PROVED BY: Hahnemann.
- ➲ DURATION: 40 days.
- ➲ COMMON NAME: Wind Flower (Anemone).
- ➲ FAMILY/KINGDOM: Ranunculaceae.
- ➲ RELATION COLD/HEAT: Hot or Chilly.
- ➲ MIASM: Psoric & Sycotic.
- ➲ TEMPERAMENT: Full of tears, slow, Phlegmatic and indecisive.
- ➲ SOURCE: Tincture of entire fresh plant when in flower.
- ➲ SPHERES OF ACTION: Female gential organs, Veins, mucous membrane of tongue, stomach, bowels.
- ➲ SUMMARY OF INDICATIONS: Anxiety states- Insomnia- Women's disorders–allergic disorders.

THERAPEUTIC PICTURE OF DRUG

C_{N-1} ➲ Ladies who are fair and beautifully-looking.

C_{N-2} ➲ Inclined to be fleshy with fine hair and blue eyes, soft and lax muscles.

C_{N-3} ➲ Anaemic and chlorotic with pale face at Puberty.

C_{N-4} ➲ Women inclined to be fleshy, with scanty and Protracted menstruation (Graph.).

M_{D-1} ➲ Weeps easily: almost impossible to detail her ailments without weeping (Weeps when thanked, lyc).

M_{D-2} ➲ Feels better by consolation.

M_{D-3} ➲ Fears in the evening of being alone, ghosts.

M_{D-4} ➲ Morbid dread of the opposite sex.

M_{D-5} ➲ Religious melancholy.

M_{D-6} ➲ Highly emotional; mentally, like an April day.

SO_1 ➲ Eyelids stick together in the mornings due to thick lacrimal discharge (Borax). Styes (Staphisagria).

SO_2 ➲ Ear-ache with thick, yellow discharge. External ear is swollen and red.

DS_1 ➲ Toothache worse in spring; at night; from picking teeth; in warm room; in warmth of bed.

DS_2 ➲ Gastric catarrh, from ice cream, fruit and pastry; Pain, as from subcutaneous ulceration.

DS_3 ➲ Pain in the stomach an hour after eating.

DS_4 ➲ All gone sensation, especially in tea drinkers.

DS_5 ➲ Diarrhoea during menses, particularly if it comes on at night.

DS_6 ➲ Diarrhoea, frequent evacuations of whitish, yellowish, sanguineous mucous, or of greenish, minced, bilious or watery and sometimes corrosive matter may contain tapeworm.

RS_1 ➲ Loose, rattling cough, worse in a heated room and at night.

FGS_1 ➲ Disordered at Puberty.

FGS_2 ➲ Delayed first menstruation Period with Painful, scanty flow.

FGS_3 ➲ Retained Placenta.

FGS_4 ➲ Menses: suppressed from getting the feet wet; too late, scanty, slimy, Painful, irregular, intermittent flow, with evening chilliness; with intense Pain and great restless and tossing about (Mag.P.); flow more during day (on lying down, kreos.).

FGS_5 ➲ Threatened abortion; flow ceases and then returns with increased forces. Pains spasmodic, excite suffocation and fainting; must have fresh air.

FGS_6 ➲ Affections in general of female genital organs; of the uterus.

FGS_7 ➲ Spasmodic Pains or drawing tension in uterus, and Pains like those of labour.

FGS_8 ➲ During Pregnancy: nausea, morning sickness; Varicose veins, bluish, < towards evening.

FGS_9 ➲ During labour: intense inertia; weeps because she is not delivered.

FGS_{10} ➲ Labour-Pains too weak, spasmodic, or ceasing.

FGS_{11} ➲ Welling of breasts, with tensive pain as if the milk rushed into them and caused Pressure, while nursing.

FGS_{12} ➲ Lumps of breasts of girls before Puberty; or escape of thin, milk-like fluid.

FGS_{13} ➲ Weeps every time child is put to breast; Pain extends into chest, neck, or down back, changes from place to place.

FGS_{14} ➲ Helps to terminate lactation, when breast feeding is over (Lac Canium).

PG_1 ➲ Fainting easily in a hot, stuffy atmosphere.

PG_2 ➲ Insomnia due to recurring thoughts, sound asleep at waking time.

PG_3 ➲ Pulsatilla is often indicated in allergies such as hayfever, bronchial asthma, eczema.

PG_4 ➲ Changeable symptoms.

PG_5 ➲ Thirstlessnes with nearly all complaints.

Modalities

Aggravation

- ➲ Heat.
- ➲ Rich, fatty food.
- ➲ Warm room.
- ➲ Twilight.
- ➲ After eating.
- ➲ Lying on the left (or painless side).

Amelioration

- ➲ Motion.
- ➲ Open air.
- ➲ Cold food and drinks, though not thirsty.
- ➲ Cold applications.

Relations

- ➲ COMPLEMENTARY: Lyc; Sil; Stann; Sul-ac.
- ➲ FOLLOWS WELL: Anac; Ant-t; Ars; Asof; Bell; Bry; Euphr; Graph; Ign; Kali-bi; Lyc; Nit-ac; Nux-v; Phos; Rhus-t; Sep; Sulph.

Pyrogenium

- ➲ PROVED BY: Drysdale.
- ➲ COMMON NAME: A product of sepsis.
- ➲ FAMILY/KINGDOM: A Nosode.
- ➲ SPHERES OF ACTION: Act on blood, heart, uterus, Skin, mucous membrane.
- ➲ SUMMARY OF INDICATIONS: Septic fevers–communicable fevers- chronic constipation.

THERAPEUTIC PICTURE OF DRUG

C_{N-1} ➲ Lean, thin, exhausted person.

M_{D-1} ➲ Full of Anxiety and insane notions.

M_{D-2} ➲ Loguacious, thinks, she is very wealthy. Restlessness.

M_{D-3} ➲ Cannot tell whether dreaming while awake or as sleep.

DS_1 ➲ Tounge large, flabby, clean, smooth as if varnished, fiery red.

DS_2 ➲ Vomiting: Persistent; brownish, coffee-ground; offensive, stercoraceous; with impacted or obstructed bowels.

DS_3 ➲ Diarrhoea; horribly offensive, brown-black, painless, involuntary.

DS_4 ➲ Constipation with complete inertia; obstinate from of impaction.

DS_5 ➲ Stool large, black, carrion like, or small black balls.

CVS_1 ➲ Pulse abnormally rapid, small, wiry, 140 to 170, cold, clammy, sweat.

CVS_2 ➲ Distinct consciousness of a heart.

CVS_3 ➲ Tired feeling around the heart.

CVS_4 ➲ Sensation as if the heart was too full.

FGS_1 ➲ Puerperal peritonitis, with extreme fetor.

FGS_2 ➲ Septicemia following Abortion.

FGS_3 ➲ Uterine Haemorrhages.

FGS_4 ➲ Menses horribly offensive.

FGS_5 ➲ Fever at each menstrual period, consequent upon latent pelvic inflammation.

FGS_6 ➲ Septic puerperal infection.

FGS_7 ➲ Pelvic calculitis.

FGS_8 ➲ Imaflammatory exudite.

FGS_9 ➲ Lochia-thin, acrid, brown, very foetid (Nit-acid) suppressed followed by chill, fever and profuse factid perspiration.

F_{R-1} ➲ Great heat with profuse, hot sweat, but sweating does not cause a fall in temperature.

F_{R-2} ➲ Coldness and chilliness; septic fevers; latent pyogenic condition.

F_{R-3} ➲ Feels hot as if he had a fever, but was only 99^{0}F., feels live 105^{0}F.

F_{R-4} ➲ Chills begins in the back; temperature rises rapidly.

F_{R-5} ➲ In all cases of fever commencing with pains in the limbs.

PG_1 ➲ The bed feels hard (Arn), Parts lain on feel sore and bruised (Bep.).

Modalities

Aggravation

- ➲ Heart's action and cough are Aggravated by motion.
- ➲ Cold, from passing plates at night.

Amelioration

- ➲ From motion.
- ➲ From heat.
- ➲ From pressure.

Relations

- ➲ COMPARE: Staphyloccin; Streptoccin; Ars; Lach; Rhus; Spin.
- ➲ COMPLEMENTARY: Bryon.
- ➲ FOLLOWS WELL: Bryo; Lach; Ruhs.-T.

Ratanhia peruviana

- COMMON NAME: Mapato.
- FAMILY/KINGDOM: Polygalaceae.
- SOURCE: Tincture of root.
- SPHERES OF ACTION: Act of Nipple of breast, Gastrointstinal tract.
- SUMMARY OF INDICATIONS: Toothache of Pregnancy of–fissures of the anus-Proctitis.

THERAPEUTIC PICTURE OF DRUG

M_{D-1} ➲ Irritable, Peevish and quarrlsome humour.

M_{D-2} ➲ Changeable mind.

DS_1 ➲ Excruciating toothache during the early months of Pregnancy, tooth feels elongated; increased by lying, compelling the patient to rise and walk about.

DS_2 ➲ Excruciating pain after stool (Nit-acid), Fissure of anus, great sensitiveness of rectum.

FGS_1 ➲ Pressure in the groins, as of a general bearing down toward genital organs followed by Leucorrhoea.

FGS_2 ➲ Leucorrhoea with itcnig in Rectum and discharge of Bloody mucus.

FGS_3 ➲ Catamenia too early and of too long duration, and too copious, pain in Abdomen and loins.

FGS_4 ➲ Metrorrhagia- uterine pain following retrocession of eruption on loins.

FGS_5 ➲ Fissure of nipples in nursing women (Graph. Sep.).

Modalities

Aggravation

- By touch.
- At night.

Amelioration

- Open air.
- By motion.

Relations

- COMPARE: Canth; Carb-ac; Iris; Sulph.
- FOLLOWS WELL: Sul; Bovis; Sep.
- ANTIDOTES: Nux-v; Camph.

Rhus toxicodendron

- PROVED BY: Hehnemann.
- DURATION: 20-30 days.
- COMMON NAME: Poison Oak.
- FAMILY/KINGDOM: Anacardiaceae.
- RELATION COLD/HEAT: Very chilly.
- MIASM: Psora.
- DIATHESIS: Rheumatic & Gouty.
- SOURCE: Tincture of fresh leaves gathered at sunset just before flowering time.
- SPHERES OF ACTION: Mucous membrane, Lymphatic glands, Muscular tissue & part of joints eg. Ligaments, tendons & fibrous tissues.
- SUMMARY OF INDICATIONS: Rheumatic disorders–Soft tissue injuries–allergy and urticaria–Skin disorders–Herpes.

THERAPEUTIC PICTURE OF DRUG

C_{N-1} ➲ Patient is very chilly, easily susceptible to cold.

C_{N-2} ➲ Adapted to womens of rheumatic diathesis.

M_{D-1} ➲ Listless sad.

M_{D-2} ➲ Thoughts of suicide

M_{D-3} ➲ Extreme restlessness [Mental & Physical both] with continuous change of Position.

M_{D-4} ➲ Fears she will die of being Poisoned (Hyos.).

M_{D-5} ➲ Great apprehension at night, cannot remain in bed.

M_{D-6} ➲ Sensorium becomes cloudy.

H_{D-1} ➲ Meningitis in exanthematous fevers, or after getting wet; tingling limbs; high fever; restlessness.

H_{D-2} ➲ Brain feels loose, when stepping or shaking the head.

H_{D-3} ➲ Stupefying headache, with buzzing; worse when sitting or lying; in the cold, in the morning, from beer; better from warmth and motion.

H_{D-4} ➲ Headache must lie down; returns from the least chagrin.

H_{D-5} ➲ Vertigo in the aged, worse when rising from lying, and from turning or stooping.

DS_1 ➲ Tongue: dry, sore, red, cracked; Triangular red tip; takes imprint of teeth (Chel; Podo).

DS_2 ➲ Nocturnal diarrhoea, with violent colic, headache, and pains in all limbs worse after on evacuation or when lying on abdomen.

DS_3 ➲ Chronic painless diarrhoea, only in morning preceded by marked commotion in the bowels.

DS_4 ➲ Diarrhoea with tearing pains running down back of the leg with every stool.

DS_5 ➲ Haemorrhoids: sore, blind; Protruding after stool, with pressing in rectum, as if everything would come out.

FGS_1 ➲ Menstrual flow light–coloured and acrid, causing biting pain in the vulva.

FGS_2 ➲ Erysipelatous inflammation of the external genitals.

FGS_3 ➲ Menorrhagia from strains; from wetting.

FGS_4 ➲ Pain as from excoriation and shootings in vagina.

FGS_5 ➲ Relieves shootings pains of cancer uteri.

FGS_6 ➲ Bearing–down pain; when standing.

FGS_7 ➲ For weeks after delivery pain in right limbs with numbness from hips to feet (varicose veins).

FGS_8 ➲ Breasts painfully distended, red in streaks, rheumatic state.

FGS_9 ➲ Amenorrhoea from getting wet; with milk in breasts.

FGS_{10} ➲ Diminished secretion (suppression) of milk; with burning over body.

MGS_1 ➲ Swelling of glands and Prepuce (balanitis), dark red erypsipelatous.

MGS_2 ➲ Scrotum becomes thick and hard, with intolerable itching.

MGS_3 ➲ Erections at night, or with desire to urinate.

LS_1 ➲ Muscular rheumatism, sciatica.

LS_2 ➲ Swelling, stiffness and paralysed sensation in joints, from sprain, over-lifting, or over-stretching.

LS_3 ➲ Rheumatic tension, drawing, tearing in limbs, during rest.

LS_4 ➲ Lameness, stiffness, and pain on first moving after rest, or on getting up in morning, better by constant motion.

LS_5 ➲ Trembling or sensation of trembling in limbs.

LS_6 ➲ The limbs on which he lied, esp. arms, go to sleep.

LS_7 ➲ Excessively cold hands and feet all day.

B_{K-1} ➲ Pains in shoulders and back, with stiffness as from a spine.

B_{K-2} ➲ Pains in small of back, better lying upon something hard.

B_{K-3} ➲ Drawing and stitches in back, esp. when seated and on stooping.

- S_{N-1} ➲ Allergy and urticaria. Itching, burning and tingling. Herpes.
- S_{N-2} ➲ Eczema: surface raw, excoriated; thick crusts, oozing and offensive.
- S_{N-3} ➲ Erysipelas; Erysipelatous inflammations.
- F_{R-1} ➲ Typhoid; tongue dry and brown; sordes; bowels loose; great restlessness.
- F_{R-2} ➲ Intermittent; chills, with a dry cough and restlessness.
- F_{R-3} ➲ Adynamic; restless, trembling.
- F_{R-4} ➲ During heat, urticaria; hydroa.
- PG_1 ➲ Adapted to womens of a rheumatic diathesis; soft tissue disorders from getting wet, sprains or strains of ligaments, muscles or tendons.
- PG_2 ➲ Stiffness and pain on first moving after rest, or on getting up in the morning, better after waking or continued motion.
- PG_3 ➲ Great thirst, with dry tongue, mouth and throat.

Modalities

Aggravation

- ➲ Before a storm.
- ➲ Cold, wet, rainy weather.
- ➲ All night, especially after midnight.
- ➲ From getting wet while Perspiring.
- ➲ During rest.
- ➲ Lying on back or right side.

Amelioration

- ➲ Warm.
- ➲ Dry weather.
- ➲ Wrapping up.
- ➲ Warm or hot food.
- ➲ Motion.
- ➲ Change of position.
- ➲ Moving the affected parts.

Relations

- ➲ COMPARE: Arn; Bry; Rhod; Nat-s; Sulph.
- ➲ COMPLEMENTARY: Bry.
- ➲ FOLLOWS WELL: Ars; Arn; Bell; Bryo Cact; Calc; Calc-p; Cham; Con; Dros; Graph; Hyos; Lach; Merc; Mur-ac; Nux-v., Phos., Puls., Sep., Sulph.
- ➲ ANTIDOTES: Ana; Bell, Bry; Camph; Coff; Crot-t; Graph; Sep; Sulph.
- ➲ INIMICALS: Apis.

Sabadilla

- ➲ PROVED BY: Stapf.
- ➲ DURATION: 20-30 days.
- ➲ COMMON NAME: Cevadilla.
- ➲ FAMILY/KINGDOM: Liliaceae.
- ➲ RELATION COLD/HEAT: Chilly.
- ➲ MIASM: Antipsoric.
- ➲ SOURCE: Tincture of seed.
- ➲ SPHERES OF ACTION: Mucous membrane of Respiratory tract Lachrymal glands and nerves.
- ➲ SUMMARY OF INDICATIONS: headache-respiratory disorders.

THERAPEUTIC PICTURE OF DRUG

C_{N-1} ➲ Light hair, fair complexion with a weak, relaxed Muscular system

M_{D-1} ➲ Delirium during intermittents (Podo).

M_{D-2} ➲ Illusion-that she is sick, that she is pregnant.

M_{D-3} ➲ When merely distended from flatus, that she has some horrible throat diseases that will be fatal.

H_{D-1} ➲ Headache from too much thinking.

H_{D-2} ➲ Headache from excessive montation, too close application or attention (Arg-n).

SO_1 ➲ Seezing in spasmodic Paroxysms; following by lachrymation, copious watery coryza-face hot and eyelids are red and burning.

RS_1 ➲ Dryness of fauces and throat

FGS_1 ➲ Menses too late, come by fits and starts. Intermit (Kreo. Puls) (due to transient and localized congestion to womb alternating with chronic anaemic state).

S_{N-1} ➲ Parchment-like dryness of skin worms.

Modalities

Aggravation

- From cold.
- Cold drink.
- At regular period.
- New and full moon.

Amelioration

- Wrapped up.
- Warm food and drink.

Relations

- COMPARE: Colo; Colch; Lyco.
- COMPLEMENTARY: Sepia.
- FOLLOWS WELL: Bry and Ran; Aco; Nux; Puls.
- ANTIDOTES: Con; Puls.

Sabina

- PROVED BY: Stapf.
- DURATION: 20-30 days.
- COMMON NAME: Savine.
- FAMILY/KINGDOM: Coniferae.
- RELATION COLD/HEAT: Hot.
- MIASM: Sycosis.
- SOURCE: Tincture of the young fresh tops of the branches.
- SPHERES OF ACTION: Especially on uterus, serous and fibrous tissue.
- SUMMARY OF INDICATIONS: Nervous disorder-Lumbar Pains-Uterine disorders-enuresis.

THERAPEUTIC PICTURE OF DRUG

C_{N-1} ➲ Chlorotic women, having tendency to miscarriage particularly in the third month.

C_{N-2} ➲ Dejection, discouragement, and sadness.

M_{D-1} ➲ Music is intolerable- produces nervousness, goes through bone and marrow (Thuja).

FGS_1 ➲ Inflammation of ovaries or uterus after abortion or premature labour.

FGS_2 ➲ Promotes expulsion of moles or foreign bodies from uterus (Canth.).

FGS_3 ➲ Tendency to miscarriage, especially at third month.

FGS_4 ➲ Ailments, following abortion or premature labour, haemorrhage from the uterus, flow partly pale red, partly clotted, wors from least motion (Sec.)

FGS_5 ➲ Pain extending from sacrum to pubes.

FGS_6 ➲ Menses: too early, too profuse, too protracted, partly fluid, partly clotted (Ferr) Pain from sacrum to pubis.

FGS_7 ➲ Discharge of blood between periods, with sexual excitement (Ambr).

FGS_8 ➲ Retained placenta from atony of uterus, intense after pain (Caul, sec).

FGS_9 ➲ Memorrhagia- During climacteric, in women who formely aborted, with early first menses.

PG_1 ➲ Drawing pains in small of back, from sacrum to pubis.

PG_2 ➲ Music is intolerable produces nervousness.

Modalities

Aggravation

- From last motion (Sec.).
- Warm air or room (Apis, Puls).

Amelioration

- In cool, open, fresh air.

Relations

➲ COMPARE:	Calc-os; Croc; Mill; Sec-Thrill.
➲ COMPLEMENTARY:	Thuja; Sepia.
➲ FOLLOWS WELL:	Thuja; Ars; Bell; Rhus; Spong; Sulph.
➲ ANTIDOTES	Con; Puls.

Sanicula aqua

- ➲ PROVED BY: Dr. J.G. Gundlach.
- ➲ COMMON NAME: Mineral Spring water (Sanicula aqua).
- ➲ RELATION COLD/HEAT: Not stamping.
- ➲ MIASM: Psoric & Sycotic.
- ➲ DIATHESIS: Scrofulous.
- ➲ TEMPERAMENT: mentally head strong and obstinate.
- ➲ SOURCE: Triturations of the evaporated salt.
- ➲ SPHERES OF ACTION: All over the body especially female sexual organs, GIT, nervous system & skin.
- ➲ SUMMARY OF INDICATIONS: Female genital disorders with skin disorders.

THERAPEUTIC PICTURE OF DRUG

C_{N-1} ➲ Sanicula child looks old, dirty, greasy & brownish.

C_{N-2} ➲ Skin about neck wrinkled, hangs in folds, scaly dandruff on scalp, eye brows and beard.

M_{D-1} ➲ Dread of downward motion (Borx.)

M_{D-2} ➲ Constantly changing his occupation.

M_{D-3} ➲ Instability of purpose.

M_{D-4} ➲ Depression; mind wanders from one subject to another, even when conversing

M_{D-5} ➲ Child headstrong and obstinate, crying and kicking, esp. 9 P.M. to 12 p.m.

M_{D-6} ➲ Head strong crossness quickly alternating with laughter and playfulness in children.

H_{D-1} ➲ Profuse sweat on occiput and in the nape of neck, during sleep.

H_{D-2} ➲ Profuse, scaly dandruff; soreness behind the ears.

DS_1 ➲ Tongue: Large, flabby, burning, must Protrude it to keep it cool; ring worm on tongue (Nat.m).

DS_2 ➲ Thirst: Drinks little and often; is vomited as soon as it reaches the stomach (Ars; Phos).

DS_3 ➲ Incontinence of urine and faeces; sphincters inefficient. (Aloe Soc.); urging from flatus, mus cross legs to prevent faeces escaping.

DS_4 ➲ Nausea and vomiting from car riding.

DS_5 ➲ Constipation with ineffectual urging.

DS_6 ➲ Impossible to evacuate the stool, which is of grayish–white balls, like burnt lime, hard and crumbling, with odour of rotten cheese; it must be removed mechanically.

DS_7 ➲ At 9.30 P.M. copious diarrhoea with urging and haste; stool yellow and fetid as after eating onions; soft, sticky, mushy stool twice each day.

FGS_1 ➲ Bearing down, as if the contents of Pelvis would escape (Prolapse).better rest.

FGS_2 ➲ Desire to support parts by placing hand against vulva, rest (Lil-t; Mux).

FGS_3 ➲ Soreness of uterus.

FGS_4 ➲ Vagina feels large.

FGS_5 ➲ Leucorrhoea with strong odour of fish brine or old cheese (Hep.).

FGS_6 ➲ A few hours after intercourse appearance of a slight watery discharge from vagina with odour of fish brine, lasting about twenty four hours; not removed by bathing.

FGS_7 ➲ During Pregnancy: swelling of lower limbs at third month, evening; swelling and stiffness of hands and feet.

FGS_8 ➲ During menses dilating pain in lower abdomen, with soreness of womb; pain in back>, when flow established; tumour size of hen's egg, left side of womb just above cervix, come on since the passing.

S_{N-1} ➲ Eczema, fissured hands and fingers.

S_{N-2} ➲ Greasy, brownish, dirty and wrinkled.

PG_1 ➲ Pain just above sacrum, before the flow and from motion; from rest.

PG_2 ➲ Constantly shifting focus of attention.

PG_3 ➲ Progressive emaciation; child looks old, dirty, greasy, and brownish.

PG_4 ➲ Child kicks off clothing even in coldest weather.

PG_5 ➲ Dread of usual work on account of weakness and exhaustion, with irresistible desire to lie down.

Modalities

Aggravation

➲ Moving arms backwards.

Relations

➲ COMPARE: Alum; Calc; Sil; Sulph; Abrot.

Sarsaparilla officinalis

- ➲ PROVED BY: Hahnemann.
- ➲ DURATION: 30 days.
- ➲ COMMON NAME: Wild Liquorice.
- ➲ FAMILY/KINGDOM: Smilaceae.
- ➲ RELATION COLD/HEAT: Cold.
- ➲ MIASM: Act three miasms.
- ➲ DIATHESIS: Lithic and scrofulous.
- ➲ SOURCE: Triturations and tincture of the dried Phizome.
- ➲ SPHERES OF ACTION: Urinary organs, gental and rectum skin, bones.
- ➲ SUMMARY OF INDICATIONS: Urinary disorders-retraction of nipples.

THERAPEUTIC PICTURE OF DRUG

C_{N-1} ➲ Lean, thin and debilitated person with dark hair and shrivelled skin which lies loose in Folds.

M_{D-1} ➲ Mental depression caused by the pains.

M_{D-2} ➲ Irritable, Impatient or changeable.

M_{D-3} ➲ Gloomy, desponding, debility.

H_{D1} ➲ Pains cause depression.

H_{D2} ➲ Pain from occiput to eyes.

H_{D3} ➲ Throbbing pain in head.

H_{D4} ➲ Vertigo, with nausea and sour risings.

SO_1 ➲ Shooting in eyes, itching like eruption on lids.

SO_2 ➲ Burning sensation in eyes and lids.

SO_3 ➲ Burning itching scabs on lobes of ears.

SO_4 ➲ Pain in nose, inflamed spots on septum.

SO_5 ➲ Words reverberate in ear.

DS_1 ➲ Burning, or cold feeling in abdomen.

DS_2 ➲ Constipation, violent urging to urinate.
DS_3 ➲ Nausea when thinking of food.
DS_4 ➲ Blood with the stool.
FGS_1 ➲ Nipple withered, small, Retracted.
FGS_2 ➲ Leucorrhoea on walking, pain at meatus urinarius after urinating.
FGS_3 ➲ Menses too late and scanty, preceded by urging to urinate, itching eruption on fore head, flow acrid.
FGS_4 ➲ During menses, gripping in pit of stomach in direction of small of back.
FGS_5 ➲ Retractions of nipples: nipples are small, atrophied, unexcitable (Sil.).
US_1 ➲ Urine-scanty, slimy, flaky, sandy, copious, passed without sensation (caust).
US_2 ➲ Passage of gravel or small calculi, Renal Colic, Stone in bladder, bloody urine.
US_3 ➲ Severe almost unbearable pain at the conclusion of urination (Beb-Vul., Euq-hye, Medo, Thuj).
US_4 ➲ Painful distension and tenderness in bladder; urine dribble while sitting, standing passes freely, air passes from urethra.
US_5 ➲ During urination air passes from bladder.
US_6 ➲ Cramp in bladder, with contractive pain.
US_7 ➲ Pain at meatus urinarius with women.
LS_1 ➲ Trembling of hands and feet.
LS_2 ➲ Rheumatic pains after gonorrhoea.
LS_3 ➲ Red spots on calves.
LS_4 ➲ Stitching in legs, especially from motion.

Modalities

Aggravation

➲ By touch, pressure motion.
➲ Going upstairs and washing.

Amelioration

➲ By warmth, Rest, cold diet and loosening garments.

Relations

➲ COMPARE:	Lyco; Nat-mur; Phospho.
➲ COMPLEMENTARY:	Mercury; Sepia; All-c.
➲ FOLLOWS WELL:	Bell; Sep; Sulph; Phos; Rhus.
➲ ANTIDOTES:	Bell; Merc; Sepia.
➲ INIMICALS:	Ac-acid.

Secale cornutum (Claviceps purpurea)

- COMMON NAME: Spurred Rye (Ergot).
- DURATION: 20-30 days.
- RELATION COLD/HEAT: Hot.
- FAMILY/KINGDOM: A Fungus [A Nosode].
- DIATHESIS: Haemorrhagic.
- MIASM: Psora.
- SOURCE: Tincture of the fresh spurs collected just before harvest.
- TEMPERAMENT: Irritable.
- SPHERES OF ACTION: Nervous system, uterine muscle, female genital, arterioles, capillaries and blood system.
- SUMMARY OF INDICATIONS: Menstrual disorders–failure of lactation.

THERAPEUTIC PICTURE OF DRUG

C_{N-1} ➲ Female patient are of very lax muscular fibre.

C_{N-2} ➲ Female patients are everything seems loose and open.

C_{N-3} ➲ Adapted to women of thin, scrawny, feeble, cachectic, appearance; irritable, nervous temperament; Pale, sunken countenance.

M_{D-1} ➲ Discouragement and timidity.

M_{D-2} ➲ Great anxiety; sadness and melancholy

M_{D-3} ➲ Mental alienation

DS_1 ➲ Inclination to colic, diarrhoea, and bloatedness of abdomen.

DS_2 ➲ Cholera Asiatica, with collapse, face sunken, distorted, particularly the mouth, crawling sensation as from ants.

DS_3 ➲ Diarrhoea of a putrid smell, with sudden prostration of strength.

DS_4 ➲ Diarrhoea: frequent brown discharges, dark-coloured; very offensive; thin, olive green; very exhausting; pernicious.

CVS_1 ➲ Pulse: small, rapid, contracted and often intermittent.

CVS_2 ➲ Violent spasmodic palpitation of heart.

CVS_3 ➲ Painful sensation over heart.

FGS_1 ➲ Menses: too profuse, and last too long; with tearing and cutting colic, cold extremities, cold sweat, great weakness and small pulse; or with violent spasms.

FGS_2 ➲ Menstrual blood: thin and black; lumpy, or brown fluid, and of disgusting smell.

FGS_3 ➲ Leucorrhoea brownish and offensive; like cream; from weakness and venous congestion.

FGS_4 ➲ Threatened abortus: more especially at the third month; with copious flow of black, liquid blood; false labor pains with bloody discharge.

FGS_5 ➲ During Pregnancy: frequent and Prolonged forcing pain, Particularly in thin, ill-conditioned women; cramp in colves.

FGS_6 ➲ During labor: Prolonged bearing down and forcing pains in the uterus; Pains irregular; Pains too weak; Pains feeble, distant or ceasing; everything seems loose and open no action; fainting fits; after labor; retained urine.

FGS_7 ➲ After pains: too long; too painful; hour-glass contraction.

FGS_8 ➲ Suppression of milk; in thin, scrawny, exhausted women; the breasts do not properly fill.

FGS_9 ➲ Puerperal fever, Putrid discharges, tympanites, coldness, suppressed urine.

FGS_{10} ➲ Swelling and warts on the cervix uteri, which is partially open.

FGS_{11} ➲ Gangrene of vaginal mucous membrane, with a dark, slate colour.

FGS_{12} ➲ Sanguineous congestion in uterus, cancer and gangrene of uterus.

FGS_{13} ➲ Suppression of milk, in thin, scraggy, exhausted women; the breasts do not engorge.

S_{N-1} ➲ Swelling and pain without inflammation; coldness, blue colour; gangrene.

S_{N-2} ➲ Skin sallow, lead-coloured, flaccid, and shrivelled.

S_{N-3} ➲ Ulcers that turn black; skin withered and gangrenous.

PG_1 ➲ Burning; in all parts of the body.

PG_2 ➲ The skin feels cold to the touch, yet the patient cannot tolerate any covering; icy coldness of the extremities.

PG_3 ➲ Loss of sensation through the body.

PG_4 ➲ For female complaints chiefly, and esp. when occurring in thin, scrawny, wrinkled females or children.

Modalities

Aggravation

- ➲ Heat.
- ➲ Warmth from covering of all affected parts.

Amelioration

- In the cold air.
- Getting cold.
- Uncovering affected parts.
- Rubbing.

Relations

- COMPLEMENTARY: Ars; Chinch; Merc-viv; Puls.
- FOLLOWS WELL: Acon; Ars; Bell; Chin; Merc; Puls.
- ANTIDOTES: Camph; Op.

Senecio aureus

- COMMON NAME: Golden Ragwort.
- SOURCE: Tincture of fresh plant in flower.

THERAPEUTIC PICTURE OF DRUG

C_{N-1} ➲ She is chlorotic, thin, debilitated.
M_{D-1} ➲ Inability to fix mind upon any one subject.
M_{D-2} ➲ Despondent.
M_{D-3} ➲ Nervous and irritable.
H_{D-1} ➲ Wave like dizziness from occiput to sinciput.
SO_1 ➲ Sharp pains over left eye, and through left temple.
FGS_1 ➲ Menses retarded, suppressed.
FGS_2 ➲ Functional amenorrhoea of young girl with backache.
FGS_3 ➲ Before menses, inflammatory condition of throat, chest and bladder.
FGS_4 ➲ After menstruation common as, these improve.
FGS_5 ➲ Anaemic dysmenorrhoea with urineary disturbances.
FGS_6 ➲ Premature and too profuse menses (Calc., Erig).
FGS_7 ➲ Awakened early by great sexual irritation, vagina full of mucus, labia swollen, itchy and burring.
FGS_8 ➲ Leucorrhoea preceded by headache, sleeplessness and irritable bladder.

Modalities

Aggravation

- At night.
- Sitting.
- In open air.

Amelioration

- Bending forward.
- At onset of menses.
- By stool.

Relations

- COMPARE: Arn; Calend; Bell.

Sepia officinalis

- PROVED BY: Hahnemann.
- DURATION: 40-50 days.
- COMMON NAME: Cuttle fish.
- FAMILY/KINGDOM: Mollusca.
- RELATION COLD/HEAT: Very chilly patient.
- MIASM: Anti-Psoric and anti-sycotic.
- TEMPERAMENT: Nervous temperament.
- SOURCE: Trituration of dried liquid contained in the ink-bag.
- SPHERES OF ACTION: Female genital organs, Nervous system, GIT, liver, Portal system and skin.
- SUMMARY OF INDICATIONS: Gynaecological disorders-Pregnancy of disorders-anxiety-lenucoderma.

THERAPEUTIC PICTURE OF DRUG

C_{N-1} ➲ In womens, male type of Pelvis.

C_{N-2} ➲ Adopted to persons of dark hair, rigid fibre, but mild and easy nature (Puls.).

C_{N-3} ➲ Cachectic yellow face, with yellow soddle across upper part of the cheeks and node; a tell tale face of Uterine ailments.

M_{D-1} ➲ Great sadness and weeping. Dread of being alone. Fear of men and of meeting friends; of Uterine troubles.

M_{D-2} ➲ Fear of indulging in sex.

M_{D-3} ➲ Weeps when narrating the symptoms.

M_{D-4} ➲ Greedy, miserly (lyc.).

M_{D-5} ➲ Sadness about one's health and her domestic affairs.

M_{D-6} ➲ Great indifference even to one's family, to those one loves best.

M_{D-7} ➲ Anxiety: with fear, flushes of heat over the face; about real or imaginary evils.

M_{D-8} ➲ Aversion to one's occupation.

H_{D-1} ➲ Headache: in terrific shocks; at menstrual nisus, with scanty flow; in delicate, sensitive, hysterical women.

H_{D-2} ➲ Stinging pain from with in outward, and upwards mostly on the left side, or in the forehead, with nausea, vomiting-migraine; worse indoors and when lying on painful side.

H_{D-3} ➲ Coldness of vertex with headache.

H_{D-4} ➲ Vertigo, with sensation of something rolling around in the head.

DS_1 ➲ Tongue foul, but become clear at each menstrual nisus, returns when flow ceases; swelling and cracking of lower lip.

DS_2 ➲ Sensitive ness of pit of stomach to touch.

DS_3 ➲ Painful sensation of emptiness in stomach and abdomen.

DS_4 ➲ Constipation during pregnancy.

DS_5 ➲ Pain in rectum during and long after stool; hard, knotty, insufficient stool, mixed or covered with mucus; involuntary straining.

FGS_1 ➲ Diseases of women, especially those occurring during Pregnancy, child birth and lactation; or diseases attended with sudden Prostration.

FGS_2 ➲ Pelivic organs relaxed.

FGS_3 ➲ Bearing down sensation as if everything would escape through the vulva. (Bell., Keros., Lit-t, Nat-C., Podo), must cross limbs to Prevent Protrusion, or press against vulva.

FGS_4 ➲ Leucorrhoea yellow, greenish, with much itching.

FGS_5 ➲ Menses too late and scanty, irregular; early and Profuse; sharp clutching Pain.

FGS_6 ➲ Violent stitches upward in the vagina, from the uterus to the Umbilicus.

FGS_7 ➲ Prolapse of Uterus and vagina.

FGS_8 ➲ Morning sickness of Pregnancy, the sight or thought of food sickness (Nux-m); the smell of cooking food nauseates (Ars., colch.).

FGS_9 ➲ Vagina Painful, especially during coition (dysparunia).

FGS_{10} ➲ Bearing down in uterus, which obstructs respiration.

FGS_{11} ➲ Colic before menses.

FGS_{12} ➲ During menses: irritability, melancholy, toothache, headache, nose-bleed, and painful weariness in limbs, or spasmodic colic and pressure towards the parts.

FGS_{13} ➲ Excoriation of nipples (which bleed and seem about to ulcerate).

FGS_{14} ➲ During Pregnancy yellow brown spot on face.

US_1 ➲ Enuresis: bed is wet almost as soon as the child goes to sleep (Kreosote).

US_2 ➲ Red, adhesive, sand in urine-haematuria.

US_3 ➲ Chronic cystitis, slow micturition with bearing down sensation above the Pubis.

US_4 ➲ Dyspnoea; worse sitting, after sleep, in room, better dancing or walking rapidly.

S_{N-1} ➲ Herpes circinatus in isolated spots on upper part of body.

S_{N-2} ➲ Itching in face, on, arms, hands, back, hips, feet, abdomen and genitals.

S_{N-3} ➲ Itching often changes to burning when scratching.

S_{N-4} ➲ Ulcers: Painless, on joints or tips of fingers or toes; itching, stinging and burning.

PG_1 ➲ All the covering of the neck feel, too tight and are constantly loosened (Lach.). Leucoderma.

PG_2 ➲ Falling of hair, after chronic headaches or at the climacteric.

PG_3 ➲ Great tendency to take cold, and sensibility to cold air, esp. in a north wind.

PG_4 ➲ Feverish shivering, syncope and afterwards corzya, after getting wet.

PG_5 ➲ Sensations: of a ball in inner parts; pain as if part would burst, were pressed or pushed as under; cramping or drawing pain in inner or outer parts.

Modalities

Aggravation

- ➲ In afternoon or evening.
- ➲ From cold air or a dry wind.
- ➲ Sexual excess.
- ➲ At rest.
- ➲ Sultry, moist weather.
- ➲ Before a thunderstorm (Psorinum).

Amelioration

- ➲ Warmth of bed.
- ➲ Hot applications.
- ➲ Violent exercise.
- ➲ Pressure.
- ➲ Cold baths.

Relations

➲ COMPLEMENTARY:	Nat-m; Nux-v.
➲ FOLLOWS WELL:	Bell; Calc; Carb-v; Con; Dros; Euphr; Graph; Lyc; Nux-v; Puls; Rhus-t; Sars; Sil; Sulph.
➲ ANTIDOTES:	Acon; Ant-c; Ant-t; Nit-s-d; Sulph; Vegetable acid.
➲ INIMICALS:	Bry; Lach.
➲ SIMILAR:	Lach; Sang; Ust.

Silicea terra

- PROVED BY: Hahnemann.
- DURATION: 40-60 days.
- COMMON NAME: Pure Silica.
- FAMILY/KINGDOM: Mineral s.
- RELATION COLD/HEAT: Extremely Chilly.
- MIASM: Psora, Syphilis & Sycosis.
- DIATHESIS: Scrofulous.
- TEMPERAMENT: Irritable and Sanguine.
- SOURCE: Trituration of Pure,precipitated silica.
- SPHERES OF ACTION: Bones, cartilages, mucous membranes, skin, nerves, glands, Eustachian tube etc.
- SUMMARY OF INDICATIONS: Gastro intestinal disorders (digestive disorders, and fissures, fistula)–chronic infections–expulsion of foreign bodies–Paronychia–osteomyelitis–silicosis–emphysema–skin disorders.

THERAPEUTIC PICTURE OF DRUG

C_{N-1} ➲ Womens of light complexion, Pale face, weakly with lax muscles.

C_{N-2} ➲ Constitution which suffer from deficient nutrition, not because of food is lacking, but from imperfect assimilation (Bar-c, Calc-carb.).

M_{D-1} ➲ Nervous, irritable, sanguine temperament.

M_{D-2} ➲ Restless, start at least noise.

M_{D-3} ➲ Anxious, yielding, fainthearted.

M_{D-4} ➲ Mental labour very difficult.

H_{D-1} ➲ Violent headache, with loss of reason.

H_{D-2} ➲ Obstinate morning headache, with chillness and nausea.

H_{D-3} ➲ Headache every seventh day.

H_{D-4} ➲ Cephalaematoma neonatorum.

H_{D-5} ➲ Sick headache–ascending from nape of neck to the vertex.

SO_1 ➲ Pressure and smarting in eyes and lids.
SO_2 ➲ Lachrymal fistula, lachrymation esp. in open air.
SO_3 ➲ Otorrhoea with great sensitiveness to cold air.
SO_4 ➲ Hardness of hearing, sometimes without noise in ear.
SO_5 ➲ Inflammation in nostrils.
SO_6 ➲ Too frequent, immoderate sneezing.
DS_1 ➲ Tough slime in the fauces.
DS_2 ➲ Swallowing difficult, as from paralysis.
DS_3 ➲ Want of appetite, excessive thirst.
DS_4 ➲ Pressure as after eating too much.
DS_5 ➲ Induration of Pylorus.
DS_6 ➲ Flatulence much rumbling.
DS_7 ➲ Inguinal hernia.
DS_8 ➲ Fistula in ano.
DS_9 ➲ Constipation–always before and during menses.
DS_{10} ➲ Stool comes down with difficulty, when partly expelled, recedes again.
FGS_1 ➲ Nipple is drawn, like a funnel (Sars.).
FGS_2 ➲ Discharge of blood from vagina every time the child takes the breast (Crot-t).
FGS_3 ➲ A milky, acrid Leucorrhoea during urination.
FGS_4 ➲ Discharge of blood between menstrual periods.
FGS_5 ➲ Itching of vulva & vagina
FGS_6 ➲ Increased menses with icy coldness of whole body.
FGS_7 ➲ Abscess of labia.
FGS_8 ➲ Vaginal cysts.
FGS_9 ➲ Herd lumps in breast
LS_1 ➲ Bones of arms feel bruised.
LS_2 ➲ Profuse sweat on hands.
LS_3 ➲ Offensive foot-sweat, with rawness between toes.
LS_4 ➲ Cramp in the calves in soles.
S_{N-1} ➲ Eruption burn only by day.
S_{N-2} ➲ Boil come in crops, tendency to boils, leave indurations.
S_{N-3} ➲ Malignant frustules.
S_{N-4} ➲ Carbuncles.
S_{N-5} ➲ Large flastry warts, suppurating.
S_{N-6} ➲ Promote & expulsion of foreign bodies from tissue.
F_{R-1} ➲ Chillness, very sensitive to cold air.

F_{R-2} ➲ Cold extremities, even in a warm room.

F_{R-3} ➲ Suffering parts feel cold.

PG_1 ➲ Sweat of hand, feet and Axillae–offensive.

Modalities

Aggravation

- ➲ During new moon.
- ➲ Uncovering of the head.
- ➲ Lying down.

Amelioration

- ➲ Warmth.
- ➲ All the symptoms except gastric, which are > by cold food (Lyco).

Relations

➲ COMPARE:	Hep; Kil-p; Ruta; Sanic.
➲ COMPLEMENTARY:	Thuja; Sanicula.
➲ FOLLOWS WELL:	Hep; Fil-ac; Lyc; Sep.
➲ ANTIDOTES:	Ac-flour; Camph; Hep.
➲ INIMICALS:	Merc.

Spongia tosta

- ➲ PROVED BY: Hahnemann.
- ➲ DURATION: 20-30 days.
- ➲ COMMON NAME: Roasted Sponge.
- ➲ FAMILY/KINGDOM: Coelentirata.
- ➲ RELATION COLD/HEAT: Chilly.
- ➲ MIASM: Psora, Syphilis & Sycotic.
- ➲ DIATHESIS: Tubercular.
- ➲ SOURCE: Tincture (20 gains in 400 drops of alcohol).
- ➲ SPHERES OF ACTION: Female sexual organs & respiratory tract, glands eg-thyroid.
- ➲ SUMMARY OF INDICATIONS: respiratory disorders–Goiter–Angina Pectoris–Orchitis.

THERAPEUTIC PICTURE OF DRUG

C_{N-1} ➲ Diseases of children and women having light hair, lax fibre, fair complexion (Brom.)

M_{D-1} ➲ Anxiety and fear.

M_{D-2} ➲ Every excitement increase the cough.

CVS_1 ➲ Valvular insufficiency-Palpitation: violent, with pain, grasping respiration; suddenly awakened after midnight, with suffocation, great alarm, anxiety.

CVS_2 ➲ Rheumatic endocarditis, loud blowing with each heartbeat.

CVS_3 ➲ Aneurism of aorta; dry, Paroxysmal cough, worse lying down.

CVS_4 ➲ Angina Pectoris; Contracting pain in chest, heat, suffocation, faintness and anxious sweat.

RS_1 ➲ The chief symptoms of this remedy is a croupy, wheezing cough.

RS_2 ➲ Sensation as if there is a plug in the larynx.

RS_3 ➲ Hoarseness of voice with soreness and burning of the air passages.

RS_4 ➲ Wakes up frightened from sleep with a sense of suffocation, loud cough, difficult breathing. The cough sounds like a saw driven through a plank (dry, breaking cough). Dryness of all the respiratory passages.

RS_5 ➲ Croup: anxious, wheezing, during inspiration (during expiration, Acon;)< before midnight (<before morning Hep).

RS_6 ➲ Throat externally swollen; suffocating attacks.

RS_7 ➲ Thyroid gland swollen even with the chin; at night suffocating spells, barking, with stinging in throat and soreness in abdomen.

FGS_1 ➲ Before menses, pain in the sacrum, hunger palpitations.

FGS_2 ➲ During menses, wakes up with suffocative spells (Cupv; Iod; Lach.)

FGS_3 ➲ Amenorrhoea, with asthma (Puls).

FGS_4 ➲ Enlargement and induration of ovaries.

MGS_1 ➲ Swelling of spermatic cord and testicles, with pain and tenderness.

MGS_2 ➲ Epididymitis and Orchitis.

PG_1 ➲ Phthisis Pulmonalis, cough, breathing, being very tight and dry.

PG_2 ➲ Excessive moral and physical dejection.

PG_3 ➲ Fits of anguish, with pain in region of heart.

Modalities

Aggravation

- ➲ Before midnight.
- ➲ Lying down (flat).
- ➲ Talking.
- ➲ Swallowing.
- ➲ Waking.

Amelioration

- ➲ Lying with head low or after eating.

Relations

- ➲ FOLLOWS WELL: Brom; Bry; Carb-v; Con; Hep; Kali-br.; Nux-v; Phos; Puls.
- ➲ ANTIDOTES: Camph.

Stannum metallicum

- ➲ PROVED BY: Hahnemann.
- ➲ DURATION: 35 days.
- ➲ COMMON NAME: Tin (Sn).
- ➲ FAMILY/KINGDOM: Minerals.
- ➲ RELATION COLD/HEAT: Chilly or Hot.
- ➲ MIASM: Psora.
- ➲ DIATHESIS: Tubercular.
- ➲ TEMPERAMENT: Irritable.
- ➲ SOURCE: Trituration of Pure Metal.
- ➲ SPHERES OF ACTION: Nervous system, Respiratory organ and female genital organ.
- ➲ SUMMARY OF INDICATIONS: Headache–Neuralgia–Chronic Chest disorder–Occupational cramps.

THERAPEUTIC PICTURE OF DRUG

C_{N-1} ➲ There is increase weakness, cachexia with sallow waxy contenance and dark rings under the eye.

M_{D-1} ➲ He is anxious, weak and irritable.

M_{D-2} ➲ Continued restlessness with Anxiety.

M_{D-3} ➲ Sad, despondent, feels like crying all the time.

H_{D-1} ➲ Headache–increase gradually to the highest point and then gradually decline (Plat.).

H_{D-2} ➲ Drawing pain in molar bones and orbits.

H_{D-3} ➲ Throbbing headache in temples.

H_{D-4} ➲ Painful shocks across the head.

SO_1 ➲ Nocturnal agglutination of lids.

SO_2 ➲ Jerking and quivering of eyes.

SO_3 ➲ Burning sensation in nose.

SO_4 ➲ Ringing in right ear.
DS_1 ➲ Ulcerated sensation in right side of throat.
DS_2 ➲ Rawness and dryness in throat without thirst.
DS_3 ➲ Bitter test of all food.
DS_4 ➲ Vomiting of bile, of mucus.
DS_5 ➲ Frequent hiccough, nausea and vomiting.
DS_6 ➲ Aching in stomach sometimes very violent.
DS_6 ➲ Sinking, gone feeling in epigastrium.
RS_1 ➲ Violent, dry cough in evening until midnight.
RS_2 ➲ Cough exited by laughing, singing, talking, worse lying on Rt. Side.
RS_3 ➲ Evening dyspnoea, must loosen the clothing.
RS_4 ➲ Chest so weak he cannot talk, empty feeling in chest.
RS_5 ➲ Haemoptysis, with tendency to Copious expectoration.
RS_6 ➲ Great sore feeling in the chest.
RS_7 ➲ Phthisis mucosa, hectic fever.
RS_8 ➲ Great weakness in chest, < from talking.
RS_9 ➲ Empty sensation in chest.
FGS_1 ➲ Menses–too early, too profuse, sadness.
FGS_2 ➲ During menses pain in malar bone.
FGS_3 ➲ Prolapsus utri–so weak she drops into chair instead of sitting down.
FGS_4 ➲ Menses early and profuse.
FGS_5 ➲ Leucorrhoea–with great debility weakness seems to proceed from chest. (Phos. Sep.).
LS_1 ➲ Paralytic pain in the shoulder-joint.
LS_2 ➲ Swelling of hand esp. in evening.
LS_3 ➲ Small red spot on back of hands.
LS_4 ➲ Limbs suddenly give out when attempting to sit down
LS_5 ➲ Typewriter's paralysis.
F_{R-1} ➲ Shivering and shuddering in morning, with coldness in hand.
F_{R-2} ➲ Chill every forenoon.
F_{R-3} ➲ Small, quick pulse.
F_{R-4} ➲ Profuse perspiration in morning.
F_{R-5} ➲ Very debilitating perspiration at night.

Modalities

Aggravation

➲ Drinking anything warm (spong).
➲ Using to voice.

- Lying on Rt. Side.
- Laughing & singing.

Amelioration

- Coughing or expectorating.
- Relieves hoarseness, Hard pressure.

Relations

- COMPARE: Ars; Calch; Nat-m; Cycl.
- COMPLEMENTARY: Pulsatilla.
- FOLLOWS WELL: Caust; Calc-carb; Phos; Sil; Sulph; Tub.
- ANTIDOTES: Puls.

Staphysagria

- ➲ PROVED BY: Hahnemann.
- ➲ DURATION: 20-30 days.
- ➲ COMMON NAME: Stavesacre.
- ➲ FAMILY/KINGDOM: Ranunculaceae.
- ➲ RELATION COLD/HEAT: Chilly.
- ➲ MIASM: Psora and sycosis.
- ➲ TEMPERAMENT: Nervous and melancholic.
- ➲ SOURCE: Tincture of the seeds.
- ➲ SPHERES OF ACTION: Genito-urinary organs, brain, mind. GIT, respiratory organs and skin.
- ➲ SUMMARY OF INDICATIONS: Psychological Problems addiction to excessive smoking Post-operative care.

THERAPEUTIC PICTURE OF DRUG

C_{N-1} ➲ Usually a young man very much weak and debilitated, with guilty and abashed look.

C_{N-2} ➲ Having wart and unhealthy skin.

M_{D-1} ➲ Impetuous, violent outbursts of passion, hypochondriacall, sad.

M_{D-2} ➲ Mental effects of onanism and sexual excesses.

M_{D-3} ➲ Very sensitive to slightest mental impressions; least action or harmless word offends (Ign.).

M_{D-4} ➲ Great indignation about things done by others or by himself; grieves about consequences.

H_{D-1} ➲ Sensation of a ball of lead in the forehead.

H_{D-2} ➲ Stupefying headache; passes off with yawning.

H_{D-3} ➲ Dull feeling of head, with inability to perform any mental labor.

SO_1 ➲ Styes, chalazae on eye lides or upper lides, one after another leaving hard nodosities in their wake. (Con., Thuja).

SO_2 ➲ Anchylops, leaving a small, hard tumor.

SO_3 ➲ Steatomer on conjunctiva Palperbranum. Polypi of conjunctive.

SO_4 ➲ Syphilitic iritis, with bursting pain in eyeball, temple and side of face.

SO_5 ➲ Arthritic opthalmia, Pains extending to teeth; eyes burn on least exertion, as if very dry, yet lachymation is constant.

DS_1 ➲ Toothache during menses.

DS_2 ➲ Gnawing, tearing in decayed teeth; shooting into ear, throbbing in temples; worse from cold drinks and touch, but not from biting on them.

DS_3 ➲ Stomach feels relaxed; desire for stimulants.

DS_4 ➲ Colic after anger; swollen abdomen in children with much flatus.

DS_5 ➲ Colic with pelvic tenesmus; severe pain following an abdominal surgery.

RS_1 ➲ Dyspnoea: with constriction; after seminal emission; towards end of coition.

RS_2 ➲ Violent cough, with expectoration of viscid mucus, in evening, after lying down.

RS_3 ➲ Croupy cough in winter, alternating with sciatica in summer; cough excited by tobacco smoke.

RS_4 ➲ Hoarseness, with accumulation of mucus, which adheres to larynx and chest.

FGS_1 ➲ Nymphomania, with sensitiveness to mental and physical impressions; mind dwells too much on sexual subjects.

FGS_2 ➲ Painful sensitiveness of genital organs (esp. when sitting), vulva so sensitive can scarcely wear a napkin (Plat.).

FGS_3 ➲ Inflammation of the ovaries with burning, stinging and pressing-drawing.

FGS_4 ➲ Menses which had ceased for a year, reappeared with cutting colic and violent rumbling at the new moon.

MGS_1 ➲ Effects of ananism: face sunken; adashed look: nocturnal emissions; backache; weak legs; organs relaxed.

MGS_2 ➲ Seminal emission followed by great chagrin and mortification; great Prostration; dyspnoea.

MGS_3 ➲ Testicles inflamed, with burning-stinging, and pressing drawing.

MGS_4 ➲ A very marked increase of sexual desire, with frequent erections, especially at night.

S_{N-1} ➲ Warts: dry Pendunculated, Cauliflower like.

S_{N-2} ➲ Eczema of head, ears, face and body; thick scabs, dry and itch violently; scraching changes location of itching.

S_{N-3} ➲ Herpes: dry, with scabs on joints; chronic with nightly twitching; burn after scratching.

S_{N-4} ➲ Inflammation of Phalanges (rheumatism).

PG_1 ➲ For the Psychological effects of sexual excess.

PG_2 ➲ Mechanical injuries from sharp-cutting instruments; Post surgical operations; stinging Pains, like the cutting of a knife.

PG_3 ➲ Craving for tobacco.

PG_4 ➲ Extreme hunger, even when stomach is full of food.

PG_5 ➲ Honeymoon cystitis. Morning sickness

Modalities

Aggravation

- Anger.
- Grief.
- Loss of fluids.
- Sexual excess.
- Indignation.
- Mortification.
- Onanism.
- Least touch on affected parts.

Amelioration

- After breakfast.
- Warmth.
- Rest at night.

Relations

- COMPLEMENTARY: Caust; Coloc
- FOLLOWS WELL: Calc; Caust; Coloc; Ign; Lyco; Nux-v; Puls; Rhus-t; Sulph.
- ANTIDOTES: Camph.
- INIMICALS: Ran-b.

Stramonium

- PROVED BY: Hahnemann.
- DURATION: 40-60 days.
- COMMON NAME: Thron Apple.
- FAMILY/KINGDOM: Solonaceae.
- RELATION COLD/HEAT: Cold.
- MIASM: Psora.
- TEMPERAMENT: Bilious.
- SOURCE: Tincture of fresh plant in flower and fruit.
- SPHERES OF ACTION: Main action on Nervous System and Mucous membrane.
- SUMMARY OF INDICATIONS: Delirium- toxic states- stammering–a phasia (dysphasia).

THERAPEUTIC PICTURE OF DRUG

C_{N-1} ➲ Young pletnoric person (Acon, Bell) especially children.
M_{D-1} ➲ In chorea, mania and fever with delirium.
M_{D-2} ➲ Desire light and company, cannot bear to be alone (Bism).
M_{D-3} ➲ Worse in dark and solitude.
M_{D-4} ➲ Disposed to talk continually (Cica, Lach) Praying, be-seeching, entreating with suppressed menses.
M_{D-5} ➲ Desire to escape, in delirium (Bell; Bry Rhus-t; Cap; Op.).
H_{D-1} ➲ Pulsating in vertex, fainting.
H_{D-2} ➲ Sensation of lightness of head.
H_{D-3} ➲ Headache, with loss of sight and hearing.
H_{D-4} ➲ Head bent backwards, boring head into pillow.
SO_1 ➲ Stammering, distorts face, makes great effort to speak.
SO_2 ➲ Inflammation of margin of lids.
SO_3 ➲ Amblyopia, confusion of letters, when reading.
SO_4 ➲ Obstruction of nose, alae nasi white, face red.

NS_1 ➲ Great inclination to lie down.
NS_2 ➲ Convulsion especially opisthotonic.
NS_3 ➲ Catalepsy, limbs can be moved by others.
NS_4 ➲ Muscles will not obey the will.
NS_5 ➲ Paralyzed limb after apoplexy.
DS_1 ➲ Hiccough, restless at night, screaming in sleep.
DS_2 ➲ Epigastrium tense, hard, painful.
DS_3 ➲ Convulsive, vomiting of mucus.
DS_4 ➲ Borborygmi and fermentation in abdomen.
DS_5 ➲ Vomiting as soon as he raise head from Pillow.
FGS_1 ➲ Nymphomania, lewd talking, sings, obscene songs, has smell of semen.
FGS_2 ➲ Menstrual flow very watery.
FGS_3 ➲ During menses loquacity, strong smell as of semen.
FGS_4 ➲ Metrorrhagia, Loquacity, singing, Praying, sometimes Passing large Coagula.
MGS_1 ➲ Onanism causing epilepsy, impotence.
MGS_2 ➲ Exalted sexual passion.
US_1 ➲ Suppression of secretion of urine.
LS_1 ➲ Hand and arms tremble.
LS_2 ➲ Spasmodic rigidity of lower limbs.
LS_3 ➲ Constant trembling of feet.
PG_1 ➲ No pain with most complaints, painlessness is characteristic (op).
PG_2 ➲ Face red and bloated.
PG_3 ➲ Whole body sensitive to touch and every movement.

Modalities

Aggravation

- ➲ In the dark, when alone.
- ➲ Looking at bright objects.
- ➲ After sleep (Apis; Op; Bell).

Amelioration

- ➲ From bright light.
- ➲ From company.
- ➲ Warmth.

Relations

- ➲ COMPARE: Bell; Hyos.
- ➲ FOLLOWS WELL: Bell; Cup; Hyos; Lyss.
- ➲ ANTIDOTES: Ac-acid; Nux; Puls; Op.
- ➲ INIMICALS: Coff.

Sulphur

- PROVED BY: Hahnemann.
- DURATION: 40-60 days.
- COMMON NAME: Brimstone.
- FAMILY/KINGDOM: Minerals.
- RELATION COLD/HEAT: Hot.
- MIASM: Antipsoric.
- DIATHESIS: Scrofulous.
- TEMPERAMENT: Nervous.
- SOURCE: Trituration of "flowers of sulphur".
- SPHERES OF ACTION: Mucous membrane, urathra, rectum, Portal system, female Reproductive organs.
- SUMMARY OF INDICATIONS: Skin disorders- Polyneuropathy– diarrhoea- liver disesase.

THERAPEUTIC PICTURE OF DRUG

C_{N-1} Especially suited to lean, stoop-shouldered person who walk and sit stooping, walk stooping like old man.

M_{D-1} Happy dreams, wakes up singing.

M_{D-2} Everything looks pretty which the patient takes a fancy, to even rags seem beautiful.

M_{D-3} Affections very selfish, no regard for other.

M_{D-4} Weak memory, especially for names.

M_{D-5} Irritable, depressed thin and weak, even with good appetite.

H_{D-1} Hammering headache on vivacious talking.

H_{D-2} Heat on crown, cold feet, frequent flushings.

H_{D-3} Painful tingling on vertex and in temples.

H_{D-4} Itching, scratching causing burning.

SO_1 Ulceration of margins of lids.

SO_2 ➲ Dryness of eyes in room, lachrymation in open air.
SO_3 ➲ Humming or hissing in ear.
SO_4 ➲ Catarrhal deafness.
SO_5 ➲ Bloody discharge when blowing the nose.
DS_1 ➲ Bitter test in morning.
DS_2 ➲ Exfoliation of membrane of mouth.
DS_3 ➲ Burning sensation and tickling on tongue.
DS_4 ➲ Burning in throat as from sour eructations.
DS_5 ➲ Loud eructations as soon as he pressure on stomach.
DS_7 ➲ Hiccough.
DS_8 ➲ Drinks much, eats little.
DS_9 ➲ Frequent unsuccessful desire for stool.
DS_{10} ➲ Alternation of constipation and diarrhoea.
DS_{11} ➲ Movement in Abdomen as of a child (Thaja, Croc).
RS_1 ➲ Difficult respiration, wants windows open.
RS_2 ➲ Much rattling of mucus.
RS_3 ➲ Coldness in throat during an inspiration.
FGS_1 ➲ Menses too late, short, scanty and difficult.
FGS_2 ➲ Memorrhagia, has not been well since her last miscarriage–"A single dose at new moon"–Lippe
FGS_3 ➲ Leucorrhorea, burning excoriating.
FGS_4 ➲ Nipple cracked and burn.
MGS_1 ➲ Fetid perspiration in parts.
MGS_2 ➲ Inflammation, swelling, and phimosis of prepuce.
MGS_3 ➲ Hydrocele, frequent pollutions, also at noon.
US_1 ➲ Retention of urine.
US_2 ➲ Rigor when urinating
US_3 ➲ Discharge of mucus from urethra.
LS_1 ➲ Rheumatic pain in shoulders, esp. the left.
LS_2 ➲ Drawing and tearing in arms and hands.
LS_3 ➲ Dropsy of knee joints.
LS_4 ➲ Burning in soles and hand at night.
S_{N-1} ➲ Voluptuous itching and tingling, with burning.
S_{N-2} ➲ Itching worse in warm bed.
S_{N-3} ➲ Skin rough, scaly, scabby.
S_{N-4} ➲ Furuncles, particularly on the nates.

Modalities

Aggravation

- Rt. Rest.
- When standing
- Warm in bed, bathing, washing.

Amelioration

- Dry, warm weather.
- Lying on Rt. Side (Rev. of stam).

Relations

COMPARE:	Psor; Tubers; Caust; Rhus-t.
COMPLEMENTARY:	Aloe; Psor; Nux.
FOLLOWS WELL:	Calc; Lyco; Sarsa; Sepia.
ANTIDOTES:	Puls; Sil; Rhus; Caust; Ars.
INIMICALS:	Ran-b.

Syphilinum

- ➲ PROVED BY: Swan.
- ➲ COMMON NAME: Syphilitic Virus.
- ➲ FAMILY/KINGDOM: A Nasode.
- ➲ MIASM: Syphilis.
- ➲ TEMPERAMENT: Melancholic.
- ➲ SPHERES OF ACTION: Brain & Spinal cord, mucous membrane, female genital organs; bones Peritoneum & skin.
- ➲ SUMMARY OF INDICATIONS: Disorders of memory–skin disorders–Neuralgic type of headaches–Paralysis of muscles–Myasthenia gravis–Alcoholism–Teeth disorders–Periarthritis.

THERAPEUTIC PICTURE OF DRUG

C_{N-1} ➲ Many different types of eruptions; Particularly copper coloured, which become blue on getting cold.

M_{D-1} ➲ Loss of memory; remembers everything previous to his illness.

M_{D-2} ➲ Apathetic; feels as if going insane or being paralyzed.

M_{D-3} ➲ Fears the night and the suffering from exhaustion on awaking.

M_{D-4} ➲ Hopeless; despair of recovery.

H_{D-1} ➲ Headache, neuralgic in character, causing sleeplessness and delirium at night; commencing at 4 P.M., worse from 10 to 11 P.M. and ceasing at day light (ceases at 11 to 12 P.M. Lyco.); falling of head hair (alop.).

H_{D-2} ➲ Pains of bones of head.

H_{D-3} ➲ Top of head feels as if coming off; stupefying cephalgia.

SO_1 ➲ Ptosis: Paralysis of the superior oblique; sleepy look from drooping lids (caus.; Graph; Gels.).

SO_2 ➲ Diplopia, one image seen below the other.

DS_1 ➲ Teeth: decay at edge of gums and facture; teeth cupped, edges serrated; dwarfed in size, coverage at their tips (Staph.), excessive salivation.

DS_2 ➲ Heartburn with pain and rawness from stomach to throat-pit, often with cough.

DS_3 ➲ Obstinate constipation for many years; rectum seemed tied up with strictures, when injections were given agony of passage was like child-bearing.

DS_4 ➲ Chronic constipations, with fetid breath, earthy complexion, gaunt appearance.

DS_5 ➲ Stools very dark offensive (infantile syphilis).

DS_6 ➲ Fissure in anus and rectum.

FGS_1 ➲ Uterus and all surrounding parts loose, soft and flabby.

FGS_2 ➲ Leucorrhoea; Profuse, Soaking through the napkins and running down to the heels (Alum.).

FGS_3 ➲ Profuse yellow leucorrhoea, <at night, in sickly, nervous children (inherited syphilis).

FGS_4 ➲ Nocturnal of right ovarian pain, preventing sleep.

FGS_5 ➲ Menstruation painful, two weeks too soon; Pink red, bright, Profuse, running free for some days; napkins wash easily.

FGS_6 ➲ Uterine and ovarian diseases with pronounced nervous disorders, especially in married women.

FGS_7 ➲ Mammae sensitive to touch, feeling sore; during menses, and at other times.

MGS_1 ➲ Aching of genitals, could not sit still for over a month.

MGS_2 ➲ Inflammation and induration of spermatic cord.

MGS_3 ➲ Chancre on penis, third in two years, all on same spot.

LS_1 ➲ Rheumatism, muscles are caked in hard knots or lumps.

LS_2 ➲ Sciatica; worse at night; better around day break.

LS_3 ➲ Rheumatism of shoulder joint, at insertion of deltoid.

LS_4 ➲ Severe pain in long bones; redness and rawness between toes.

S_{N-1} ➲ Maculae; copper-coloured.

S_{N-2} ➲ Raddish-brown eruption, with a disagreeable odor.

S_{N-3} ➲ Pemphigus, looking like a pock, often confluent and persistently reappears.

PG_1 ➲ All symptoms are worse at night (Merc), from sun down to sunrise.

PG_2 ➲ Pain from darkness to day light; begin with twilight and end with daylight. (Merc. Phyt.).

PG_3 ➲ Craving for alcohol, in any form.

PG_4 ➲ Epileptic convulsions after menses.

PG_5 ➲ Great prostration and debility in morning.

Modalities

Aggravation

➲ At night.

➲ Sundown to sunrise.

- Seashore.
- In summer.

Amelioration

- Inland and mountains.
- During the day.
- Moving about slowly.

Relations

- COMPARE: Merc; Kali-i; Nit-ac; Aur; Alum.
- ANTIDOTES: Camph.

Tarentula

- ➲ PROVED BY: Nunez.
- ➲ COMMON NAME: Spanish Spider.
- ➲ FAMILY/KINGDOM: Aranoidiceae.
- ➲ SOURCE: Tincture of the living spiders.
- ➲ SPHERES OF ACTION: Nervous system, genito-urinary system.
- ➲ SUMMARY OF INDICATIONS: Paralysis–Chorea–Parkinsonism–Hyperaesthesia.

THERAPEUTIC PICTURE OF DRUG

M_{D-1} ➲ Ungrateful discontented.

M_{D-2} ➲ Sudden alteration of mood.

M_{D-3} ➲ Must constantly busy herself or walk.

M_{D-4} ➲ Sensitive to music.

M_{D-5} ➲ Guided by whims.

H_{D-1} ➲ Headache by noise, touch, strong light.

FGS_1 ➲ Vulva dry and hot, with much itching.

FGS_2 ➲ Profuse menstruation, with frequent erotic spasm.

FGS_3 ➲ Dysmenorrhoea, with very sensitive ovaries.

FGS_4 ➲ Sexual excitement extreme even to mania Nymphomania.

FGS_5 ➲ At every menstrual nisus, throat, mouth and tongue intolerably dry, especially when sleeping (Nux-m).

PG_1 ➲ Restlessness, could not keep quite in any position.

PG_2 ➲ Though walking aggravates all symptoms (Rev. of Rhus-t, Ruta).

Modalities

Aggravation

- ➲ Motion, change of weather.
- ➲ Contact, noise.

Amelioration

- Open air, music.
- Bright colours.
- Rubbing affected parts.

Relations

- COMPARE: Agr; Ars; Cuprum; Phos.
- COMPLEMENTARY: Ars.
- ANTIDOTES: Lach.
- SIMILAR: Apis; Lach; Platira; Nay; Theridion.

Thlaspi bursa pastoris

- ➲ COMMON NAME: Shepherd's Purse.
- ➲ FAMILY/KINGDOM: Cruciferae.
- ➲ SOURCE: Tincture of fresh flowering plant.

THERAPEUTIC PICTURE OF DRUG

FGS_1 ➲ Metrorrhagia; with uterine colic; in haemorrhagic chlorosis; in sequelae of absortion or labour.

FGS_2 ➲ Premature menstruation; first day she hardly had a shaw, second day a haemorrhage with severe colic and expulsion of clots, flow lasted eight to fifteen days, left a state of exhaustion which was not recovered from before the next period came on; this proved very profuse, next less so.

FGS_3 ➲ Haemorrhages; with violent uterine colic and cramps; consequent on abortion; at critical age; with cancer of cervix; or fibroids.

FGS_4 ➲ Too frequent and copious menstruation, especially in persons of a relaxed constitution.

FGS_5 ➲ Haemorrhages dark, with clots.

FGS_6 ➲ Leucorrhoea: bloody, dark, foetid, before and some days after menses, which were profuse and dark.

FGS_7 ➲ Haemorrhages after abortion.

FGS_8 ➲ Following an attack of jaundice, after menses a discharge of brownish-green blood, with obscure abdominal pains; cervix swollen and soft but not ulcerated.

PG_1 ➲ Profuse passive haemorrhage from every outlet of the body; blood dark and clotted.

Relations

➲ COMPARE: Sinapis, Trillium, Viburnum, Ustilago.

Thuja occidentalis

- PROVED BY: Hahnemann.
- DURATION: 60 days.
- COMMON NAME: White Cedar (three of life).
- FAMILY/KINGDOM: Coniferae.
- RELATION COLD/HEAT: Chilly.
- MIASM: Sycosis.
- TEMPERAMENT: Lymphatic.
- SOURCE: Tincture of a fresh green twings.
- SPHERES OF ACTION: skin and genito-urinary organs. Nervous system esp. brain etc.
- SUMMARY OF INDICATIONS: headache–Skin disorders–dandruff–warts–vaccinosis.

THERAPEUTIC PICTURE OF DRUG

C_{N-1} ➲ Hydrogenoid constitution of grauvogl.

C_{N-2} ➲ Patient having dark hair and dark complexion, unhealthy, oily, greasy skin, bearing warty excrescence.

C_{N-3} ➲ Dirty brownish spots all over the body.

M_{D-1} ➲ Insane women will not be touched or approached.

M_{D-2} ➲ Fixed ideas, as if a strong person were at her side, as if soul and body were separated.

M_{D-3} ➲ Emotional sensitiveness, music, causes weeping and trembling.

M_{D-4} ➲ Senentation is if body esp. limbs, were made at glass and would break easily.

H_{D-1} ➲ Headache: as if a nail had been driven into the Parietal bone. (coffea cruda, Ignatia amara).

H_{D-2} ➲ Boring through temples.

H_{D-3} ➲ Headache worse from tea.
H_{D-4} ➲ White, scaly dandruff, hair dry and falling out.
H_{D-5} ➲ Nervous, sycotic or syphilitic headache.
SO_1 ➲ Acute and subacute inflammation of sclera.
SO_2 ➲ Chronic otitis, pressive pain behind ears.
SO_3 ➲ Fluent coryza, with cough and hoarseness.
DS_1 ➲ Aphthae in mouth.
DS_2 ➲ Condylomata under tongue.
DS_3 ➲ Taste in mouth sweet as sugar, with gonorrhoea.
DS_4 ➲ Ulceration in throat and mouth like chancres.
DS_5 ➲ Induration of stomach, swelling of pit of stomach.
DS_6 ➲ Stitches in the hypochondria.
DS_7 ➲ Intussusception of intestines.
DS_8 ➲ Constipation which continues several days.
RS_1 ➲ Sputa green, taste like old cheese.
RS_2 ➲ Spasm of lungs from drinking cold water.
FGS_1 ➲ Vagina very sensitive causes prevent coition (plat-by dryness of Lyco; Lyss; Nat-m.).
FGS_2 ➲ Abdomen, as if an animal were crying, motions, if something alive, protrudes here and there like arm of faetus (Cro-s, Sulph.).
FGS_3 ➲ Profuse Leucorrhoea thick and greenish.
FGS_4 ➲ Severe pain in left ovary and left inguinal region.
FGS_5 ➲ Warty excrescence on vulva and Perineum.
MGS_1 ➲ Gonorrhoeal rheumatism.
MGS_2 ➲ Chronic induration of testicles.
MGS_3 ➲ Condylomata on glans and prepuce.
MGS_4 ➲ Fig like warts on inner side of prepuce.
US_1 ➲ Bladder feels paralyzed, has no power to expel urine.
US_2 ➲ Stitches from rectum to bladder.
US_3 ➲ Cloudy sediment in urine.
LS_1 ➲ Trembling of hand and arm when writing.
LS_2 ➲ Ganglion of wrist.
LS_3 ➲ Stitches above heel in tendo Achillis.
S_{N-1} ➲ Pemphigus painful.
S_{N-2} ➲ Bleeding fungous growth.
S_{N-3} ➲ Nail crippled, brittle and soft.
S_{N-4} ➲ Eruption on only covered parts.

S_{N-5} ➲ Small-pox stage of maturation.
S_{N-6} ➲ Condylomata, warts, seedy, pediculated.
F_{R-1} ➲ Shivering, with yawning, after midnight.
F_{R-2} ➲ Chill without thirst.

Modalities

Aggravation

- At night.
- At 3 A.M. and 3 P.M.
- From cold, damp air.

Amelioration

- In open air.
- Warmth.
- By movement, pressure.

Relations

➲ COMPARE:	Cannabis; Sativa; Staph.
➲ COMPLEMENTARY:	Ars; Nat-s; Sabina; Sil; Medo.
➲ FOLLOWS WELL:	Medorrhinum; Mercurius sal Nit-Acid.
➲ ANTIDOTES:	Camph; Cham; Cocc; Puls; Sulph.

Tilia Europaea

- COMMON NAME: Liden

THERAPEUTIC PICTURE OF DRUG

FGS_1 ➲ Intese, sore feeling around the uterus.

FGS_2 ➲ Bearing down pain with hot sweat, but without relief.

FGS_3 ➲ Profuse slimy Leucorrhoea when walking. (Bov; Carb-an; Graph.).

FGS_4 ➲ Soreness and hyperemia of the external genitals. (Thuj.; Sulph.).

FGS_5 ➲ Pelvic inflammation, typanites, abdominal tenderness and hot sweat which does not relieve.

PG_1 ➲ Sensation of a gauze before the eyes (calc; caust. nat-m.).

PG_2 ➲ Much sneezing, with fluent coryza.

PG_3 ➲ Neuralgia (right to left), with a veil before the eyes confused, with dimness of vision.

Modalities

Aggravation

- Afternoon and evening.
- In a warm room.
- Heat of bed.

Amelioration

- Cool room.
- Motion.

Relations

- COMPARE: Lil-t; Bell.

Trillium pendulum

- PROVED BY: H. Minton.
- FAMILY/KINGDOM: Smilaceae.
- COMMON NAME: Wake Robin.
- SOURCE: Tincture of the fresh root.
- SUMMARY OF INDICATIONS: Haemorrhages- menstrual disorders.

THERAPEUTIC PICTURE OF DRUG

M_{D-1} ➲ Melancholy with sadness.

M_{D-2} ➲ Irritable, Anguish, agitation and toosing about.

M_{D-3} ➲ Impossible to keep still.

FGS_1 ➲ Displaced uterus, with consequent menorrhagia, flow profuse.

FGS_2 ➲ Gushing of bright red blood from uterus, at the least movement, later, blood pale from anaemia.

FGS_3 ➲ Menses often come on after overexertion, too-long a ride, etc., profuse flow.

FGS_4 ➲ Leucorrhoea: bloody, with great prostration, yellow, creamy, profuse, between menses.

FGS_5 ➲ Lochia suddenly becomes sanguinous.

FGS_6 ➲ Dribbling of urine after labor.

FGS_7 ➲ Uterine haemorrhages with sensation as though hips and back were falling to places, better tight bandages.

PG_1 ➲ Flooding, with fainting

PG_2 ➲ Epistaxis, profuse, passive bright red.

PG_3 ➲ Faint, dim Sight, palpitation, abstruction and noise in ears.

Modalities

Aggravation

- Motion.
- Over exertion.

Amelioration

- Tight bandaging (strapping).

Relations

COMPARE:	Chin; Calc; Ham; Ust; Sang.
COMPLEMENTARY:	Calc-Phos.
ANTIDOTES:	Nux-v.
SIMILAR:	Cinchona (China); Bell; Cal-Carb; Mille; Lach; Sep; Sulph; Thal-bur-Pas; Ust-may.

Tuberculinum bacillinum

- ➲ PROVED BY: Burnett.
- ➲ COMMON NAME: Pus (with bacilli) from tubercular abscess.
- ➲ FAMILY/KINGDOM: A nosode.
- ➲ RELATION COLD/HEAT: Highly Chilly.
- ➲ MIASM: Pseudo–Psora.
- ➲ DIATHESIS: Tubercular & Scrofulous.
- ➲ TEMPERAMENT: Nervous.
- ➲ SOURCE: A glycerine extract of a Pure cultivation of tubercle bacilli (human).
- ➲ SPHERES OF ACTION: Skin, GIT, glands & lungs.
- ➲ SUMMARY OF INDICATIONS: Tuberculosis–Chronic infections–Anorexia–Continued fever–Mental depression–Hyperhidrosis.

THERAPEUTIC PICTURE OF DRUG

C_{N-1} ➲ Persons who are very precocious mentally but weak physically.

C_{N-2} ➲ Adapted to the light complexioned, narrow–chest subjects with blue eyes.

C_{N-3} ➲ Who are tall, slim and active, but rapidly emaciate, especilly children.

M_{D-1} ➲ Contradictory characteristics of Tub. are mania and melancholia insomnia and sopar.

M_{D-2} ➲ Irritable, especially on waking up.

M_{D-3} ➲ Depressed, melancholic.

M_{D-4} ➲ Fear of dogs, animals especially.

M_{D-5} ➲ Desire to use foul language, curse and swear.

H_{D-1} ➲ Intense pain, as if an iron band was around the head.

H_{D-2} ➲ School-girls headache: worse by study or even slight mental exertion.

H_{D-3} ➲ Plica Polonica: nocturnal hallucinations, wakes up frightened.

DS_1 ➲ Eructations and sensation of fullness over stomach.

DS_2 ➲ Discrete papular rash over chest and abdomen.

DS_3 ➲ Diarrhoea with Pinching and burning pains.

RS_1 ➲ Tuberculosis outgrowth.

RS_2 ➲ General infillration of mucous membrane of larynx, high red colour, brighter than normal.

RS_3 ➲ Cough, secretion of Phlegm, especially by walking, with sticking pains in lungs and Palpitation.

FGS_1 ➲ Severe pains in breast in evening at beginning of menstruation.

FGS_2 ➲ Menstruation with pains in lumbo-sacral and ovarian region.

FGS_3 ➲ Sticking pain in lower abdomen; Pains in lumbo-sacral region <when walking.

FGS_4 ➲ Blood lumpy, menstruation lasting more days than usual; menstruation antepones eight days.

FGS_5 ➲ Sensation of heart in genitalia externa, with increased leucorrhoea.

FGS_6 ➲ Menstruation returns fourteen days after parturition.

FGS_7 ➲ Menses: too early, too profuse and too long-lasting; slow in commencing.

S_{N-1} ➲ Great bronze Patches on the forehead and temples.

S_{N-2} ➲ Itching all over the body in the evening in bed; changing place after rubbing.

S_{N-3} ➲ Erythematous eruption like measles or scarlatina.

PG_1 ➲ A family history of tubercular affections.

PG_2 ➲ Symptoms ever changing; disorders affecting are organ then another.

PG_3 ➲ Emaciation rapid and pronounced; emaciation with a good appetite (Abro., Calc.carb; Con-mac; Iod; Nat-m).

PG_4 ➲ Cachexia, continued chronic fever.

PG_5 ➲ Takes cold easily without knowing how or where; seems to take cold "every time she takes breath of fresh air" (Hep.).

Modalities

Aggravation

- ➲ Motion.
- ➲ Music.
- ➲ After sleep.

Amelioration

- ➲ Open air.

Relations

- ➲ COMPLEMENTARY: Bell; Calc; Hydr; Psor; Sulph.
- ➲ FOLLOWS WELL: Bar-c; Calc; Calc-p; Sil.
- ➲ ANTIDOTES: Camph.

Urtica Urens

- PROVED BY: Burnett.
- COMMON NAME: Stinging Nettle.
- FAMILY/KINGDOM: Urticaceae.
- SOURCE: Thincture of the fresh plant in flower.
- SPHERES OF ACTION: Skin, mucous membrane, Mammae, genito-Urinary organs, spleen and joint.
- SUMMARY OF INDICATIONS: Agalactia- lithiasis–rheumatism gout-urticaria-kin disorders- Pruristus–oedema–burns and scalds.

THERAPEUTIC PICTURE OF DRUG

H_{D-1} ➲ Neuritis, vertigo, headache.

DS_1 ➲ Diarrhoea due to chronic disease of the large intestines characterised by secretion of mucus.

FGS_1 ➲ Diminished secretion of milk.

FGS_2 ➲ Arrests flow of milk after weaning.

FGS_3 ➲ Excessive swelling of breasts.

FGS_4 ➲ Uterine Haemorrhage.

FGS_5 ➲ Leucorrhoea acrid and excoriating.

FGS_6 ➲ Pruritus vulvae, with stinging, itching and oedema.

LS_1 ➲ Pain of acute gout, shoulder and pain in other joints.

S_{N-1} ➲ Urticaria, burning, heat with formication; violent itching.

S_{N-2} ➲ Herpes labialis with sensation of heat and itching.

S_{N-3} ➲ Erythema, with burning and stinging.

S_{N-4} ➲ Burns & scalds, chicken-pox (Dulcamara). Angioneurotic oedema.

Modalities

Aggravation

- Cool Moist air.

- Cold bathing.
- By touch.

Amelioration

- By rubbing.
- From lying down.

Relations

- COMPARE: Agn; Apis Bell; Ars; Ust; Sulph; Hep.
- COMPLEMENTARY: Nat-mur.
- ANTIDOTES: Apis; Nut-v; Camph.

Ustilago maydis

- ➲ PROVED BY: Burt.
- ➲ COMMON NAME: Corn-smut.
- ➲ FAMILY/KINGDOM: Fungi.
- ➲ SPHERES OF ACTION: Skin, Hair, Nails.

THERAPEUTIC PICTURE OF DRUG

M_{D-1} ➲ Depression of spirits in afternoon.

M_{D-2} ➲ Very sad, cries frequently, exceedingly prostrated from exual abuse; sleep restless.

M_{D-3} ➲ The day seemed like a dream.

M_{D-4} ➲ Melancholia; depression of sprits; oppression and faintness in a warm. An aversion to or < from warmth in general.

M_{D-5} ➲ Partial or complete loss of control over the functions of vision and deglutition.

M_{D-6} ➲ Great irritability, mental weakness and depression.

H_{D-1} ➲ Headache: all the morning; at 7 A.M.; in evening, worse forehead and walking.

H_{D-2} ➲ Vertigo at climax is with Profuse menstruation.

H_{D-3} ➲ Scald-head, watery serum oozing from scalp.

DS_1 ➲ Haematemesis, Passive-venous, accompanied by nausea, which is better by vomiting.

DS_2 ➲ Periodical cutting in umbilical and hypogastric regions at 6 P.M., worse at 8 p.m. by a constipated stool, afterwards grumbling pains in whole abdomen.

FGS_1 ➲ Vicarious menstruation.

FGS_2 ➲ Ovaries burn, painful and swollen (ovaritis).

FGS_3 ➲ Profuse menses after miscarriage; discharge of blood from the slightest Provocation; bright red; Partly clotted.

FGS_4 ➲ Ooging of dark blood, clotted, forming long black strings.

FGS_5 ➲ Uterus hypertrophies (fibroids).

FGS_6 ➲ Cervix bleed easily.

FGS_7 ➲ Postpartum haemorrhage.

FGS_8 ➲ Flabby condition of the uterus.

FGS_9 ➲ Congestion of varicous parts, especially at climacteric.

PG_1 ➲ Faint spells beginning in epigastrium, with small pains in hypochordrium and bowels.

PG_2 ➲ Neuralgic pain in forehead, hands and feet.

Relations

➲ COMPARE: Sec; Sab; Zea-ita.

Veratrum album

- PROVED BY: Hahnemann.
- DURATION: 20-30 days.
- COMMON NAME: White Hellebore.
- FAMILY/KINGDOM: Melanthaceae.
- RELATION COLD/HEAT: Chilly.
- MIASM: Psora.
- TEMPERAMENT: Nervous and Sanguine.
- SOURCE: Tinchtare of the root-stocks collected early in June before flowering.
- SPHERES OF ACTION: Blood, Vascular system, Nervous System.
- SUMMARY OF INDICATIONS: Acute gastroenteritis-dysmenorrhoea-alcoholism- excessive smoking.

THERAPEUTIC PICTURE OF DRUG

C_{N-1} ➲ Persons, who are habitually cold and deficient in vital reaction.
C_{N-2} ➲ Face Pale, blue, collapsed, features sunken, Hippocratic.
M_{D-1} ➲ Thinks she is pregnant or will soon be delivered.
M_{D-2} ➲ Mania with desire to cut and tear everythings esp. clothes (tarent).
M_{D-3} ➲ Delusion of impending misfortunes.
H_{D-1} ➲ Scalp very sensitive, with headache.
H_{D-2} ➲ Plica polonica.
H_{D-3} ➲ Vertigo esp. when walking.
SO_1 ➲ Lachrymation with redness of eye.
SO_2 ➲ Nose grows more pointed, seems longer.
SO_3 ➲ Deafness, as from obstruction in ears.
DS_1 ➲ Rising with taste of food.
DS_2 ➲ Vomiting of mucus at night, mucus green in colour.
DS_3 ➲ Painful contraction of abdomen, when vomiting.
DS_4 ➲ Swelling of abdomen, abdomen hard and inflamed.

DS_5 ➲ Inflammation of intestine.

DS_6 ➲ Violent expulsion of flatus upwards and downwards.

DS_7 ➲ Stools, watery, greenish, mixed with flakes, gushing, profuse, rice-water discharge, with tonic cramp, Asiatic cholera.

CVS_1 ➲ Strong palpitation of heart, with chorea.

CVS_2 ➲ Pulse irregular feeble.

RS_1 ➲ Chronic bronchitis in the aged.

RS_2 ➲ Rattling in chest, much mucus in bronchial tubes.

RS_3 ➲ Cough on entering warm room from cold air.

RS_4 ➲ Convulsive stage of whooping cough.

FGS_1 ➲ The women is in a cold sweat, feel faints and collapse occurs.

FGS_2 ➲ Menses too early, exhausting profuse.

FGS_3 ➲ Dysmenorrhoea, with coldness, purging, cold sweat.

FGS_4 ➲ Sexual mania precedes menses.

FGS_5 ➲ Strangulated prolapsed vagina, with cold sweat, exhausting vomiting and diarrhoea.

LS_1 ➲ Neuralgia in chranchial plexus, as if beaten.

LS_2 ➲ Cramp in calus.

LS_3 ➲ Feet icy cold.

LS_4 ➲ Sciatica, pain like electric flashes.

Modalities

Aggravation

- ➲ From least motion.
- ➲ After drinking.
- ➲ Before and during menses.
- ➲ After fright.
- ➲ Night.
- ➲ During stool.

Amelioration

- ➲ Walking.
- ➲ Warmth.
- ➲ From walking about.

Relations

- ➲ COMPARE: Arn; Ars; Cupr; Ipec and podo
- ➲ COMPLEMENTARY: Arn; Carb-V.
- ➲ FOLLOWS WELL: Acon; Ars; Arn; Arg-n; Bell; Puls; Phus; Sulph; Camph; Chin; Coff; Puls.

Veratrum Viride

- PROVED BY: BURT.
- COMMON NAME: Green Hellebore.
- FAMILY/KINGDOM: Melanthaceae.
- SOURCE: Tincture of fresh root gathered in autumn.
- SPHERES OF ACTION: Heart, nerves, joint blood vessels, Pneumo-gastric nerve, lungs and joints.
- SUMMARY OF INDICATIONS: Rheumatism-gout-traumatic arthritis-acute rheumatic fever-meningitis.

THERAPEUTIC PICTURE OF DRUG

C_{N-1} ➲ Persons full blooded, Plethroix, with bloated and lived face.

M_{D-1} ➲ Quarrelsome and delirious.

M_{D-2} ➲ Depression and Prostration.

M_{D-3} ➲ Puerperal mania: Silent, suspicious, fears being poisoned.

H_{D-1} ➲ Sunstroke: fullness in head, throbbing arteries; increased sensitiveness to sounds; buzzing in the ear; double or partial vision.

H_{D-2} ➲ Headache from nape of neck, with vertigo, dim vision, dilated pupils.

H_{D-3} ➲ Congestion to head: from high living, abuse of stimulants, during dentition.

NS_1 ➲ Opisthotonic convulsions in anaemic subjects from exhausting diarrhoea.

NS_2 ➲ Paralysis; tingling in limb; cerebral hyperaemia.

NS_3 ➲ Convulsions: dim vision; basilar meningitis; head retracted; child on verge of spasms.

FGS_1 ➲ Menstrual colic or dysmenorrhoea; much nausea and vomiting; Plethora; Cerebral congestion.

FGS_2 ➲ Amenorrhoea from exposure; chill, complete suppression of discharge, heavy pressive aching in uterus region; intense pain in head with heat and throbbing arteries; mind wandering, sobbing; tendency to hysteric spasms.

FGS_3 ➲ Puerperal fever, sudden suppression of milk and lochia; quick, weak or hard, bounding pulse.

- FGS_4 ➲ Mastitis with great arterial and nervous excitement.
- FGS_5 ➲ Congestion of Pelvic organs, tenderness of uterus.
- PG_1 ➲ Violent Pains accompanying an inflammation meningitis.
- PG_2 ➲ Acute rheumatism, high fever, full, hard, rapid pulse. Severe pains in joints and muscles (Bryo. Sali-ac.).
- PG_3 ➲ Gout, traumatic arthritis.

Modalities

Aggravation

- ➲ Morning on waking.
- ➲ Going from warm to cold.
- ➲ After exposure.

Amelioration

- ➲ By Pressure.
- ➲ By rubbing.

Relations

- ➲ COMPARE: Gels; Bapt; Bell; Acon; Ferr-P.
- ➲ ANTIDOTES: Nux; Hot Strong coffee.

Viburnum opulus

- ➲ PROVED BY: H.C. Allen.
- ➲ COMMON NAME: Cramp bark.
- ➲ FAMILY/KINGDOM: Caprifoliaceae.
- ➲ SOURCE: Tincture of the fresh bark.
- ➲ SPHERES OF ACTION: Female genital organ uterus ovaries and other genital organ.

THERAPEUTIC PICTURE OF DRUG

C_{N-1} ➲ Suited to tall, slender, dark or fair haired Hysterical subjects.

M_{D-1} ➲ Depressed.

M_{D-2} ➲ Unable to concentrate mind on usual mental labor.

FGS_1 ➲ Ovarian Region feels heavy and congested.

FGS_2 ➲ Aching in sacrum and pubes, with pain in anterior museles of thigh.

FGS_3 ➲ Spasmodic and membranous dysmenorrhoea.

FGS_4 ➲ Leucorrhoea, excoriating smarting and itching of gentals.

FGS_5 ➲ Frequent and very early miscarriage, causing seeming sterility.

FGS_6 ➲ Pains from back to loins and womb worse early morning.

FGS_7 ➲ Menses too late, scanty, lasting a few hours, offensive in odour, with crampy pains, cramps.

FGS_8 ➲ Cramp extended down tnighs (Bell).

FGS_9 ➲ Bearing down pain before menses.

FGS_{10} ➲ Often prevents miscarriage.

FGS_{11} ➲ Leucorrhoea- thin, yellow-white colourless, excoriating.

PG_1 ➲ Constant nausea, relieved by eating.

PG_2 ➲ Sudden cramps and colic pains.

Modalities

Aggravation

- From movement.
- Before menses.
- In worm room.
- Lying on affected side (Puls.).

Amelioration

- Lying down.
- In open air (Puls).

Relations

- COMPARE: Cauloph; Act rac; Gels; Sepia; Secale; Xantho.

Viscum album

- COMMON NAME: Viscum album.
- FAMILY/KINGDOM: Loranthaceae.
- SOURCE: Tincture of bruised leaves or whole plant.

THERAPEUTIC PICTURE OF DRUG

M_{D-1} ➲ Incoherent talk and spectral illusions.
M_{D-2} ➲ Keeping waking in night thinking the most horrible things.
M_{D-3} ➲ Imaginable.
M_{D-4} ➲ Felt inbad temper when pain in chest was on Great Depression.
FGS_1 ➲ Haemorrtage, with pain, blood partly Clot and bright red.
FGS_2 ➲ Climacteric complaints (lach, Sulph).
FGS_3 ➲ Pain from sacrum into Pelvis with tearing, shooting pains from above downwards.
FGS_4 ➲ Retained placenta (Secale).
FGS_5 ➲ Chronic endometritis.
FGS_6 ➲ Metrorrhagia
FGS_7 ➲ Ovaralgia especially left.
PG_1 ➲ Pheumatic deafness.
PG_2 ➲ Pheumatism with tearing pain.
PG_3 ➲ Feeling of suffocation when lying on left side.

Modalities

Aggravation

- By motion.
- Stormy weather
- Winter, Weather.
- In bed.

Amelioration

- By pressure.

Relations

- COMPARE: Bell; Stram; Plumb; Calc; Secale; Puls; Rhus.
- FOLLOWS WELL: ACO.
- ANTIDOTES: Camph; Chin.

Xanthoxylum Fraxineum

- ➲ COMMON NAME: Prickly ash.
- ➲ FAMILY/KINGDOM: Rutaceae.
- ➲ MIASM: Psoric and Syphilific.
- ➲ TEMPERAMENT: Nervous.
- ➲ SOURCE: Tincture of fresh bark.
- ➲ SPHERES OF ACTION: Nervous system and mucous membrane and female genital system.

THERAPEUTIC PICTURE OF DRUG

C_{N-1} ➲ Specially for the nervous women.

C_{N-2} ➲ Womens who are thin, emaciated.

M_{D-1} ➲ Nervous, frightened feeling.

M_{D-2} ➲ Mental depression and weakness.

M_{D-3} ➲ Easily startled, hysterical.

M_{D-4} ➲ Indifference and malaise.

M_{D-5} ➲ Did not care if she lived or died.

M_{D-6} ➲ Seems entirely void of ideas.

FGS_1 ➲ Menstrual flow: too early and profuse; Pains down thighs; scanty and retarded.

FGS_2 ➲ Menses eight days before time; flow increased red; bearing-down pain and pain in right ovarian region.

FGS_3 ➲ Leucorrhoea; Profuse, milky-white.

FGS_4 ➲ Great increase of leucorrhoea during time when menses should appear.

FGS_5 ➲ Ovarian Pain: with scanty and retarded menses; extending down genito-crural nerves; and sacral Pains during Pregnancy.

FGS_6 ➲ Severe contant aching Pain in right ovarian region, radiating to hip, thights, and back, with occasional shouts, making her catch her breath.

FGS_7 ➲ Constant headache, during menses at which time she also suffered agonizing pains in Pelric region.

FGS_8 ➲ Amenorrhoea for five months, with severe pains in right ovary constant headache; bearing down and tension in hypogastic region.

FGS_9 ➲ Sharp, cutting pain in right orarian region, extending about hip and down thigh, awoke her.

FGS_{10} ➲ Dysmenorrhaea: with agonizing Pains, driving Patient almost distracted.

PG_1 ➲ Pricking sensation, shocks as from electricity.

PG_2 ➲ Body felt as though it were elastic and stretches itself out.

PG_3 ➲ Mucous membrane smarts as from Pepper.

PG_4 ➲ Paralysis of the left side following spinal disorders.

PG_5 ➲ Hemiplagia: Numbness of the left side; impairment of nerves of motion.

Modalities

Aggravation

➲ In the morning 4 A.M.

Relations

➲ COMPARE: Gnaph; Cimic.

Zincum metallicum

- PROVED BY: Franz.
- DURATION: 30-40 days.
- COMMON NAME: Zinc (Zn.).
- FAMILY/KINGDOM: Minerals.
- SOURCE: Trituration of metal.
- SPHERES OF ACTION: Corebro–spinal system, blood, digestive system, urino-genital organ.
- SUMMARY OF INDICATIONS: Nervous Patient-spinal disorders-menstrual disorder.

THERAPEUTIC PICTURE OF DRUG

C_{N-1} ➲ Person suffering from defective vitality, brain or neural power wanting too weak develop menstrual function.

M_{D-1} ➲ Very sensitive to noise.

M_{D-2} ➲ Weak memory.

M_{D-3} ➲ Averse to work, to talk.

M_{D-4} ➲ Lethargic, stupid.

M_{D-5} ➲ Fears arrest on account of a supposed crime.

M_{D-6} ➲ Melancholy.

H_{D-1} ➲ Hemicrania, worse after dinner; tearing and stinging.

H_{D-2} ➲ Feels as if he would fall to the left side.

H_{D-3} ➲ Pressure on top head worse after dinner; frequent dizziness, then nausea and vomiting of bile; face pale; costive; cerebral depression.

H_{D-4} ➲ Meningitis: bore head into the pillow.

H_{D-5} ➲ Brainfag, headaches in overtaxed school children; forehead cool; base of brain hot.

NS_1 ➲ Spasms: child cross before attack, body hot, restless at night, fidgety feet, right side twitched; Pale children, during teething.

NS_2 ➲ Beginning of locomotor ataxia, when lightning–like pains are marked and intense.

NS_3 ➲ Twitching in various muscles–The whole body jerks during sleep.

NS_4 ➲ Chorea, depressed spirits, health suffers; caused by fright; suppressed eruptions, worse after wine.

FGS_1 ➲ Nymphomania of lying in women, also before menses.

FGS_2 ➲ Incessant and violent fidgety feeling in feet or lower extremities, must move them constantly.

FGS_3 ➲ Menses flow more at night (Bov.).

FGS_4 ➲ Dry cough before and during menses.

FGS_5 ➲ Irresistable sexual desire at night, desire for onanism.

FGS_6 ➲ Amenorrhoea, with alternately red and pale face.

FGS_7 ➲ Cutting pain succeeded by leucorrhoea.

FGS_8 ➲ Pruritus valvae causes masturbation.

FGS_9 ➲ Varicose veins of external genitals, with fidgety feet.

MGS_1 ➲ Drawing in of testicles, up to the spermatic cord.

MGS_2 ➲ Spermatorrhoea; emissions without dreams, face pale, sunken, blue rings around eyes.

MGS_3 ➲ Hair falls off from genitals.

MGS_4 ➲ Easily excited; the emission, during and embrance, is too rapid; or, difficult and almost impossible.

MGS_5 ➲ Long-lasting and violent erections.

B_{K-1} ➲ Spinal irritation with Prostration; numbness of lower limbs.

B_{K-2} ➲ Burning pressure upon spine above small of back.

B_{K-3} ➲ Burning along whole spine, worse when sitting.

B_{K-4} ➲ Violent, long-lasting ache about last lumbar vertebrae.

LS_1 ➲ Tearing in limbs, worse when over-heated or when taking exercise.

LS_2 ➲ Incessant and violent fidgety feeling in feet or lower extremities; must move them constantly.

LS_3 ➲ Weakness and trembling of extremities.

LS_4 ➲ Nervous, fidgety movement of the feet; after retiring and during sleep.

PG_1 ➲ Hunger- Ravenous about (11 or 12 A.M.) (Sulph) Great greediness when eating.

PG_2 ➲ Always feels better every way as soon as the menses begin to flow, it relives all-her sufferings.

PG_3 ➲ Chilbains, painful, increased from rubbing.

PG_4 ➲ Excessive nervous moving of feet in bed from hours after retiring, even when asleep.

PG_5 ➲ Feet sweaty and sore about toes; foetid offensive foot-sweat; very nervous.

PG_6 ➲ Spinal affection: burning along the length of spine; backache, increases from sitting, decreases by walking about (Cobal, Puls-nig, Rhu-tox).

Modalities

Aggravation

- ➲ All symptoms are aggravated by drinking wine, taking even a small quantity of Alcohol

Amelioration

- ➲ By urinating of back.
- ➲ By emissions.
- ➲ By menstrual flow.

Relations

- ➲ COMPARE: Hell; Tub.
- ➲ COMPLEMENTARY: Puls.
- ➲ FOLLOWS WELL: Ing; Sulph; Puls; Sep.
- ➲ ANTIDOTES: Camph; Hep; Ign.
- ➲ INIMICALS: Cham; Nux; Vinum.

Multiple Choice Questions

Q.1. Great aversion to being alone, Pain stitiching, darting, worse during rest and lying on affected side, bag like swelling between the upper eyelids and eye brow. Toothache only when eating, remedy will be-

(a) Bismuth (b) Kali-carb
(c) Staphisigria (d) Bryonia

Q.2. Fits of uncontrollable weeping and profound melancholic delusions. Loss of memory, forgets how to talk, night terror of children, somnambulism, hand and fingers in constant motion, fidgety hands, remedy will be-

(a) Zincum (b) Nat-mur.
(c) Kali-brom (d) Kali-phos.

Q.3. First stage of all febrile disturbances and inflammations before exudation set in headache better by cold application, haemorrhages: bright red blood from orifice, remedy will be-

(a) Aconite (b) Ferrr-phos.
(c) Belladonna (d) Ipecac.

Q.4. Adenomata, the gland are inlarged and of a stony hardness, mammae, testicles, usually painless, sometime darting pain, induration and swelling of external glands with a sense of numbness after contusions or bruises, this symptoms shows by the remedy-

(a) Calc-Flor. (b) Carbo-an.
(c) Conium-mac. (d) Phytolacca.

Q.5. Symptom alternate sided, throat, ovaries etc, or wander about Glistering Part. Glistening, throat, ulcers etc. oversensitive full of imagination, horrid a snakes vermin, as if floating etc desire upto the milk, remedy will be-

(a) Pulsatilla (b) Kali-bich.
(c) Lac-can. (d) Nat-mur.

Q.6. Frequent and extreme changes in sensation, sudden, from the greatest hilarity to the deepest despondency, excessive happy, affectionate, wants to kiss every body, the next moment in a rage, remedy will be-

(a) Ignitia (b) Crocus sativa
(c) Nux-moxchata (d) Nat-mur.

Q.7. Aching, tired, heavy, weak and sore, overpowering aching, nerve, exhausting, dull, drowsy and dizzy. Tremore, or twitches of side muscles heavy drooping eyelids, vision double. Dread of following. Headache dull heavy, band like occipital to over eyes, remedy will be-

(a) Acid-Phos. (b) Gelsemium
(c) Arnica (d) Nux-Mos.

Q.8. Spasm, tremor, jerks, cramps etc or active mania, alternating with, or ending in depression, narcosis, with angular or clutching motions, carphology-subsultus etc. Piks fingers. Eclampia.... Many bewildosing aberrations, confusion, delirium mania, erotic, exposes genils, remedy will be-

(a) Platina (b) Stramonium
(c) Veratrum-alb. (d) Hyocyamous

Q.9. Profuse, foul, hot acrid discharge, sputum, eructations etc, redden the part rawness. Burning like fire. Pulsation, general haemorrhage, passive, brown, dark, lumpy discharges, menses etc., remedy will be-

(a) Mag-carb. (b) Kreosote
(c) Sulphur (d) Borax

Q.10. Worse night, emotions, violent exertion, eating, drinking, vital losses, sweats, quinine, eggs, heat and cold. Sudden motions, raising arms, better gentle motions, slight bleeding, leaning head on something, remedy will be-

(a) China (b) Acid-phos.
(c) Ferr-met. (d) Carbo-veg.

Q.11 A person is great debilited after overlifting and it face, cheeks and lips are blue, remedy will be-

(a) Carbo-Ani. (b) Carro-veg.
(c) Antim-tart. (d) Phosp-acid.

Q.12. A person is melancholic, indolent when lived in house, red cheeks and can hot sleep, remedy will be-

(a) Bryonia (b) Capsicum
(c) Hyoscyamus-Nig. (d) Aconite

Q.13. Sexual desire increase in both sexes, preventing sleep, tenacious mucus in the air passage and erythema due to sunburn select the remedy-

(a) Bovista (b) Kali-bich.
(c) Canth-vers (d) Nat-mur.

Q.14. A person when sitting than feel sitting on a ball. Person is very fright full in nature, inability to recall any thought. Answer is-

(a) Ana-card. (b) Can-ind.
(c) Lac-can. (d) All of these

Q.15 If the external wound is with or without loss of substance, a very lot of blood loss from wound, Exhausted from loss of blood what will be choice-

(a) Calendula-off. (b) China-off.
(c) Hammemalis-v. (d) All of these

Q.16 A person when awake in the morning by eye is not opened but when he/she open the eye or even slight thinking than diarrhoea start, medicine is-

(a) Bryonia (b) Cal-phos.
(c) Sulphar (d) China

Q.17 A person feel great anxiety from horse back riding. Eyelashes agglunated in the morning excessively nervous, easily frightend by a cry, medicine is-

(a) Arg-nit. (b) Baryta-carb.
(c) Antim-crud. (d) Borax

Q.18. Throat and larynx feel raw and sore on swallowing or caughing total loss of voice with professional singer, remedy will be-

(a) Arg-nit. (b) Arg-met.
(c) Causticum (d) Capsicum

Q.19 The medicine which is used in treatment of Jaundice-

(a) Carduus (b) Kalmegh
(c) Chelidonium (d) All

Q.20 Which belongs to the Trio's of burner-

(A) Arsenic album (b) Sulphur
(c) Phosphorus (d) All

Q.21 One of them is trio's of Sleeplessness medicine-

(a) Nux-Moschata (b) Antimonium-tart.
(c) Opium (d) All

Q.22. The remedy which cure the Aphthae (Punch like cutting) round scar in mouth-

(a) Kali Bichromicum (b) Borex
(c) Mer-sol. (d) All

Q.23 The medicine which is used in treatment of Boils which is painful and hypersensitive-

(a) Heper-Sulph. (b) Merc- Sol.
(c) Silicea (d) All

Q.24. One of them is Thirstlessness medicine-

(a) Pulsatilla (b) Apis-Mel.
(c) Aethusa Cyanapium (d) All

Q.25. There is great dryness and parched mouth without thirst-

(a) Pulsatilla (b) Merc-Sol.
(c) Bryonia (d) None

Q.26 The medicine which is not helpful in cholera-

(a) Arsenic Album (b) Camphora
(c) Veratrum Album (d) None of them

Q.27 Which is not characteristic symptoms of Arsenic Album-

(a) Restlessness (b) Burning
(c) Weakness (d) Stinging Pain

Q. 28 The symptoms alternate constipation and diarrhoea: Lienteria is found in-

(a) Abrotanum (b) Bryonia
(c) Pulsatilla (d) Belladonna

Q.29 Cholera like symptoms at the commencement of menstruation are not found in-

(a) Ammonium Carb. (b) Bovista
(c) Veratrum Album (d) Bryonia

Q.30 Discharge from nose and all mucous membranes very tough, stringy, tenacious in found in-

(a) Bovista (b) Kali Bichrome
(c) Hydrastis (d) Graphitis
(e) All of them

Q.31 Impatence: Penis SMALL, COLD, RELAXED old men with strong desire but imperfect erections falls asleep during an embrace, the characteristic symptoms are found in-

(a) Carbo-Veg. (b) China
(c) Lycopodium (d) None

Q.32. The aggravation period of Natrum Mure is-

(a) From 4-8 P.M. (b) At 10 OR 11 A.M.
(c) From 4-9 P.M. (d) After mid night

Q.33 A great fear and anxiety of mind with great nervous excitability afraid to go out to go into a crowd where there is any excitement to cross the street, remedy will be-

(a) Aconite (b) Helleborus
(c) Bryonia (d) Gelsemium

Q.34 Sudden loss of memory everything seems to be in a dream. Patient is greatly troubled about his forget-fullness confused until for business medicine is-

(a) Anacardium (b) Argentum-Met.
(c) Aconite (d) Aurum Met.

Q.35. Irresistible desire to talk in rhymes or repeated verses, answer is-

(a) Abrotanum (b) Anacardium
(c) Antim-crud. (d) Sulphur

Q.36 Constant picking at the nose until it bleed, boring with the finger into the side of nose. Picks lips until they bleeds-

(a) Aurum-Met. (b) Aurum-triph.
(c) Arsenic album (d) Bryonia alba.

Q.37 Memory deficient, forgetful inattentive, child can not be tought because they cannot remember threatened idiocy-

(a) Bryonia (b) Baryta-Carb.
(c) Thuja (d) Silicea

Q.38 Dread of down wards motion-

(a) Gelsemium (b) Borex
(c) Sanicula (d) All of the above

Q.39 Mental condition rapidly, in an almost incredibly short time change from joy to sorrow from laughing to weeping-

(a) Ignatia (b) Nux Moschata
(c) Coffea (d) All of the above

Q.40 Mentally restless but physically too week to move cannot rest in any place, changing place continuously- wants to be moved from one bed to another, and lies now here, now there, medicine will be-

(a) Arsenic (b) Aconite
(c) Sulpher (d) Bryonia

Q.41 Hasty-eating and drinking-

(a) Belladonna (b) Hepersulph
(c) Coffea (d) Above all

Q. 42 Lascivious Mania: Immodesty, will not be covered, picks of clothes, exposes the person, signs abscene, songs, lies naked in bed and chaters, medicine will be-

(a) Bellodonna (b) Helleborus
(c) Hyoscymus (d) Heper Sulph

Q.43 Illusion of a mouse moving/running from under her chair-

(a) Lac-caninum (b) Aethusa
(c) Actea-Recemosa (d) All of the above

Q.44 Sleepy but can not sleep-

(a) Belladonna (b) Chamomilla
(c) Opium (d) All above

Q.45 Burning of soles at night puts feet out of bed-

(a) Pulsatilla (b) Medorrhinum
(c) Sulphur (d) All of the above

Q.46 Hair becomes frowsy and tangled-splits sticks, together a the tip-

(a) Borex (b) Phosphorus
(c) Nat-Mur. (d) Argentum Nitricum

Q.47 Great falling of hair after chronic headache or at climacteric age-

(a) Pulsatilla (b) Silicea
(c) Sepia (d) Platina

Q.48 Catarrhal dull headache, with coryza, worse in evening better in open air, worse on returning to warm room, remedy will be-

(a) Euphrasia (b) Pulsatilla
(c) Allium cepa (d) All of the above

Q.49 Severe headache before and during menses-

(a) Kreosote (b) Sepia
(c) Above both (d) None

Q.50 Headache: after a fall upon occiput, with sensation as if being lifted up high into the air, great anxiety lest she should fall from the height.

(a) Arnica (b) Ruta
(c) Hypericum (d) Ledum-Pal.

Q.51 Intense congestion of Brain from delayed or suppressed menses, headache in place of menses -

(a) Lachesis (b) Pulsatilla
(c) Bryonia (d) Glonoine

Q.52 Headache: Intense as if thousand of needles where pricking in the brain-

(a) Gelsemium (b) Bryonia
(c) Tarentula (d) Tabacum

Q.53 Fear of RAIN is the characteristic feature of -

(a) Bufo (b) Elaps
(c) Both above (d) None.

Q.54 A remedy of terrors, cannot bear solitude or darkness, must have light and company. Dread of darkness. Devout, earnest, beseeching and useless talking religious insanity-

(a) Belladonna (b) Hyoscyamus
(c) Stramonium (d) Lachesis

Q.55 Flushes of heat, aversion of water, dry, unhealthy hair and skin, red orifices, sinking feeling at stomach about 11 a.m. complains that relapse.

(a) Sepia (b) Phosphorus
(c) Sulphur (d) Nat-mur.

Q.56 Crying infants, who being crying immediately after birth-

(a) Chammomilla (b) Syphilinum
(c) Cina (d) Borex

Q.57 Vaccinosis, never well since vaccination, vagina very sensitive prevents sex-

(a) Platina (b) Staphisagria
(c) Silicea (d) Thuja

Q.58 Desire to travel, does not wants to remain in one place long-

(a) Tuberculinum (b) Pulsatilla
(c) Chamomilla (d) Medorrhinum

Q.59 A perfect picture of collapse with extreme coldness, blueness & weakness. Cold perspiration on the forehead with nearly all complains-

(a) Camphora (b) Carbo-veg.
(c) Muriatic Acid (d) Veratrum Album

Q.60 Epilepsy, feels a glow that rises up from feet to head. Rheumatic deafness. Feeling of a burning cool under the right shoulder is a key symptom.

(a) Sulphur (b) Phosphorus
(c) Sangunaria (d) Viscus Album

Q.61 Restless feet in continued motion, can not keep them still. Lameness, weakness, trembling & twitching of various muscles.

(a) Gelsemium (b) Zincum met.
(c) Agaricus (d) Stramonium

Q.62 Sensation–As if something alive creeping under skin. As of sparks of fire feeling on different parts. Fuzzy feeling in limbs. As if sacrum would be forced out, medicine is-

(a) Secale Cor. (b) Lac Caninum
(c) Belladonna (d) Sepia

Q.63 Pain from right kidney downward. Severe pain at conclusion of urination. Child screams before & while passing urine. Can pass urine only when standing. Urine scanty, slimy, slaky, sandy, pus, bloody, please select the remedy-

(a) Sarsaparilla (b) Berberis
(c) Cantharis (d) Apis

Q.64 Boenninghausen's give croup power in order–

(a) Aco. → Spong. → Hep-s. → Spong. → Hep-s.
(b) Aco. → Hep-s. → Hep-s. → Spongia → Spongia
(c) Aco. → Spong. → Hep-s. → Spong. → Spongia
(d) Aco. → Hep-s. → Spong. → Hep-s. → Spong.

Q.65 Which of the following is Sanicula symptoms-

(a) Must cross leg to prevent stool from escaping
(b) Does not pass urine at standing
(c) Pass urine while sitting & bending backward
(d) Tormented about her salvation

Q.66 Which of the following is Sanicula symptoms-

(a) Wanted to lies on something hard
(b) Wanted to lies on cold soft bed
(c) Bed feel to hard & wanted soft bed
(d) None of the above

Q.67 Which of the sabal-serrulata symptoms.

(a) Excessive desire for light & dark both
(b) One breast was much smaller than the other
(c) Children grow too rapidly
(d) None of the Above.

Q. 68 Headache of Silicea patient is ameliorated by–

(a) Pressure (b) Wrapping up warmly
(c) Profuse Urination (d) All of the above

Q. 69 Body painfully sensitive to touch, part touched feels chilly, is the characteristic symptoms of -

(a) Camphor (b) Silicea
(c) Spigelia (d) Stannum-met.

Q.70 Expectoration relieve hoarseness is one of the red line symptoms of–

(a) Stannum-met. (b) Arg-met.
(c) Kali-carb. (d) Nat-carb.

Q. 71 Ailment of staphisagria patient are from–

(a) Onanism (b) Sexual excess
(c) Anger & Chagrin (d) All of the above

Q. 72 Sulphur patient complain diarrhoea usually at–

(a) Night (b) Day time
(c) Morning (d) Evening

Q. 73 Obstinate constipation for year is one of the characteristic symptom of-

(a) Alumina (b) Alumen
(c) Bry-alb. (d) Symphilinum

Q. 74 Vertigo on operating the eye is one of the red line symptoms of–

(a) Thuja-occi. (b) Bryo-alb.
(c) Tabacum (d) None of the above

Q. 75 Sexual excitement extreme even to mania is one of the characteristic symptoms of–

(a) Graphites (b) Mercurius
(c) Puls-Nig. (d) None of the above

Q. 76 Coition prevented by extreme sensitiveness of vagina is one of the characteristic symptoms of–

(a) Selenium (b) Murex-pur.
(c) Arg-Nit. (d) Thuja-occ.

Q. 77 Sensation of great coldness in head is one of the characteristic symptoms of–

(a) Calc-Carb. (b) Psorinum
(c) Valeriana (d) Graphitis.

Q. 78 Diarrhoea for painful coitus followed by bleeding per vagina are–

(a) Ars-alb. & Arg-nit. (b) Crot-tig. & Trombidium
(c) Alumina and alumen (d) Nux-vom. & Ign-amar.

Q. 79 Burning in throat as from coal of fire or red hot iron is one of the characteristic symptoms of–

(a) Phytolacca-dec. (b) Sepia
(c) Psorinum (d) Aconit- Nap.

Q. 80 Petroleum patient complains of diarrhoea only at–

(a) Night (b) Daytime
(c) Afternoon (d) Morning

Q. 81 "Sudden hoarseness which is aggravated from walking against wind" is one of the characteristic Peculiar symptoms of–

(a) Euphrasia (b) Hepar-sulph.
(c) Nux-mosch. (d) All of the above

Q. 82 Mark the medicine which has Ascending emaciation with Lienteria-

(a) Nat-Mur. (b) Sanicula
(c) Abrotanum (d) Tuberculinum

Q. 83 Choose most appropriate medicine which has intense thirst during dropsy, no thirst in fever, lying on belly & cough on inhalation & antidotes carbolic acid-

(a) Amm-Carb. (b) Spongia
(c) Apocy-Cann. (d) Acetic Acid.

Q. 84 Click the medicine which has Great Fear & Anxiety fear of crossing the road & music makes her sad & about it Hahnemann says–wherever fear, anxiety, restless meets altogether you must choose it?

(a) Sabina (b) Nat-Carb.
(c) Arsanic (d) Aconite

Q. 85 Predict the correct medicine–Abortion at 3rd month, left sided inflammary pain, illusion of mouse running under her chair & aggr. during menstruation.

(a) Sabina (b) Ustilago
(c) Actaea Racemosa (d) Lachesis

Q. 86 If there is haemorrhoids blind, painful rarely bleeding with lumbosacral bachache it may be–

(a) Aesc-Hipp. (b) Nux-V.
(c) Aloe-Soc. (d) Sulphur

Q. 87 Select the mediine–Herpetic eruption on nose with complete abs. Of thirst, children can't tolerate milk & vomit it in curd form-

(a) Mag-Carb. (b) Sanicula
(c) Aeth-Cyn. (d) Calc-Carb.

Q. 88 Complaints appear diagnonally upper left & lower right, pain in Lumber & sacral region & sense of ice-cold needless here piercing the skin-

(a) Agaricus-M. (b) Aes-Hipp.
(c) Ambra-G. (d) Phosphorus

Q. 89 Choose the correct medicine for–Reduce power of insight, has to read a sentence twice before confirmed & complete impotence & coldness of Genitalia-

(a) Caladium (b) Agnus Castus
(c) Lycopodium (d) Phosph.

Q. 90 Headache ceases during menses, flow disappear then retures nasal polpus, Acrid coryza & blend lawymal discharge effieacious in rubbed sore feet-

(a) Alli-Cepa. (b) Euphrasia
(c) Bell. (d) Nat-Mur.

Q. 91 Colic; cutting pain before & during stool, diarrhoea immediately after eating, blue haemorrhoids, flatus offensive & insecurity of rectum.

(a) Mercurius (b) Nux-V.
(c) Aloe-Soc. (d) Alumina

Q. 92 Inactivity of Rectum, constipation–no desire until large acumulation; great straining, leucorrhoea running down to heels-

(a) Bryonia (b) Anac.
(c) Alumina (d) Puls.

Q. 93 Leucorrhoea–Blue thick, presence of others during stool is unbearable, ineffectual desire-

(a) Ambra-Gr. (b) Nux-V.
(c) Nat-Mur. (d) Caustium

Q. 94 Smelling bottle lady, who have nose bleeding when washing the face from left nostril & cholera like symptom at commencement of menses-

(a) Bovista (b) Kreosotum
(c) Verat-alb. (d) Amm- Carb.

Q.95 Obstinate constipation–crumbling stools requires great effort crumbling, no two stools alike, & leucorrhoea–white of egg after every urination-

(a) Amm. Mur (b) Pulsatilla
(c) Nat-Mur. (d) Mag-Mur.

Q. 96 Loss of memory, everything seems in a dream. Headache relived by eating. All five sensation, great desire for stool but with effort, desire passes away without evacuation-

(a) Lac-can. (b) Puls.
(c) Anacardium (d) Medorrhinum.

Q. 97 Alternate constipation & diarrhoea with thick white coated tongue. Desire for acid & pickles-

(a) Sulphur (b) Bryonia
(c) Antim-Crud. (d) Arsanic-alb.

Q. 98 Thirstlessness in every complaints except fever with burning, stinging pain, oedema under the eyes-

(a) Pulsatilla (b) Sulphur
(c) Apis-Mel. (d) Kali-Carb.

Q. 99 Dropsy with thirst, acute hydrocephalus, constant & voluntary motion of one arm & one leg & amenorrhoea in young girls with bloating/ dropsical extension of abdomen & extremities-

(a) Acetic acid (b) Apocy-Cam.
(c) Calc-Phos. (d) Bryonia

Q.100 Bowels are disturbed by any changes in living, consequently heart burn, wind colic, copious flow of saliva. Pain is however mostly in hip region as well as in iliac muscle-

(a) Alli-Sativa (b) Acetic Acid
(c)Nat-Mur. (d) Alli-Cepa

Answer Sheet

1-b	2-c	3-b	4-c	5-c	6-b	7-b	8-d	9-b	10-c
11-a	12-b	13-c	14-c	15-a	16-a	17-d	18-b	19-d	20-d
21-d	22-a	23-a	24-d	25-a	26-d	27-a	28-a	29-d	30-e
31-c	32-b	33-a	34-a	35-c	36-b	37-b	38-d	39-d	40-a
41-d	42-c	43-d	44-e	45-d	46-a	47-c	48-d	49-c	50-c
51-d	52-c	53-c	54-c	55-c	56-b	57-d	58-a	59-d	60-d
61-b	62-a	63-a	64-a	65-a	66-a	67-b	68-d	69-c	70-a
71-d	72-c	73-d	74-c	75-d	76-d	77-c	78-c	79-a	80-b
81-d	82-c	83-d	84-d	85-c	86-a	87-c	88-a	89-b	90-a
91-c	92-c	93-a	94-d	95-a	96-c	97-c	98-c	99-b	100-a.

Bibliography

Allen, H.C. *Allen's Keynotes.*

Boericke, William. *New Manual of Homoeopathic Materia Medica & Repertory.*

Choudhary. *A Study of Materia Medica.*

Clark, J.H. *Dictionary of Practical Materia Medica in 3 Vols.*

Dubey, S.K. *Textbook of Materia Medica.*

Dunhomm, C. *Lecture on Materia Medica.*

Farrington, E.A. *A Clinical Materia Medica.*

Gross. *Comparative Materia Medica.*

Hahnemann, Samuel. *Materia Medica Pura.*

Hansen, O. *A Textbook of Materia Medica & Therapeutics.*

Hering, C. *Condensed Materia Medica*

Jayasurya, Anton. *Clinical Homoeopathy.*

Juliar, O.A. *Dictionary of Homoeopathic Materia Medica.*

Kent, J.E. *Lecture on Homoeopathic Materia Medica.*

Lippe, A.D. *Textbook of Materia Medica.*

Mohanti, B. *New Textbook of Homoeopathic Materia Medica.*

Nash, E.B. *Lecture in Homoeopathic Therapeutics.*

Tyler, M.L. *Homoeopathic Drug Picture.*

Vithoulkas, G. *Materia Medica Viva.*

Woodward, A.W. *Constitutional Therapeutics.*

Yasgur. *Homoeopathic Dictionary.*